Comprehensive Intraaortic Balloon Counterpulsation

D1275729

Comprehensive Intraaortic Balloon Counterpulsation

Susan J. Quaal, PhD, RN, CVS, CCRN

Associate Clinical Professor
University of Utah Health Sciences;
Cardiovascular Clinical Specialist
Veterans Affairs Medical Center
Salt Lake City, Utah

SECOND EDITION

with 319 illustrations

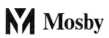 Mosby

A Harcourt Health Sciences Company

St. Louis London Philadelphia Sydney Toronto

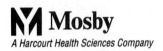

A Harcourt Health Sciences Company

Publisher: Alison Miller
Acquisitions Editor: Robin Carter
Editorial Assistant: Jeanne Allison
Project Manager: John Rogers
Production Editor: Chuck Furgason
Manufacturing Supervisor: Mary Stueck
Designer: Susan Lane
Cover Illustration: Eric Lubbers

SECOND EDITION

Printed in the United States of America

Mosby, Inc.
11830 Westline Industrial Drive
St. Louis, Missouri 63146

Library of Congress Cataloging-in-Publication Data

Quaal, Susan J.
    Comprehensive intraaortic balloon counterpulsation / Susan J.
Quaal.— 2nd ed.
        p.   cm.
    Rev. ed of. : Comprehensive intra-aortic balloon pumping. 1984.
    Includes bibliographical references and index.
    ISBN 0-8016-6656-2
    1. Intra-aortic balloon counterpulsation.   2. Heart failure-
-Treatment.   3. Heart failure—Nursing.   I. Quaal, Susan J.
Comprehensive intra-aortic balloon pumping.   II. Title.
    [DNLM: 1. Counterpulsation.   2. Intra-Aortic Balloon Pumping.   WG
168 Q103c 1993]
    RC684.I58Q3 1993 617.4′ 12—dc20
    DNLM/DLC   92-48411

00 01 02 CL/DC 9 8 7 6 5 4 3

Consultants

C. Richard Conti, MD
Palm Beach Heart Association Eminent Scholar (Cardiology)
Professor of Medicine
Director, Division of Cardiovascular Medicine
University of Florida
Gainesville, Florida

Joseph S. Janicki, PhD
Director of Research Services in Cardiology
Professor of Medicine
University of Missouri at Columbia
Columbia, Missouri

Adrian Kantrowitz, MD
Senior Cardiac Surgeon, Sinai Hospital of Detroit
Professor of Surgery, Wayne State University School of Medicine
President, L. Vad Technology, Inc.
Detroit, Michigan

Spyridon D. Moulopoulos, MD, DSc (Hon)
Professor, University of Athens School of Medicine
Department of Clinical Therapeutics
Athens, Greece

Joan Vitello-Ciccu, MSN, RN, CCRN, CS
Clinical Nurse Specialist
Surgical Critical Care
University Hospital at Boston University Medical Center
Boston, Massachusetts

Sidney Wolvek, MA
Director Scientific Research
Cardiac Assist Division
Datascope Corporation
Oakland, New Jersey

Contributors

Kathleen Beaver, BSN, RN
Senior Associate
Clinical Support Services
Datascope Corporation
Montvale, New Jersey

Cynthia A. Cadwell, BSN, RN
Application Specialist
Boston Scientific Cardiac Assist
Mansfield, Massachusetts

Raul R. Cardona, MD
Surgical Research Associate
Sinai Hospital of Detroit and L. VAD Technology Inc.
Detroit, Michigan

Bernice Coleman, MS, RN
Cardiovascular Clinical Specialist
Cardiovascular Surgery/Thoracic Transplantation
Cedars-Sinai Medical Center & Doctoral Student, UCLA
Los Angeles, California

Daniel J. Diver, MD
Assistant Professor of Medicine
Harvard Medical School
Associate Director of Invasive Cardiology
Cardiovascular Division
Beth Israel Hospital
Boston, Massachusetts

Paul S. Freed, MS
Director, Biomedical Engineering Research and Development
L. VAD Technology Inc.
Detroit, Michigan

Theresa M. Gaffney, BSN, RN
Senior Product Manager
Bard Cardiopulmonary Division
CR Bard Inc.
Tewksbury, Massachusetts

Patricia C. Garison, RN
Scientific Writer and Technical Consultant
Westford, Massachusetts

William Gee, MD
Director, Vascular Laboratory
Lehigh Valley Hospital
Allentown, Pennsylvania

Terrance M. Hartnett, BA
VP Education Affairs
Clinical Perfusionists, Inc.
Annapolis, Maryland

Debra W. Hartigan, BSN, RN
Former Manager of Clinical Support
Kontron Instruments
Everett, Massachusetts

Debra L. Joseph, BSN, RN
Director, Clinical Support Services
Datascope Corporation
Montvale, New Jersey

Janet Kalina, BSN, RN
Former Clinical Specialist
Kontron Cardiovascular
Everett, Massachusetts

Adrian Kantrowitz, MD
Senior Cardiovascular Surgeon, Sinai Hospital of Detroit
Professor of Surgery, Wayne State University School of Medicine
President, L. VAD Technology Inc.
Detroit, Michigan

Pamela Kasold, BSN, RN, CCRN
Clinical Education Manager
St. Jude Medical
Chelmsford, Massachusetts

Sydney S. Lange, MSN, RN, CCRN
Faculty Associate
University of Texas Health Science Center & Staff Nurse Medical ICU
Spring Branch Medical Center
Houston, Texas

Gary B. Mertlich, MS, RN
Flight Nurse Air Med
University of Utah
Salt Lake City, Utah & Doctoral Student
Case Western Reserve University
Cleveland, Ohio

Spyridon D. Moulopoulos, MD, DSc (Hon)
Professor, Department of Clinical Therapeutics
University of Athens School of Medicine
Athens, Greece

James F. Reed III, PhD
Director, Research Department
Lehigh Valley Hospital Center
Allentown, Pennsylvania

Kathleen Rolston, BSN, RN, CCRN
Clinical Specialist
Cardiac Assist Division
Boston Scientific Corporation
Mansfield, Massachusetts

George Tyson, MD
Cardiovascular Surgeon
Lakeland Regional Medical Center
Lakeland, Florida

L. George Veasy, MD
Professor of Pediatrics
University of Utah Medical Center
Salt Lake City, Utah

Marie G. Witham
Research Intern
Lehigh Valley Hospital Center
Allentown, Pennsylvania

Tom Wrublewski
Manager Research & Development Group
Cardiac Assist Division
Boston Scientific Corporation
Mansfield, Massachusetts

To

Datascope, Kontron, Boston Scientific Corporation, and St. Jude Medical

In appreciation for many years of support
and generous sharing of their expertise and resources.

Foreword

Twenty five years have elapsed since the first clinical application of intraoartic balloon counterpulsation (IABC) with an elongated air chamber. It is difficult to estimate the exact number of procedures occurring each year. It is certain, however, that hundreds of thousands of patients have profited from IABC. It is also obvious that the indications have broadened during the last years. A large number of more seriously ill patients with coronary heart disease are being treated with surgical operations or interventional procedures, and mechanical assistance "back-up" is becoming more and more necessary. Furthermore, a number of patients require IABC as a bridge-to-heart transplantation or as a ventricular assistance device. There are indications that use of IABC will increase even further in the future.

Although an impressive number of other cardiac assistance devices have been introduced, IABC has remained the least traumatic, especially since the construction of transdermal, small diameter balloon catheters. Nevertheless, in spite of the simplicity of the technique and application of newer equipment modifications, IABC remains a novel and unusual interference with the circulatory system's hemodynamics. Clinicians responsible for interfacing patient with IABC must be well versed in basic physiological principles of blood circulation, hemodynamics of heart failure and circulatory insufficiency, and the effect of other parameters such as medications on the cardiovascular system. Clinicians must also be aware of critical technical details regarding equipment and specific patient management in the application of IABC.

This book indeed provides all the information needed to present comprehensive IABC patient management in a detailed and thorough way. It is with great pleasure that I recommend it strongly to everyone working with IABC. This second edition is offering state-of-the art information, where even a small detail may prove to be life-saving. Susan J. Quaal has done a wonderful job.

S.D. Moulopoulos, MD, DSc (Hon)

Preface

Ten years have passed since the original printing of the first edition. This second edition reflects the wealth of expanded knowledge regarding the field of intraaortic balloon counterpulsation (IABC) that has accrued during the interim. Entering its third decade, IABC is the most commonly used cardiac assistance device and has evolved into a discipline nearly unto itself. Major advancements have been made in instrumentation, which has now become very user friendly, and in balloon design and insertion techniques. New concepts such as ocular pneumoplethysmography, in conjunction with IABC, balloon size selection, "real timing," and weaning options are presented. This edition addresses many clinical questions regarding patient management and hemodynamic support of the IABC patient. Additional new topics include IABC in the community hospital setting, total quality management, pulmonary artery IABC, pediatric adaptation, and air transport. The reader will also have the opportunity to be enlightened with a detailed history of balloon pumping and a view of future directions.

Susan J. Quaal

Susan J. Quaal

Acknowledgments

It is with sincere appreciation that I acknowledge my indebtedness to:

†**Leo Schamroth,** MD, DSc, Professor Emeritus, University of Witwatersrand School of Medicine and Chief Physician Baragwanath Hospital, Johannesburg, South Africa, who was a very dear friend and mentor. This book began with Professor Schamroth reviewing the early chapters as we sat around his dining room table at his home in Johannesburg, just a month before he passed away.

Willem Kolff, MD, PhD, and Distinguished Professor of Medicine and Surgery, University of Utah Health Sciences. It has been a great honor and privilege to come under his tutelage.

Marg Self, RN, formerly Senior Coordinator of Advanced Clinical Research, Datascope Corporation, who has selflessly shared her invaluable expertise with me since I first began learning about IABC. She is the most knowledgeable nurse about IABC in the entire world.

Barbara Breslin, Territory Manager, Kontron Instruments, who has provided tremendous personal assistance throughout the years.

The many excellent employees of Datascope, Kontron, St. Jude Medical, and Boston Scientific Corporation, who have always been most generous in responding to my every request.

Robin Carter, Chris Kuehne, Jeanne Allison, Chuck Furgason, and John Rogers at Mosby–Year Book for their excellent editorial and production assistance.

All my colleagues who offered constructive criticism on the first edition, and thus helped to strengthen this second edition.

---

†Deceased

Contents

PART ONE
THE MYOCARDIAL PUMP

1   **Physiological fundamentals relevant to balloon counterpulsation** 3
Susan J. Quaal

2   **Myocardial excitation and contraction** 26
Susan J. Quaal

3   **Myocardial energetics** 37
Susan J. Quaal

4   **An overview of heart failure** 41
Susan J. Quaal

5   **Pharmacological management of myocardial pump failure** 65
Susan J. Quaal

PART TWO
CLINICAL APPLICATION OF INTRAAORTIC BALLOON COUNTERPULSATION (IABC)

6   **Basic principles of IABC** 93
Susan J. Quaal

7   **Interactive hemodynamics of IABC** 101
Susan J. Quaal

8   **Indications** 118
Susan J. Quaal

9   **Contraindications** 144
Susan J. Quaal

10   **Complications associated with IABC** 146
Sydney S. Lange

11   **Ocular pneumoplethysmography in IABC**   165
James F. Reed III, William Gee, and Marie G. Witham

12   **Balloon insertion techniques**   171
Susan J. Quaal

13   **Sheathless balloon insertion**   199
Daniel J. Diver

14   **Intraaortic balloon size selection**   207
Terrance M. Hartnett and Theresa Gaffney

PART THREE
INTERFACING COUNTERPULSATION TO THE PATIENT'S CARDIAC CYCLE

15   **Supportive hemodynamic monitoring**   217
Susan J. Quaal

16   **Conventional timing using the arterial pressure waveform**   246
Susan J. Quaal

17   **Conventional timing practice exercises**   260
Susan J. Quaal

18   **Real timing**   281
Cynthia A. Cadwell and George Tyson

19   **Use of the balloon pressure waveform in conjunction with the augmented arterial pressure waveform**   295
Janet Kalina

PART FOUR
PATIENT MANAGEMENT

20   **Nursing care of the IABC patient**   313
Susan J. Quaal

21   **IABC patient case studies**   343
Susan J. Quaal

22   **IABC in the community hospital setting**   357
As derived by Susan J. Quaal

23   **A total quality management IABC program**   683
Susan G. Osguthorpe

24   **Weaning from IABC**   398
Adrian Kantrowitz, Raul R. Cardona, and Paul S. Freed

PART FIVE
IABC INSTRUMENTATION

25   **The historical account**   411
As derived by Susan J. Quaal

26   **St. Jude Medical Inc., Cardiac Assist Division Model 700 IABP Control System**   430
Pamela Kasold

27   **Datascope Systems 95 and 90T**   447
Debra L. Joseph and Kathleen Beaver

28   **Kontron KAAT-II and Model 7000**   463
Debra W. Hartigan

29   **Boston Scientific Corporation Cardiac Assist Series 3001**   483
Kathleen Rolston and Tom Wrublewski

30   **Bard H-8000**   495
Patricia C. Garison and Theresa M. Gaffney

PART SIX
IABC IN SPECIAL SITUATIONS

31   **Ambulatory IABC**   517
Susan J. Quaal

32   **Pulmonary artery balloon counterpulsation**   520
Bernice Coleman

33   **Pediatric adaptation in balloon pumping**   531
L. George Veasy

34   **Air transport**   535
Gary B. Mertlich and Susan J. Quaal

35   **Balloon pumping and beyond**   552
Spyridon D. Moulopoulos

PART ONE

THE MYOCARDIAL PUMP

Physiological fundamentals relevant to balloon counterpulsation

Susan J. Quaal

Essential to an understanding of physiological benefits derived from intraaortic balloon counterpulsation (IABC) is a foundation of normal cardiac anatomy and physiology. Specifically, the series circuit arrangement of right and left heart pumps and the intricate dynamics of left pump function must be appreciated. Working in a series circuit, these two pumps provide the force necessary to propel venous blood into the pulmonic circulation and oxygenated blood into the systemic circulation (Fig. 1-1). IABC may be employed when the left ventricle fails to provide an adequate pumping effort.

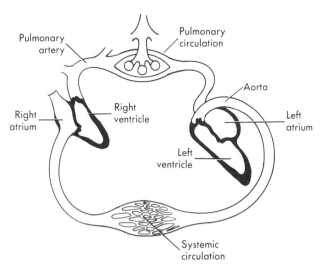

Fig. 1-1. Normal cardiopulmonary circulation. Right and left ventricles are in series circuit with pulmonary and systemic circulations.

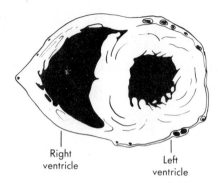

Right
ventricle   Left
                             ventricle

Fig. 1-2. Cross section of ventricular musculature. Left ventricular wall is three times as thick as right ventricle.

The pulmonary circuit is a low-pressure system, offering little resistance to blood flow from the right ventricle. Conversely, the high-pressure systemic circulation presents considerably greater resistance to left ventricular blood flow. Therefore right ventricular work load is much lighter than that of the left, and right ventricular wall thickness is only one third that of the left ventricle (Fig. 1-2). A review of left ventricular function is necessary before proceeding to a discussion of the physiological action of balloon pumping because the principal goal of balloon assistance is to reduce left ventricle work. Normal left ventricular performance expectations must first be reviewed. Concepts of preload and afterload apply to both right and left heart pumps, but the discussion that follows is restricted to a definition applicable to the left ventricle and balloon counterpulsation. We begin with a rudimentary and brief review of the duties of each heart chamber and then concentrate on principles specific to left ventricular function.

THE HEART
Right atrium

The right atrium functions as a conduit to transport systemic blood returned through the vena cava and coronary sinus to the right ventricle (Fig. 1-3, A). Right atrial venous return flows passively through the tricuspid valve into the right ventricle. An additional 20% of ventricular filling occurs during atrial contraction; this added contribution to cardiac output is termed the *atrial kick*.

Right ventricle

Work required of the right ventricle is modest compared to demands placed on the left ventricle. Normally the pulmonary bed offers little resistance to right ven-

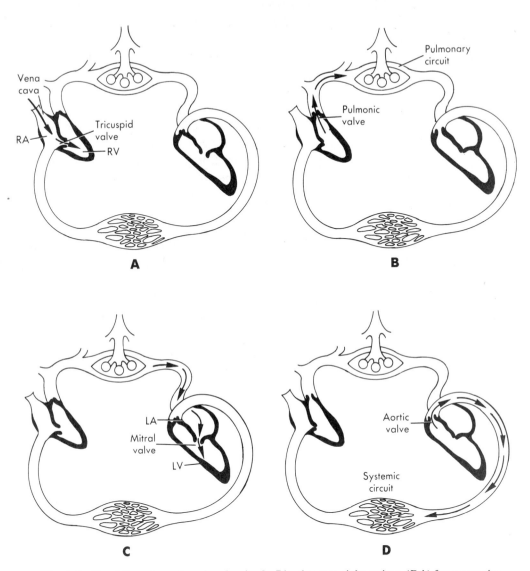

Fig. 1-3. Blood flow through series circuit. **A,** Blood enters right atrium *(RA)* from superior vena cava, inferior vena cava, and coronary sinus and flows passively to right ventricle *(RV)* through tricuspid valve. **B,** Blood volume is propelled from *RV* through pulmonic valve and out into lungs. **C,** Oxygenated blood flows from lungs via four pulmonary veins to left atrium *(LA)*, through mitral valve, and into left ventricle *(LV)*. **D,** High pressure generation by *LV* finally propels blood through aortic valve and out into aortic and systemic circulation during ventricular systole.

tricular contraction (Fig. 1-3, B). Resistance may drastically increase in the presence of a pulmonary embolism, which could cause massive right ventricular failure. The most common cause of right ventricular failure, however, is left ventricular failure. A look at the series circuit arrangement lends appreciation for the influence left-sided failure exerts on the right side.

Left atrium

The left atrium passively empties oxygenated blood received from the lungs via four pulmonary veins, through the mitral valve, and into the left ventricle (Fig. 1-3, C).[6] Since no true valves separate pulmonary veins from the left atrium, elevation of left atrial pressure is reflected retrogradely into the pulmonary vasculature.

Left ventricle

High pressure generation is a requirement of left ventricular function to overcome the systemic circulation resistance and to propel blood through the aortic valve and into the peripheral arterial tree (Fig. 1-3, D). Contributing to development of high pressure during left ventricular contraction is the circular shape and thick musculature of this chamber (see intramyocardial wall tension, p. 19). The intraventricular septum also contributes to the powerful compression sustained during contraction.[9]

Conduction system

Synchronized contraction and relaxation of the previously mentioned chambers follow an inherent rhythmicity of the cardiac muscle. Fig. 1-4 illustrates the conduction network. The highest level of automaticity lies in the sinoatrial (SA) node located in the right atrial posterior wall, immediately beneath the point of entry of the

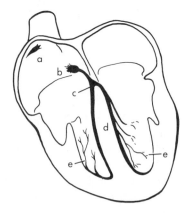

Fig. 1-4. Conduction system of heart. *a*, SA node; *b*, AV node; *c*, bundle of His; *d*, bundle branches; *e*, Purkinje fibers.

superior vena cava. Once the impulse is discharged from the SA node, it travels first to the atria, causing them to depolarize and contract; it then propagates to the atrioventricular (AV) node, where it is delayed a few hundredths of a second before passing through the bundle of His, bundle branches, and Purkinje network. This delay of the impulse in the AV node allows blood to flow from atria to ventricles before ventricular contraction.[12,21]

Depolarization and repolarization: action potential

Electrochemical activity precedes mechanical contraction. Intracellular and extracellular fluids are electrolyte solutions composed of negative and positive ions. Ion fluxes across the cell membrane shift electrical charges, which cause depolarization and repolarization. Depolarization of the myocardial cell occurs when the inside of the cell becomes less negative. Repolarization is the process by which the cell returns to its resting state. These changes in electrical potential across the cell membrane constitute what is referred to as the *cardiac action potential*. Insertion of a microelectrode into the cell allows the recording of this action potential (Fig. 1-5).

Five phases are characteristic of a myocardial cell action potential. Briefly, when the microelectrode is introduced into the myocardial muscle cell (nonpacemaker cell), the graph reading plunges to about −90 millivolts. Phase 0 represents rapid cellular depolarization. Phases 1 through 3 represent the three stages of repolarization, and phase 4 is the period of electrical diastole. Phase 4 of the myocardial fiber differs from a pacemaker cell in that the myocardial fiber requires some sort of stimulus to jar the cell membrane to cause an ion flux—hence depolarization. A pacemaker cell is therefore self-perpetuating and continuously generating new action potentials during phase 4.[14]

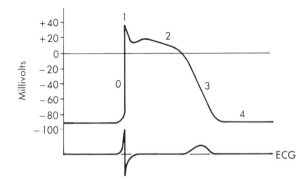

Fig. 1-5. Myocardial cell action potential. Phase 0, rapid influx of sodium (depolarization); phases 1 to 3, stages of repolarization; phase 4, electrical diastole.

Ventricular systole and diastole

Understanding systolic and diastolic phases of the cardiac cycle is important to later chapters in which the physiological outcome of intraaortic balloon inflation and deflation and timing of this inflation-deflation sequence in proper synchronization with the cardiac cycle are discussed. Physiologically, systole is considered to begin approximately with closure of the AV valves and to end approximately with their opening.[10] The breakdown of ventricular systole and diastole has been approached in several ways. More important is an understanding of the events that occur during ventricular contraction and relaxation. Both systole and diastole are described in terms of early and late phases (Fig. 1-6). In early diastole, mitral and tricuspid valves are open, and blood entering the atria through venous channels flows passively and rapidly into the ventricles through the open AV valves. Finally the atria

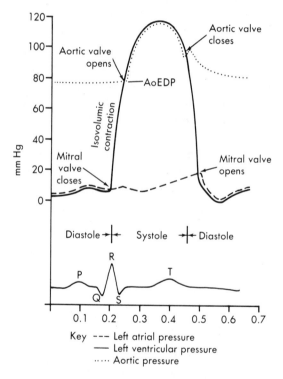

Fig. 1-6. Electrical and mechanical cycles of left heart. P wave is noted (atrial depolarization) to immediately precede the atrial pressure wave generated by atrial contraction. QRS complex represents ventricular depolarization, which is followed by left ventricular contraction and rise of left ventricular pressure to 120 mm Hg during peak systole. Systole begins with QRS complex and ends with T wave. Diastole begins with T wave and ends with onset of QRS complex. Aortic pressure curve is represented as 120 mm Hg in systole and 80 mm Hg in diastole. (*AoEDP,* Aortic end-diastolic pressure.)

contract, contributing an additional 20% to ventricular volume. At this point, the ventricular filling phase reaches a plateau. Such an interval of unchanging ventricular volume is termed the *period of diastasis*. In early systole the papillary muscles are excited and begin to contract. Shortening papillary muscles exert traction on the chordae tendinae, drawing the AV valves into apposition. Since all four valves are closed, the contracting muscles elevate ventricular pressure but do not change ventricular volume. Thus the interval during which ventricular pressure rises to a level sufficient to open the semilunar valves by overcoming aortic end-diastolic pressure is termed *isovolumic contraction*. This is an extremely important phase of the cardiac cycle to understand in relation to balloon counterpulsation, and it is discussed later in greater detail. As soon as ventricular pressure exceeds the aortic end-diastolic pressure, the aortic valve opens, and ventricular ejection into the systemic circulation occurs.[2,3,20]

Blood flow

Ventricular systole causes a propulsion of blood from the left ventricle to the systemic circuit. During ventricular relaxation, or diastole, this driving force is absent, but blood flow to the peripheral tissues continues. The elastic proximal aorta and large arteries stretch to accommodate cardiac stroke volume in systole.[1] This permits much of the force imparted to the blood by ventricular contraction to be stored as potential energy in the elastic arterial wall. When the heart relaxes and intravascular pressure falls, these stretched aortic fibers recoil, maintaining a pressure head (Fig. 1-7). Runoff into the peripheral tissues continues in diastole under the pressure head created by energy released from the aorta, now termed kinetic energy. Temporary storage of stroke volume during the ejection period is termed the *Windkessel effect*. This effect serves to smooth out the flow of blood in the circulation so that flow continues during diastole. Without the Windkessel effect, the blood would reach the tissues in spurts.[3,18]

Determinants of cardiac output

Cardiac output is the product of heart rate and stroke volume. Stroke volume, the volume of blood pumped by the ventricle per beat, averages 70 ml in the adult. Thus at a heart rate of 70 beats per minute, the cardiac output would equal 4900 ml per minute. Stroke volume, which represents myocardial performance, is dependent on the following four distinct but interrelated variables: preload, afterload, contractility or inotropic state of the heart, and heart rate (Fig. 1-8).[6,25]

Preload: Frank-Starling law of the heart. In 1884 Howell and Donaldson[8] presented their findings that the heart possesses an intrinsic mechanism by which its output is adjusted to the venous input. This concept, known as preload, suggests that ventricular fiber length before contraction (fiber stretch caused by end-diastolic volume) determines strength of the contraction. The capacity of the intact ventricle

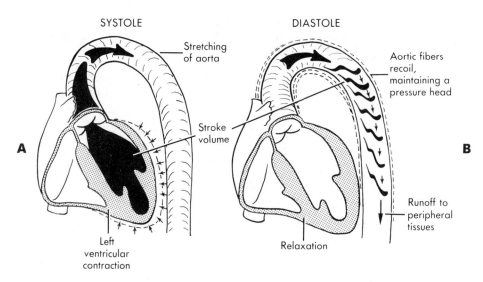

Fig. 1-7. Windkessel effect. **A,** Ventricular systole—elastic proximal aorta and large arteries stretch to accommodate cardiac stroke volume. Force imparted to blood by ventricular contraction is stored as potential energy in elastic arterial wall. **B,** Ventricular diastole—fibers in aorta, which were stretched in systole, now recoil, maintaining a pressure head. Runoff into peripheral tissues continues in diastole under this pressure head created by stored elastic energy in the aorta.

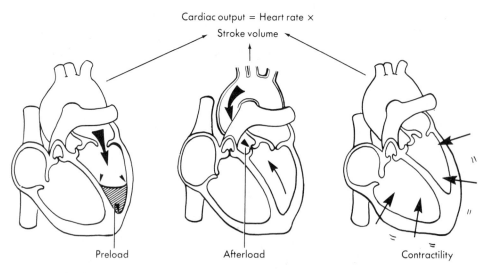

Fig. 1-8. Cardiac output equals heart rate times stroke volume. Factors influencing stroke volume are preload, afterload, and contractility (see text for discussion).

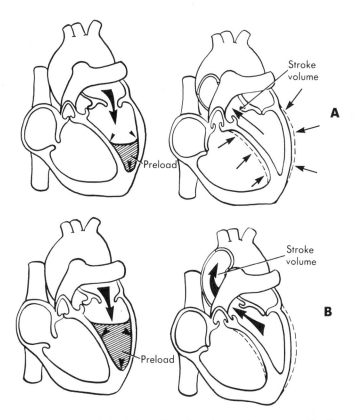

Fig. 1-9. A, Increased preload (end-diastolic volume) stretches contractile fibers just before systole, enabling left ventricle to contract with greater vigor. **B,** Additional preload results in even greater stroke volume ejected during systole.

to vary its force of contraction on a beat-to-beat basis as a function of end-diastolic fiber length constitutes the *Frank-Starling law of the heart*.[5,22] When cardiac muscle fibers are stretched before contraction because of increased end-diastolic volume, a greater contractile effort ensues[2] (Fig. 1-9). Simplistically this concept can be illustrated by examining the water pressure effect generated with release of balloons containing two different amounts of water before release (Fig. 1-10). Increasing water volume before release of the balloon nets a greater force of pressure generated when the balloon is released.

The gain falls off when myocardial fibers are stretched beyond "physiological limits"; further stretching fails to produce a positive effect on the force of ventricular contraction (Fig. 1-11). Because end-diastolic fiber length and intraventricular pressure are normally related to each other, it is common in clinical practice to monitor the left ventricular end-diastolic pressure or pulmonary artery wedge pressure (PAWP) as representative of left ventricular fiber length. In a normal Starling curve

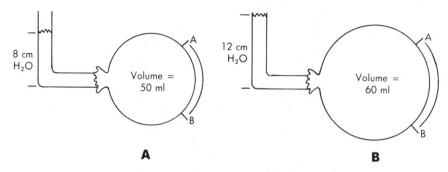

Fig. 1-10. Effect of preload on ensuing ventricular systole, using analogy of balloon filled with water and attached to manometer (*A*). Balloon is filled with 50 ml of water. On release, 8 cm of water pressure is generated (*B*). Balloon is now filled with 60 ml of water. Added stretch is placed on balloon wall (tangent *A* to *B*). On release of balloon, 12 cm of water pressure is generated.

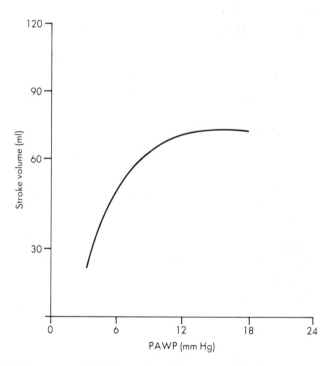

Fig. 1-11. Starling's curve of the heart. Increasing preload (pulmonary artery wedge pressure, *PAWP*) results in greater force of contraction in systole, but only to a certain physiological point. Thereafter, increasing end-diastolic volume does not facilitate greater force of contraction, and eventually with continued added stretch on fibers, the ventricle may fail.

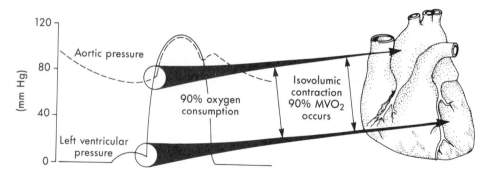

Fig. 1-12. Isovolumic contraction—early systolic phase of cardiac cycle. All four heart valves are closed, and left ventricle is required to generate enough pressure to overcome aortic end-diastolic pressure to open the aortic valve. Systolic ejection then follows. Approximately 90% of myocardial oxygen consumption (MVO$_2$) occurs during isovolumic contraction.

very slight changes in fiber length, produced by small changes in left ventricular end-diastolic pressure, are associated with significant increases in stroke volume. In many cases a patient's myocardial muscle appears to operate chronically at the maximal projection length. Therefore it is unable to significantly respond to increased filling or stretch with a greater force of contraction.[1,2,11,13,15]

Afterload. Resistance to left ventricular ejection is termed the *afterload* component of cardiac work. Major contributors of left ventricular afterload are aortic impedance and peripheral vascular resistance. Aortic end-diastolic pressure represents the pressure resistance the left ventricle must overcome to push open the aortic valve during isovolumic contraction (Fig. 1-12).[13,20] Aortic end-diastolic pressure is an extremely important landmark in balloon counterpulsation; the net outcome is to produce a lowering of this aortic end-diastolic pressure. Approximately 90% of myocardial oxygen consumption occurs during this isovolumic phase as the heart works against the afterload. Anticipated physiological improvement to the patient with balloon assistance would be to reduce afterload and myocardial oxygen consumption during isovolumic contraction.

Contractility. Contractility refers to changes in the force of myocardial contraction and is a function of the interaction between contractile elements (actomyosin crossbridges, Chapter 3) at the cellular level. By definition, contractility refers to alterations in the force of contraction that occur independently of myocardial fiber length. Contractility may be increased by sympathetic stimulation that may occur with endogenous production of catecholamines or with those exogenously administered in the form of epinephrine, norepinephrine, isoproterenol, dopamine, or calcium. These drugs effect an increase in inotropic (increased force of contraction) performance of the heart muscle. Myocardial contractility may be decreased by hypoxemia and by the following drugs: propranolol, quinidine, procainamide, lidocaine, and barbiturates.[2,6,19]

Heart rate. Acceleration of the frequency of contraction increases stroke volume at any given level of filling. This phenomenon is termed the *staircase* or *Bowditch effect*. However, reduction in duration of diastole at rapid heart rates can interfere with ventricular filling time, ultimately limiting the rise in cardiac output associated with tachycardia.[7,16] The intraaortic balloon is inflated in diastole. A decreased diastole (increased heart rate) shortens duration of balloon inflation.

Factors influencing vascular resistance

Braunwald[2] identified major stimuli that are responsible for alterations in vessel caliber and therefore vascular resistance: (1) metabolic, hormonal, or chemical substances that are carried in the blood or released locally and (2) the autonomic nervous system.

Metabolic, hormonal, or chemical substances. A decrease of oxygen, increase in potassium, or increase in osmolality produces vasodilation. Conversely, systemic release of norepinephrine and epinephrine by the adrenal medulla, as occurs in stressful situations, can initiate potent vasoconstriction (Chapter 4).

Autonomic nervous control of the heart. Intrinsic pacemaker systems enable the heart to operate without any nervous influences. However, efficacy of the heart's action can be changed by tonic influence of the autonomic nervous system. The heart interconnects with the autonomic nervous system via parasympathetic (vagi) and sympathetic nerves (Fig. 1-13). Sympathetic fibers originate in the spinal cord (T1-L2) and articulate with the heart via the cervical sympathetic ganglia. Sympathetic nervous fibers supply both atria and ventricles. Norepinephrine is the mediator, and its effect on the heart is to increase the force of contraction and heart rate by its stimulation of the sinus node. Sympathetic system–induced tachycardia decreases the period of diastole and coronary artery filling time.

Parasympathetic fibers originate in the medulla and reach the heart via the vagus nerve. Stimulation of the vagi causes the hormone acetylcholine to be released, slowing rate of impulse discharge from the sinus node and conduction of the impulses through the AV node.[3,9,10,12]

Myocardial oxygen use: supply and demand

If the heart is deprived of oxygen for only a few minutes, mechanical activity ceases. Metabolic processes of contraction are almost totally aerobic; the heart extracts 75% to 80% of the arterial oxygen content of coronary blood. Thus the balance between oxygen supply and demand is so intricate that the demands of accelerated myocardial work can only be provided by augmenting coronary blood flow through vasodilation, since extrapolation is already extraordinarily high[17] (Fig. 1-14).

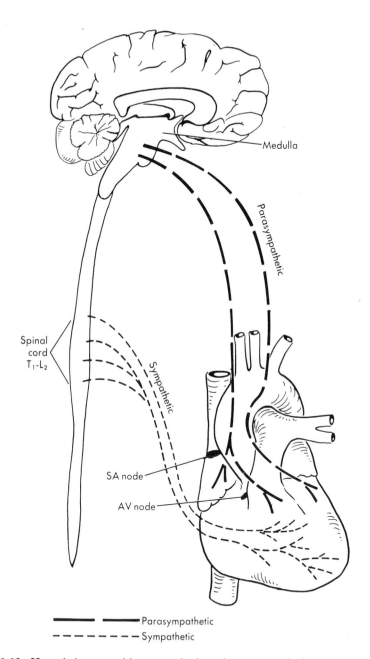

Medulla

Parasympathetic

Spinal
cord
T_1-L_2

Sympathetic

SA node

AV node

——— ——— Parasympathetic
— — — — — — Sympathetic

Fig. 1-13. Heart is innervated by sympathetic and parasympathetic nervous systems.

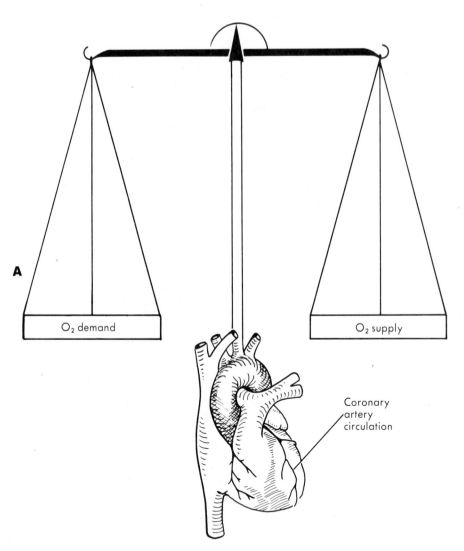

A

O₂ demand

O₂ supply

Coronary
artery
circulation

Fig. 1-14. Myocardial oxygen supply and demand. **A,** Normally, oxygen supply meets demand required to perform myocardial work.

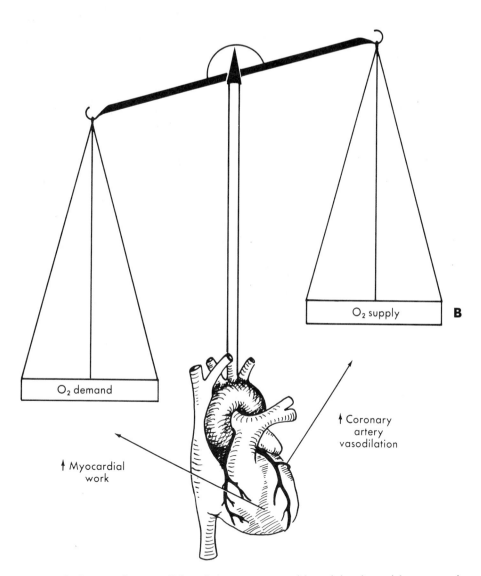

Fig. 1-14. B, Increased myocardial work (as may occur with peripheral arterial vasoconstriction) increases oxygen demand. Coronary artery vasodilation may occur as compensatory mechanism to increase perfusion and myocardial oxygen delivery.

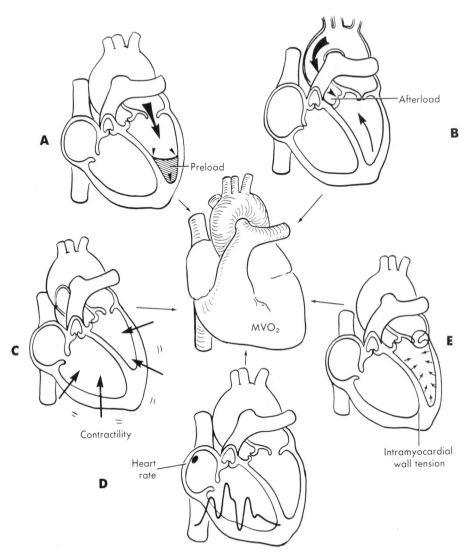

Fig. 1-15. Determinants of myocardial oxygen consumption (MVO$_2$). **A,** Preload. **B,** Afterload. **C,** Contractility. **D,** Heart rate. **E,** Intramyocardial wall tension (determined by pressure generated by contracting ventricle in systole and radius of ventricular cavity).

Myocardial oxygen consumption

Determinants of myocardial oxygen consumption are expressed in Fig. 1-15. Afterload, preload, contractility, and heart rate have been previously discussed. Intramyocardial wall tension is determined by the following: (1) pressure generated by the contracting ventricle in systole and (2) size of the ventricular cavity. During isovolumic contraction, ventricular radius decreases, which builds tension that contributes to the left ventricle overcoming the aortic end-diastolic pressure (afterload). An expansion of the chamber radius (cardiac dilation) nets an increased *intramyocardial wall tension.* Therefore a dilated heart requires more oxygen than a normal heart.[2,6]

Coronary circulation

Fig. 1-16 depicts a cutaway view of the left ventricle and aorta, representing anatomical locations of the coronary arteries. Orifices of the right and left coronary arteries are located within the sinuses of Valsalva in the aorta, immediately above the aortic valve. These sinuses of Valsalva appear as pockets just above the aortic valve cusps. During diastole, blood flows into and distends the sinuses and then flows out into the right and left coronary arteries. Right and left main coronary arteries and their subdividing branches are illustrated in Fig. 1-17. Arising from the aortic anterior surface, the right coronary artery passes diagonally toward the right side of the heart and descends in the groove between the right atrium and ventricle (the AV

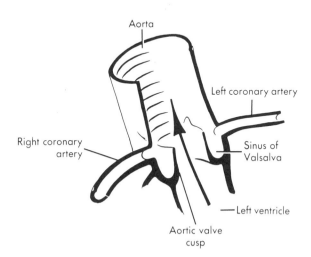

Fig. 1-16. Cutaway view of left ventricle and aorta, representing anatomical location of coronary arteries. Orifices of right and left coronary arteries are located within sinuses of Valsalva, which arise from aortic walls, immediately above aortic valve.

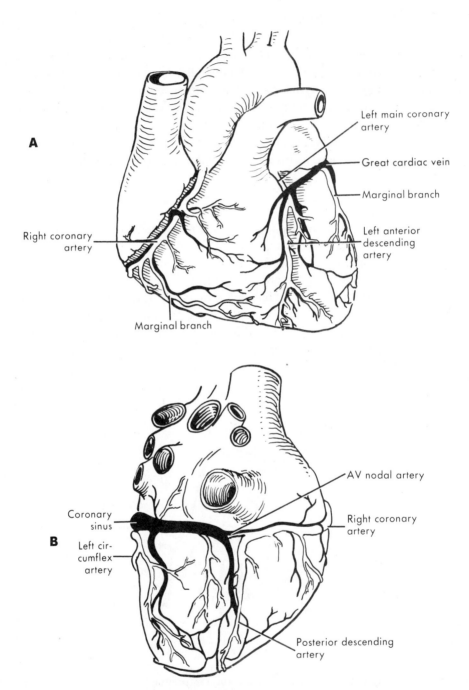

A

Left main coronary artery

Great cardiac vein

Marginal branch

Left anterior descending artery

Right coronary artery

Marginal branch

B

AV nodal artery

Right coronary artery

Coronary sinus

Left cir- cumflex artery

Posterior descending artery

Fig. 1-17. Coronary arteries and veins. **A,** Anterior view. **B,** Posterior view.

Table 1-1.   Right coronary artery subdivisions

Anterior branches	Area supplied
Conus	Outflow tract of right ventricle (infundibulum)
Marginal	Anterior and posterior right ventricle
Posterior branches; transverses high across the posterior heart along the intraventricular groove that separates the two ventricles	Crux of the heart (juncture of the AV and intraventricular grooves)
Posterior descending	Posterior interventricular septum; supplies adjacent areas of the right and left ventricles
Obstruction to blood flow of the right coronary artery =	Inferior myocardial infarction

groove). Table 1-1 lists right coronary artery subdivision. In about 80% of the population the right coronary artery supplies the posterior descending coronary vessel. The right coronary is then said to be *dominant*. In the remaining 20%, the posterior descending vessel arises from the terminal portion of the left coronary artery, which is then termed a *predominant left coronary system*.[6,7,12]

Arising from the posterior surface of the aorta and left of the sinus of Valsalva is the left coronary artery. The short stub of a main left vessel soon divides into the following two major vessels: the anterior descending branch and the circumflex branch. Subdivisions and areas of the heart supplied by these tributary vessels are listed in Table 1-2.

Venous coronary circulation (Fig. 1-17). Once blood has circulated through the rich network of coronary capillaries, about 90% returns to the right atrium through

Table 1-2.   Left coronary artery subdivisions

Branch	Area supplied
Left Anterior Descending Branches	
Septal	Anterior part of interventricular septum
Anterior branches	Anterior surface of left ventricle
Diagonal branch	Supplies lateral margin of left ventricle
Obstruction to blood flow of anterior descending branch	Anterior, anterior-septal, or anterior-lateral myocardial infarction
Circumflex Branches	
Marginal	Posterior surface of left ventricle
Obstruction to circumflex branch =	Posterior myocardial infarction

Data from Hurst JW et al, eds: *The heart*, ed 5, New York, 1982, McGraw-Hill.

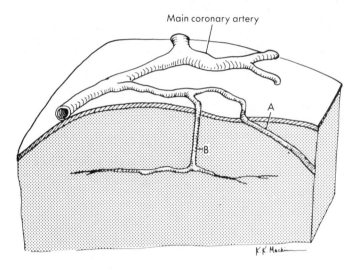

Fig. 1-18. Intramyocardial distribution of coronary arteries (*A*). Epicardial arteries arise at acute angles from main coronary vessels to supply epicardial surface of heart (*B*). Smaller vessels branch at oblique angles from main coronary vessels that penetrate deeper into myocardium and endocardium (intramural arteries).

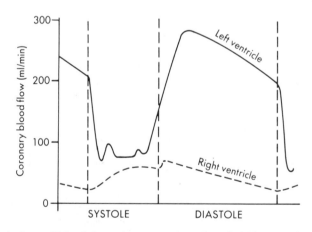

Fig. 1-19. Phasic flow of blood through coronary arteries of right and left ventricle. (From Guyton A: *Textbook of medical physiology*, ed 5, Philadelphia, 1976, WB Saunders.)

the coronary sinus; the remainder returns through thebesian vessels that empty directly into the right atrium.

Phasic coronary blood flow. Blood flows from the main coronary artery vessels through branches over the outer surface of the heart and then into smaller arteries in the cardiac muscle.[17] The outer, epicardial layer of the heart is supplied with blood from coronary branches that arise at acute angles from the main coronary branches (Fig. 1-18). Smaller vessels also branch at right angles from right and left coronary arteries, which penetrate into the myocardium and endocardium (intramural arteries). The heart muscle is supplied with an unusually rich network of capillaries, but blood flow through this rich network is phasic with systolic and diastolic cycles of myocardial contraction. In contrast to blood flow in other portions of the circulation, perfusion through coronary arteries is generally greater in diastole than in systole. Fig. 1-19 illustrates coronary capillary circulation in systole and diastole. Strong compression of cardiac muscle around the deeply embedded coronary capillaries creates a marked rise in coronary vascular resistance and a phasic reduction in blood flow. During diastole, the cardiac muscle relaxes completely and no longer obstructs blood flow.

Chilian and Marcus[4] at the University of Iowa studied phasic coronary circulation. During controlled conditions, the percentage of total coronary blood flow velocity occurring during diastole per cardiac cycle was significantly greater ($p \leq 0.05$) in the intramural artery (septal—92%) than in the epicardial artery (left anterior descending—75%). Phasic blood velocity pattern in penetrating coronary arteries was found to be different from large epicardial arteries. Blood flow velocity during midsystole was retrograde in the intramural vessel and antegrade in the epicardial vessel. During vasodilation, following nitroglycerin, the mid-systolic retrograde flow component of the intramural artery persisted, despite large increases (300% to 400%) in the mid-systolic antegrade flow of the epicardial artery.

The right ventricular coronary capillary circulation also undergoes phasic changes in perfusion. However, the force of right ventricular contraction is significantly less than the left ventricle. Therefore phasic reduction in coronary flow is relatively mild compared to the left ventricle.

Autoregulation of coronary blood flow. Coronary blood flow is controlled by the process of autoregulation within the coronary bed. Autoregulation is an intrinsic mechanism, maintaining a balance between local myocardial oxygen supply and demand. Myocardial tissue hypoxia is the most potent stimulus for increasing coronary blood flow and oxygen supply through vasodilation. Conversely, a reduction in oxygen demand produces a decrease in coronary blood flow through vasoconstriction.[1,11]

Collateral circulation. When a gradual narrowing of a coronary artery occurs, intercoronary communications (collateral flow) are established (Fig. 1-20). Major areas of anastomotic connections are at the posterior surface, where the terminal portions

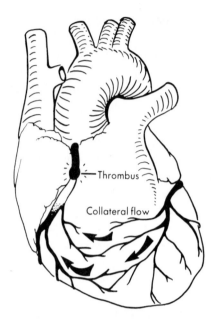

Fig. 1-20. Collateral coronary circulation. A thrombus or atherosclerotic lesion can obstruct blood flow through main coronary vessel. Intertributary communication allows flow to be re-established distal to area of occlusion via blood flow through collateral vessels.

of the right coronary artery and left circumflex branch unite and at the heart's apex, where the terminal portion of the anterior and posterior descending and marginal branches of the right coronary artery all converge. Collateral flow, communication in blood flow to the narrowed vessel from an alternative branch, is then established.

REFERENCES

1. Alpert NR et al: Heart muscle mechanics, *Annu Rev Physiol* 41:521, 1979.
2. Braunwald E et al: The contraction of the normal heart. In Braunwald E: *Heart disease: a textbook of cardiovascular medicine*, ed 4, Philadelphia, 1992, WB Saunders.
3. Burton AC: *Physiology and biophysics of the circulation*, ed 2, Chicago, 1972, Mosby–Year Book.
4. Chilian WM and Marcus ML: Phasic coronary blood flow velocity in intramural and epicardial coronary arteries, *Circ Res* 50:775, 1982.
5. Frank O: On the dynamics of cardiac muscle, *Am Heart J* 58:282, 1959. (Translated by Chapman CB and Wasserman E.)
6. Guyton AC: *Textbook of medical physiology*, ed 8, Philadelphia, 1991, WB Saunders.
7. Hirsch EF: The innervation of human heart. IV. (1) The fiber connections of the nerves with the perimysial plexus (Gerlach-Hofmann); (2) The role of nerve tissues in the repair of infarcts, *Arch Pathol* 75:378, 1963.
8. Howell WH and Donaldson F Jr: Experiments upon the heart of the dog with reference to maximum volume of blood sent out by the left ventricle in a single beat, *Philos Trans R Soc Lond (Biol)* 175:139, 1884.
9. James TL et al: Anatomy of the heart. In Hurst JW et al, eds: *The heart*, ed 7, New York, 1990, McGraw-Hill.

10. Katz AMP: *Physiology of the heart*, New York, 1977, Raven Press.
11. Little RC: *Physiology of the heart and circulation*, Chicago, 1977, Mosby–Year Book.
12. Little RC, ed: *Physiology of atrial pacemakers and conductive tissue*, Mount Kisco, NY, 1980, Futura Publishing.
13. Mahler F et al: Effects of changes in preload, afterload, and inotropic state on ejection and isovolumic phase measures of contractility in the conscious dog, *Am J Cardiol* 36:626, 1975.
14. Marriott HJL and Conover M: *Advanced concepts in arrhythmias*, ed 2, St. Louis, 1989, Mosby–Year Book.
15. Mirsky I et al: *Cardiac mechanics: physiological, clinical and mathematical considerations*, New York, 1974, John Wiley & Sons.
16. Mitchell JH et al: Intrinsic effects of heart rate on left ventricular performance, *Am J Physiol* 205:411, 1963.
17. Pasyk S et al: Systemic and coronary effects of coronary artery occlusion in the unanesthetized dog, *Am J Physiol*, 220:646, 1971.
18. Rushmer RF: *Cardiovascular dynamics*, ed 5, Philadelphia, 1993, WB Saunders.
19. Sarnoff SJ: Myocardial contractility as described by ventricular function curves: observations on Starling's law of the heart, *Physiol Rev* 35:107, 1955.
20. Schlant RC and Sonnenblick EB: Pathophysiology of heart failure. In Hurst JW et al, eds: *The heart*, ed 7, New York, 1990, McGraw-Hill.
21. Sommers JR and Johnson EA: A comparative study of Purkinje fibers and ventricular fibers, *J Cell Biol* 36:497, 1968.
22. Starling EH: *The Linacre lecture on the law of the heart*, London, 1918, Longmans, Green and Co.
23. Wiggers CJ: Determinants of cardiac performance, *Circulation* 4:485, 1951.

CHAPTER 2

Myocardial excitation and contraction

Susan J. Quaal

Understanding fundamental mechanisms of contraction of the normal and failing heart is essential to a textbook on intraaortic balloon counterpulsation (IABC). Impaired contractile function, resulting in cardiac failure, is a precipitating factor that may necessitate IABC. Myocardial contraction is a result of the integrated function of its individual contractile elements. This chapter defines myocardial ultrastructure functional activities during the contraction process.

MYOCARDIAL ULTRASTRUCTURE

Myocardial ultrastructure, as described by Fawcett and McNutt,[1] is illustrated in Fig. 2-1. The myocardium is composed of longitudinal series of bundles of myocardial cells that interdigitate with each other to form a fiber, *the myofibril*. Most of these fibers are arrayed parallel to one another with *mitochondria*, the energy source for contraction, sandwiched between myofibrils.

Within the cell, myocardial ultrastructure consists of the following organelles: cell membrane or sarcolemma, intercalated disk, sarcomeres, myofibrils, actin, myosin, tropomyosin and troponin proteins, sarcotubular system, and mitochondria.[2]

Sarcolemma (cell membrane)

The *sarcolemma* separates intracellular constituents from extracellular fluid. Numerous vesicles are found immediately external to and within the membrane as well as within the cell cytoplasm. These vesicles are termed *pinocytotic*, capable of absorbing liquids by phagocytosis, and are presumably involved in cellular metabolism. Functions ascribed to the sarcolemma are (1) separation of intracellular and extracellular environments, (2) membrane transport activity as necessary for cellular metabolism, (3) active maintenance of cellular ionic composition, and (4) transmembrane movement of ions, producing electrical currents that are manifested on the electrocardiogram.[3,4]

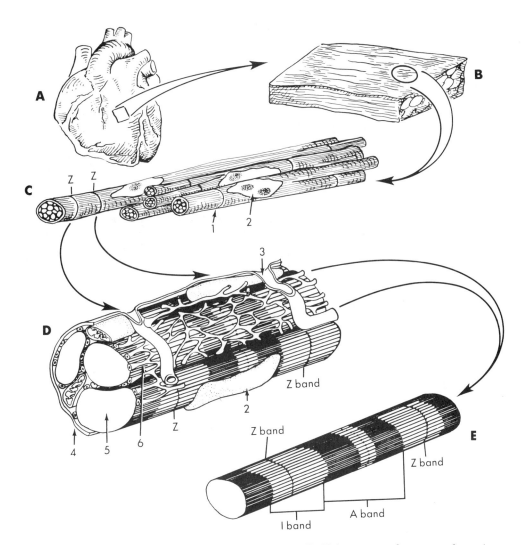

Fig. 2-1. Microscopic structures of heart muscle. **A** to **B,** Enlargement of segment of ventricular myocardium. **C,** Myofibril (*1*), intercalated disk (*2*), and mitochondria. **D,** Microscopic ultrastructure (*3*), T tubule, (*4*) sarcolemma, (*5*) myofibril, and (*6*) sarcoplasmic reticulum. **E,** Enlargement of myofibril. (See text for discussion.)

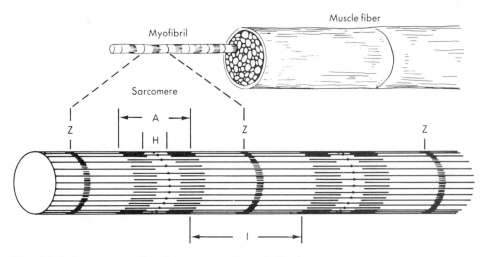

Fig. 2-2. Ultrastructure of working myocardial cell, illustrating Z band (separates each contractile unit or sarcomere), I band (actin filaments), A band (overlapping of myosin filaments from actin filaments), and H zone (region occupied only by myosin filaments).

Intercalated disk

Electron microscopic examination reveals that each cell is separated by an *intercalated* disk. Therefore cells of the working myocardium are not an anatomical *syncytium* (a group of cells in which the protoplasm of one cell is continuous with that of adjoining cells). However, these boundaries offer little electrical resistance so that the myocardium is considered a functional syncytium. In working myocardial cells, myofibrils insert into the region of the intercalated disk. The disk must therefore possess great strength to support forces generated by repeated myofibril contraction.[3,5,6]

Myofibrils

Each cardiac muscle fiber contains a group of branching longitudinal, striated strands approximately 1 μm in diameter, termed *myofibrils*. They exhibit a characteristic pattern of light and dark transverse bands and are subdivided into a series of repeating contractile units, the *sarcomeres*, by a dark, transverse line (*Z band*) (Fig. 2-2). The sarcomere functions as the cell's contractile unit and is ideally suited to structural aspects of contraction as a result of its elongated shape.[7,8]

Sarcomeres exhibit a band appearance because they are composed of an ordered array of two different overlapping protein filaments, *actin* (thin) and *myosin* (thick). Actin filaments extend in both directions from the Z band that produces a light area (*I band*) (Fig. 2-2), so called because it rotates polarized light under the electron mi-

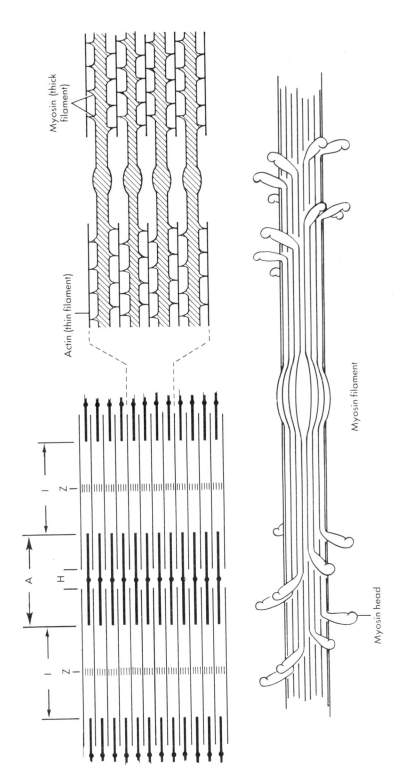

Fig. 2-3. Organization of thick myosin filaments of sarcomere.

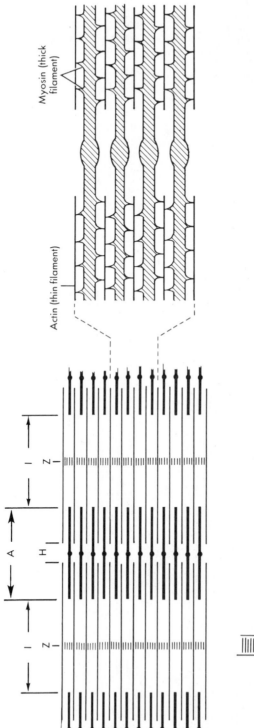

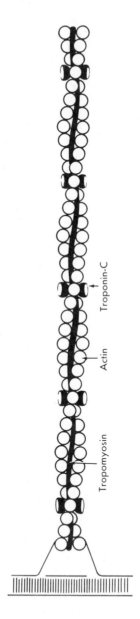

Fig. 2-4. Organization of helically arrayed double-strand thin actin filaments of sarcomere. Troponin and tropomyosin proteins lie in helical grooves.

croscope. Myosin fibrils overlap onto the actin filaments, which gives rise to a darker, transverse band (A band). The central light area (*H zone*) of the A band represents regions occupied only by the myosin filaments.[9,10]

Myosin filaments

Myosin (thick) filaments extend throughout the A band, from one A-I band boundary to the next (Fig. 2-3). Myosin is a rod-shaped molecule with a globular enlargement at one end. Localized in this globular head are two important biological properties.

1. Myosin has the ability to hydrolyze the polyphosphate chain on adenosine triphosphate (ATP), thereby releasing chemical energy.
2. Myosin heads come together with the actin filaments to form cross-bridges in a sliding mechanism that results in contraction.[9,11]

Actin, tropomyosin, troponin proteins

Thin filaments are composed of the following three proteins: *actin, tropomyosin*, and *troponin*. The actin protein is much smaller than myosin. Unlike myosin, which is a highly asymmetrical structure, actin forms a slightly ovoid shape. Thin actin filaments are helically arranged like a double string of beads twisted together (Fig. 2-4). Tropomyosin has no biological properties. Similar to the myosin molecule tail, tropomyosin was found to be a coiled tail.[12] Troponin is the receptor for calcium and acts to modulate interaction between actin and myosin through alterations in tropomyosin.[5,13]

The troponin complex is now recognized to be made up of three proteins. *Troponin-I*, like tropomyosin, has the ability to inhibit the interaction of actin and myosin. *Troponin-T* serves to bind the troponin complex to tropomyosin, and *troponin-C* contains the binding site for calcium.[13,14] Therefore the major effect of the troponin-tropomyosin complex is to inhibit the ability of actin to interact with myosin.

Sarcotubular system

Membrane-limited microtubules, the *sarcotubular system*, fill cardiac muscle interfibrillar spaces. The network is composed of two elements: (1) a transverse component called the *T system* and (2) a longitudinal component, the *sarcoplasmic reticulum (SR)* (Fig. 2-1).

The *T-tubule system* originates from invaginations along the surface of the sarcolemma. This transverse tubular system provides an extension of the sarcolemma into the cell. Tubular content is therefore continuous with the extracellular fluid, possibly has a similar ionic content, and may be involved in movement of substrates into the cell and removal of cellular metabolic end products.[15,16]

The SR is an entirely intracellular system of tubules that forms a membrane-limited network around each myofibril. A single T tubule passes between two myofibrils, each of which is encircled by an SR system. This point of close association of the two systems is called a *triadic junction*,[6] although direct membrane continuity has not been observed.

The sarcotubular system plays an important role in electrochemical coupling involved in initiation and regulation of contraction and relaxation. Calcium is thought to be bound within the sarcotubular system, specifically in a portion of the SR called the *terminal cisternae*.[12,17,18] When an action potential courses over the surface of a cardiac muscle fiber, a wave of depolarization spreads passively along the membranes of the sarcotubular system. This leads to a release of bound calcium, which then diffuses within the SR toward the A-band region of the sarcomere, where it is involved in activation of cardiac contraction.[14]

Mitochondria

Between 25% and 50% of the entire myocardial mass is composed of *mitochondria*. These cylindrical bodies are found arranged systematically between and in close approximation to parallel rows of sarcomeres (see Fig. 2-1). Oxidative phosphorylation, the process by which ATP is produced with the energy contained in carbohydrates, lipids, and proteins, occurs within the mitochondria. The exact mechanism for transfer of ATP from the mitochondrion to the myofibril is not known. The great number of mitochondria in the myocardium is commensurate with a massive demand for energy by the continuously contracting heart muscle, in contrast to conduction tissue, where only 10% of its volume is occupied by mitochondria.[2,18-20]

PROPERTIES OF MYOCARDIAL MUSCLE
Excitation and contraction

Katz[21] described properties of myocardial muscle contraction observed during myosin head interaction with actin to form cross-bridges. These properties include: (1) adenosine triphosphate (ATP) hydrolysis and liberation of energy, (2) physiochemical changes in which the chemical energy derived from ATP hydrolysis is converted to mechanical work, and (3) regulation of contraction by the regulatory proteins, tropomyosin and troponin (dependent on the cellular levels of calcium).

Depolarization and release of calcium

Calcium triggers the contractile process by reversing the inhibitory effect of the regulatory protein, troponin-C. Following ventricular or individual myocardial cell membrane depolarization, the electrical impulse propagates through the transverse tubules into the cell (Fig. 2-5). Depolarization causes calcium to be released from its

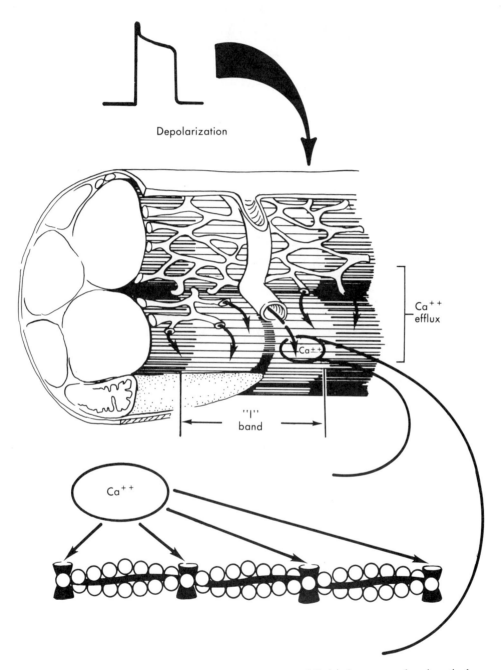

Fig. 2-5. Depolarization of myocardial cell and release of Ca^{++} from sarcoplasmic reticulum and T tubules.

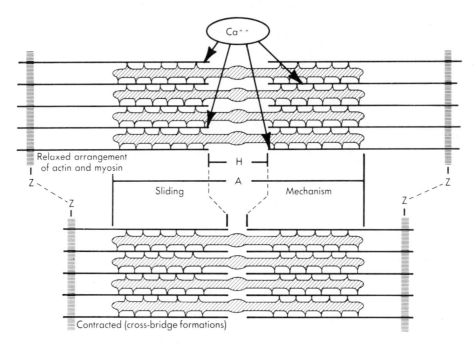

Fig. 2-6. Actin filaments drawn into A band (sliding over myosin filaments) to form cross-bridges.

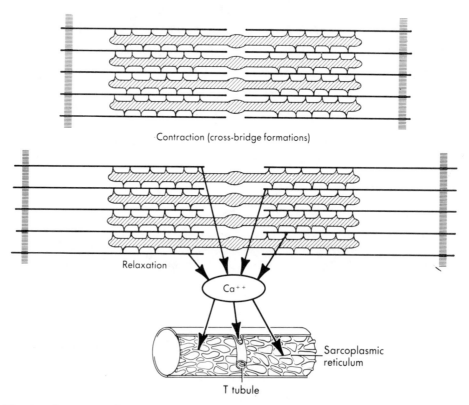

Fig. 2-7. Relaxation of actin and myosin cross-bridges (Ca^{++} sequestered back into sarcoplasmic reticulum and T tubules).

stores in the T-tubule system and sarcoplasmic reticulum.* Calcium then migrates to the thin acting filaments and binds with troponin-C. Calcium therefore removes the inhibition that is present, and a cross-bridge is formed.[22-24]

Formation of actin and myosin cross-bridges

Theories of myocardial muscle contraction have been simplified by introduction of the Huxley sliding filament hypothesis of contraction.[25] Calcium binds to troponin-C and causes tropomyosin to shift out of the way allowing a physical interaction to develop between myosin heads and the activated actin filaments. Myosin heads then hydrolyze ATP and form cross-bridges. Attachment of myosin filaments to a binding site on the appropriate actin filament draws actin filaments into the A band in a sliding mechanism and reduces sarcomere length, which is the process of contraction (Fig. 2-6). Cross-bridges systematically detach from reactive sites, return to their original configuration, and reattach to new reactive sites on the actin filaments, thus beginning a new cycle of ATP splitting. Repeated attachments of the cross-bridges to the actin filaments are believed to occur.[26] Cross-bridges are thought to attach to actin filaments, swivel to a new position, release, reattach to a new site, and repeat the process in rapid succession.[27-30]

Relaxation

Repolarization of the cell membrane is associated with myocardial relaxation, which is initiated by an unknown stimulus. Calcium is sequestered back into the sarcoplasmic reticulum. Recapture of calcium by the sarcoplasmic reticulum requires use of energy from the splitting of ATP. This removal of calcium from the troponin-binding sites results in inhibition of ATP hydrolysis, breaking of the cross-bridge attachments, and finally relaxation of the muscle (Fig. 2-7).[31,32]

REFERENCES

1. Fawcett DW and McNutt NS: The ultrastructure of the cat myocardium; capillary muscle, *J Cell Biol* 43:1, 1969.
2. Hurst JW: *The heart,* ed 7, New York, 1990, McGraw-Hill.
3. Fawcett DW: Physiologically significant specializations of the cell surface, *Circulation* 26:1105, 1962.
4. Robertson JD: The molecular structure and contact relationships of cell membranes, *Prog Biophys Mol Biol* 10:343, 1960.
5. Katz AM: Contractile proteins of the heart, *Physiol Rev* 50:63, 1970.
6. Kawamura K and James TN: Comparative ultrastructure of cellular junctions in working myocardium and the conduction system under normal and pathologic conditions, *J Mol Cell Cardiol* 3:31, 1971.
7. Johnson EA and Sommer JR: A strand of cardiac muscle: its ultrastructure and the electrophysiological implications of its geometry, *J Cell Biol* 33:103, 1967.
8. Moore DH and Rustu H: Electron microscopic study of mammalian cardiac muscle cell, *J Biophys Biochem Cytol* 3:261, 1957.

---

*The mitochondria contain ample stores of calcium. Its release, however, is too slow to be effectively used to trigger contraction.

9. Noble D: Application of Hodgkin-Huxley equation to excitable tissue, *Physiol Rev* 46:1, 1966.
10. Rushmer RF: *Cardiovascular dynamics*, Philadelphia, 1976, WB Saunders.
11. Spiro D and Sonnenblick EH: The structural basis of the contractile process in heart muscle under physiological and pathological conditions, *Prog Cardiovasc Dis* 7:295, 1965.
12. Bond E: Physiology of the heart. In Underhill S et al: *Cardiac nursing*, Philadelphia, 1982, JB Lippincott.
13. Ebashi S: Regulatory mechanism of muscle contraction with special reference to the Ca-troponin-tropomyosin system. In Campbell PN and Dickens F, eds: *Essays in biochemistry*, vol 10, London, 1974, Academic Press.
14. Sonnenblick EH and Stam AC Jr: Heart excitation, conduction and contraction, *Annu Rev Physiol* 31:647, 1968.
15. Simpson FO: The transverse tubular system in mammalian myocardial cells, *Am J Anat* 117:1, 1965.
16. Simpson FO and Dertelis SJ: The fine structure of sheep myocardial cells; subsarcolemmal invaginations and transverse tubular system, *J Cell Biol* 12:91, 1962.
17. Ebashi S and Lipmann F: Adenosine triphosphate linked concentrations of cations in a particular fraction of rabbit muscle, *J Cell Biol* 14:389, 1962.
18. Weeks L: Cardiovascular physiology. In Kinney MR et al: *AACN's clinical reference for critical care nursing*, New York, 1981, McGraw-Hill.
19. Fawcett DW: Mitochondria. In Briller SA and Conn J, eds: *The myocardial cell: structure, function and modification by cardiac drugs*, Philadelphia, 1966, University of Pennsylvania Press.
20. Rendi R and Valter AE: Possible location of phospholipids and structural protein in mitochondrial membranes, *Protoplasma* 63:200, 1967.
21. Katz AM: *Physiology of the heart*, New York, 1977, Raven Press.
22. Gergely J: Some aspects of the role of the sarcoplasmic reticulum and the tropomyosin-troponin system in the control of muscle contraction by the calcium ions, *Circ Res 35* (suppl 3):74, 1974.
23. Peachy LD: The role of transverse tubules in excitation contraction coupling in striated muscles, *Ann NY Acad Sci* 137:1025, 1966.
24. Reuter H and Beeter GW: Calcium current and activation of contraction in ventricular myocardial fibers, *Science* 163:399, 1969.
25. Huxley HE and Hanson J: Changes in the cross striation of muscle during contraction and stretch and their structural interpretation, *Nature* 173:973, 1964.
26. Rushmer RI: *Cardiovascular dynamics*, Philadelphia, 1976, WB Saunders.
27. Barany M: ATPase activity of myosin correlated with speed of muscle shortening, *J Gen Physiol* 50:6, 1962.
28. Braunwald E, Ross J Jr, and Sonnenblick EH: *Mechanism of contraction of the normal and failing heart*, ed 1, Boston, 1968, Little, Brown & Co.
29. Katz AM and Brady AY: Mechanical and biochemical correlates of cardiac contraction, *Mod Concepts Cardiovasc Dis* 40:39, 1971.
30. Weeks L: Cardiovascular physiology. In Kinney MR et al: *AACN's clinical reference for critical care nursing*, New York, 1981, McGraw-Hill.
31. Huxley HE: The mechanism of muscular contraction, *Science,* 164:1356, 1969.
32. Langer GA: Heart: excitation-contraction coupling, *Annu Rev Physiol* 35:55, 1973.

CHAPTER 3

Myocardial energetics

Susan J. Quaal

CARDIAC METABOLISM

The heart normally functions as an aerobic organ, converting metabolic energy to intracardiac pressure that is necessary to produce ventricular ejection; the net result is perfusion of blood to tissues and vital organs. Myocardial energetics is a process of metabolism of nutrients that are delivered to the myocardial muscle and turn into a usable energy source needed during ventricular systole.

With an adequate oxygen supply, myocardial cells extract free fatty acids and glucose, among other substrates, from the blood and oxidize them to pyruvate, which is catabolized in Krebs' cycle. Adenosine triphosphate (ATP) is generated via Krebs' cycle, which provides a necessary energy source for myocardial contraction (Fig. 3-1).[1,2]

Activation of contractile elements in early systole produces a longitudinally oriented tension within the muscle fibers in the same manner that a stretched rubber band placed around a tube occludes the lumen. Tension increases, but muscle length remains constant. This early systolic phase is termed *isometric contraction*. Shortening of the ventricular myocardium occurs later as the aortic and pulmonic valves open, and blood is ejected (i.e., *isotonic contraction*).[3-4] Tension that develops during this transfer of metabolic energy to ventricular pressure is affected by ventricular volume. Displacement of volume during systole constitutes what is termed *cardiac work*.

Cardiac work

Physics terminology describes work as energy transfer that occurs when a mass is moved or a volume is displaced. External and internal work are involved in myocardial transfer of energy from its metabolic substrate to the pressure developed in contraction.

External work. Relating ventricular volume and pressure to the cardiac cycle graphically illustrates the principle of left ventricular external work (Fig. 3-2). During the isovolumic phase of ventricular contraction (*A* to *B*), pressure increases, but

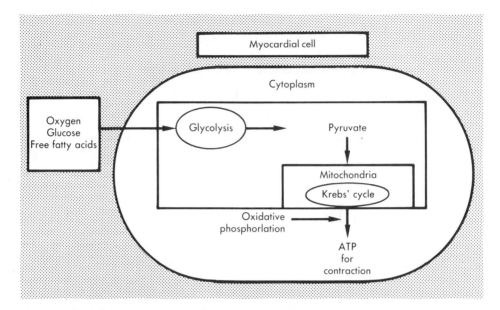

Fig. 3-1. Myocardial metabolism in presence of adequate oxygen. Among other substances, glucose and fatty acids are extracted from blood by myocardial cell and oxidated to pyruvate. Oxygen then enables oxidation of pyruvate to adenosine triphosphate (ATP) during Krebs' metabolic cycle, which occurs in mitochondria of cell.

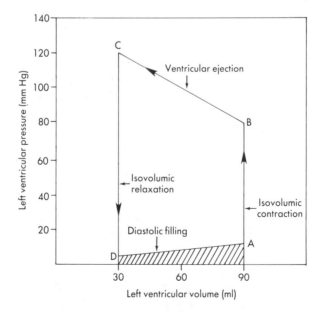

Fig. 3-2. Schematic representation of relationship between left ventricular pressure and volume during complete cardiac cycle. (See text for discussion.)

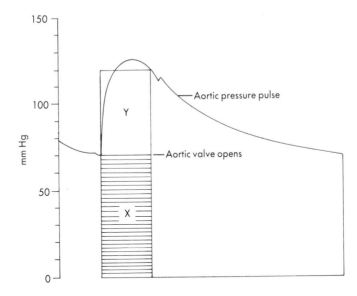

Fig. 3-3. Schematic representation of static (*X*) and dynamic work (*Y*) involved with ventricular ejection. Static work is isometric effort that occurs as left ventricle generates and sustains pressure necessary to push open aortic valve. Dynamic work occurs during ejection itself. (From Little RC: *Physiology of the heart and circulation*, ed 2, Chicago, 1981, Mosby–Year Book. [Modified from Wiggers CJ: *Circulatory dynamics*, New York, 1952, Grune & Stratton.])

volume remains unchanged. Ventricular volume decreases rapidly during ventricular ejection (*B* to *C*), whereas pressure continues to rise. Ventricular pressure falls rapidly after aortic valve closure during isovolumic relaxation (*C* to *D*). Finally ventricular volume rises with only a small increase in pressure (*D* to *A*). The area bounded by the loop *ABCDA* represents the pressure-volume work (i.e., the external work of the left ventricle).[5]

Static and dynamic external work. Static work refers to the development and maintenance of ventricular pressure before opening of the aortic valve. Dynamic work occurs during the process of ventricular ejection. Little[4] beautifully describes division of external cardiac work into static and dynamic components by an analogy to forces involved in pouring a pail of water over a fence. Static effort is constituted by lifting the pail of water to a height equal to or slightly above the top of the fence. Additional energy (dynamic) must be used to tip the pail so that water pours out over the fence.

Static and dynamic work can be graphically illustrated by drawing a horizontal line at the level of the diastolic pressure of an aortic pressure pulse (Fig. 3-3). Static work encompasses the effort involved in raising the ventricular pressure to a level sufficient to open the aortic valve and then holding that pressure for the duration of systole. Static work is therefore an isometric effort that requires a large amount of energy. Dynamic work involves systolic ejection.

Internal work. Energy dissipated in the form of heat or used to open and close valve cusps and to carry out the normal basal tissue activity is termed *internal cardiac work*.[4]

REFERENCES

1. Huxley HE: The contraction of muscle, *Sci Am* 199:66, 1958.
2. Katz AM: *Physiology of the heart*, New York, 1977, Raven Press.
3. Bond EF: Physiology of the heart. In Underhill S et al: *Cardiac nursing*, Philadelphia, 1982, JB Lippincott.
4. Little RC: *Physiology of the heart and circulation*, ed 2, Chicago, 1981, Mosby–Year Book.
5. Burton AC: *Physiology and biophysics of the circulation*, ed 2, Chicago, 1972, Mosby–Year Book.

CHAPTER 4

An overview of heart failure

Susan J. Quaal

Intraaortic balloon counterpulsation (IABC) has been used as an effective intervention for management of heart failure (HF). Therefore an overview of HF is useful before the tutorial chapters on IABC. The Centers for Disease Control estimate that approximately 2.3 million individuals are affected with chronic HF. Nearly 400,000 people in the United States develop HF each year, and this number is likely to increase as greater numbers of patients who might have died of an acute myocardial infarction are surviving, but with compromised ventricular function.[1] Approximately 1000 individuals die daily from HF.[2] As a consequence the number of hospitalizations for HF has increased more than threefold during the past 15 years. This disorder now represents the most common medical discharge diagnosis for patients over the age of 65 years (Fig. 4-1).[3]

Kannel[4] analyzed 34 years of follow-up from the Framingham Study, which provided insight into the prevalence, incidence, secular trends, prognosis, and modifiable risk factors for the occurrence of HF in a general population sample. HF was found to afflict about 1% of individuals in their fifth decade, rising progressively with age. About 10% of people in their 80s are afflicted (Fig. 4-2). HF was greater in men than in women due to a higher incidence of coronary artery disease, which confers a fourfold increased risk of HF. Within 2 years of diagnosis 37% of men and 33% of women died. The 6-year mortality rate was 82% for men and 67% for women, corresponding to a mortality rate fourfold to eightfold greater than the general population for the same age. Sudden death occurred in 28% of men with HF and 14% of women.[4]

PATHOPHYSIOLOGY

HF pathophysiology is complex; the amount of new information that continues to be published attests to its attraction for basic science and clinical medicine re-

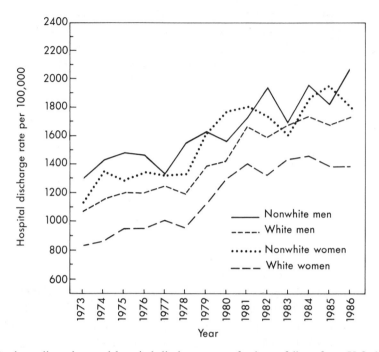

Fig. 4-1. Age-adjusted annual hospital discharge rates for heart failure from U.S. hospitals, 1973-1986, National Hospital Discharge Survey, by sex-race group. (From Chung TO: *Am J Med* 91:409, 1991.)

Age:	50-59	60-69	70-79	80-89
Person-bienniums	20520	19298	8994	2084
Person-bienniums with CHF	166	451	438	190
Percent prevalence	0.8	2.3	4.9	9.1

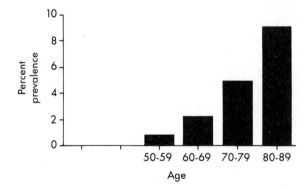

Fig. 4-2. Prevalence of heart failure by age. A 34-year follow-up experience from the Framingham Study in men and women combined. (From Kannel WB, Belanger AJ: *Am Heart J* 121:951, 1991.)

searchers and also to the fact that many essential aspects of HF are still poorly understood.

Definition

HF is not a specific disease, but rather the inability of the heart to pump blood commensurate with body tissue metabolic needs. Delivery of oxygen and nutrients becomes inadequate, leading to cellular dysfunction and imminent organ failure. Systemic blood flow and cardiac output decrease, resulting in further deterioration and impairment of cardiac function.[1]

A more clinical definition of HF has been offered by Packer: "Congestive heart failure represents a complex clinical syndrome characterized by abnormalities of left ventricular function and neurohormonal regulation, which are accompanied by effort intolerance, fluid retention, and reduced longevity."[5] Braunwald[6] described the wide spectrum of clinical physiological states included in these two definitions. Rapid impairment of cardiac function can occur secondary to a massive myocardial infarction, or sudden onset of a tachyrhythmia or bradyrhythmia. A more gradual, but progressive state of HF may occur when the heart is subjected to pressure or volume overload for a prolonged period.

HF should be differentiated from the state of "circulatory congestion" consequent to abnormal salt and water retention, without disturbance of cardiac function. Another related, yet differentiated condition is "circulatory failure," in which an abnormality of blood volume or concentration of arterial oxygenated hemoglobin causes inadequate cardiac output. Braunwald[7] clarified that "myocardial failure," "HF," and "circulatory failure" are not synonymous, but refer to progressively broader entities. Myocardial failure, when sufficiently severe, always produces HF, but the converse is not necessarily the case because a number of conditions in which the heart is suddenly overloaded (e.g., acute aortic regurgitation secondary to acute infective endocarditis) can produce HF in the presence of normal myocardial function. Also, conditions such as tricuspid stenosis and constrictive pericarditis, which interfere with cardiac filling, can produce HF without myocardial failure. HF always produces circulatory failure, but the converse is not the case because a variety of noncardiac conditions (e.g., hypovolemic shock or extremely severe anemia, beriberi, and other high-output states) can produce circulatory failure at a time when cardiac function is normal or only slightly impaired."

Causes and precipitating factors

HF may be a result of (1) underlying causes, (2) fundamental causes, or (3) precipitating factors.[8] Underlying causes comprise structural abnormalities (congenital or acquired) of the pericardium, myocardium, cardiac valves, or peripheral and coronary vessels. These causes lead to myocardial insufficiency or an increased hemodynamic burden that results in HF. Fundamental causes are physiological or biochemical mechanisms that cause impaired cardiac contraction. Precipitating factors account for about 50% of the episodes of HF and include dysrhythmias, inappropriate changes in drugs or treatment (such as increasing salt intake or gaining weight), systemic infection, pulmonary embolism, stressors (emotional, physical, environmental, or sociocultural), cardiac inflammation and infection, untreated illness, or development of a secondary form of heart disease.[8]

Dysrhythmias impede cardiac output through several mechanisms. Bradydysrhythmias can depress cardiac output. Reducing the number of beats per minute without increasing stroke volume will reduce cardiac output. Tachydysrhythmias cause a reduction in ventricular filling time and increase myocardial demand. Increased heart rates may further raise the elevated atrial pressure, thus contributing to a more severe decrease in cardiac output. Atrioventricular (AV) dissociation eliminates the atrial kick, which impairs ventricular filling, thus raising atrial pressure and lowering cardiac output. Total body metabolic needs are increased with a systemic infection through mechanisms of coughing, fever, and tachycardias, which increase the hemodynamic load of the heart.[9]

Psychophysiological stressors induced by physical activity, emotions, environment, or sociocultural factors can cause cardiac decompensation. Anemia, hyperthyroidism, and high-output states in the presence of underlying heart disease are also precipitating causes of HF.

Causes of HF from the Framingham study. Preponderant causes of HF found in the Framingham study were long standing hypertension and coronary heart disease. Those with hypertension or receiving antihypertensive treatment included 76% of the men and 79% of the women. Approximately 46% of men and 27% of women had a history of coronary heart disease. Rheumatic heart disease was a cause in only 2% to 3%.[4]

Indicators of impaired function

Whitman[10] described several intrinsic measurable factors of impaired myocardial function that arose from the Framingham Study.[4] An enlarged heart, electrocardiographic (ECG) abnormalities, poor vital capacity, and rapid heart rate were associated with an increased risk of developing HF. In the asymptomatic patient these symptoms represented deteriorating myocardial function. HF increased progressively with heart rates >85 in both men and women. The risk of HF in men with heart rates >85 was nearly doubled at all blood pressure levels (Fig. 4-3). In asymptomatic individuals a low or falling vital capacity, perhaps reflective of pulmonary vascular engorgement resulting from left ventricular dysfunction, was associated with a risk of HF in both smokers and nonsmokers. ECG abnormalities associated with an increased risk for HF included left ventricular hypertrophy (LVH), intraventricular conduction disturbance, and nonspecific repolarization abnormalities. Left ventricular hypertrophy by ECG criteria contributed more significantly to the

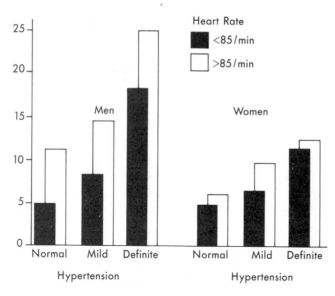

Fig. 4-3. Risk of heart failure by hypertensive and heart rate status: 34- year follow-up from Framingham Study. Subjects 35 to 94 years. (From Kannel WB, Belanger AJ: *Am Heart J* 121:951, 1991.)

incidence of HF. Although risk of HF associated with ECG-LVH was independent of blood pressure, the risk increased in patients who experienced combined ECG-LVH and hypertension. Kannel[4] suggested that the risk of heart failure associated with ECG-LVH may be reduced by correction of hypertension. He cautioned that "ECG-LVH must be regarded as a grave prognostic sign for impending heart failure in the course of hypertension and coronary artery disease."

Modifiable predisposing risk factors

Predisposing risk factors for HF as delineated by Kannel[4] from the Framingham Study included hypertension, diabetes, cigarette smoking, obesity, poor total to high-density lipoprotein (HDL) cholesterol ratio, and hematocrit level. Hypertension was a major contributing factor, increasing the risk of HF by about threefold. Diabetes predisposed patients to HF because of its associated complications (accelerated coronary atherosclerosis, hypertension, and obesity). Diabetes increased the risk of HF from twofold to sevenfold, with a greater impact in women than men. Kannel stated "Diabetes was observed to predispose to heart failure whether or not there is interim overt coronary heart disease and does so independent of the often associated hypertension. This suggests that some form of diabetic cardiomyopathy exists."

Both low and high hematocrit levels were a significant risk factor for HF in women. Cigarette smoking moderately increased the HF risk in younger men and older women. Total to HDL cholesterol ratio was powerfully related to the rate of occurrence of HF in both sexes. Obesity was also a significant contributor, especially in women.

Systolic heart failure

Systolic HF refers to a defect in stroke volume ejection during systole, in which an impaired inotropic state is present and poses an impedance to forward blood flow. Systolic myocardial dysfunction is precipitated by prolonged pressure overload, i.e., hypertension, prolonged volume overload, or loss of muscle from an acute myocardial infarction.[11-13] Systolic HF is caused by both the chronic loss of contracting myocardium secondary to myocardial necrosis and the acute loss of contractility induced by a transient episode of ischemia.[6] The ventricle becomes stiff, ischemic, and volume overloaded; ejection fraction (EF) decreases.[10]

Survival data from the first Veterans Administration Cooperative Vasodilator-Heart Failure Trial (V-Heft I) study confirmed that patients with HF and a normal EF have a better prognosis than those with a low EF (19% vs. 8% mortality).[14] A shortcoming of the V-Heft trial was the absence of Doppler data to assess the presence and severity of mitral or aortic regurgitation, which may lead to normal calculations of EF in the presence of impaired systolic function (SF).

A more recent study conducted at Loyola University Medical Center[15] investigated the impact of impaired vs. preserved SF on survival of patients with HF. Mean EF of the impaired SF group was $15 \pm 5\%$ and $40 \pm 13\%$ for the preserved SF group. By the end of 48 months, 36 patients in the impaired group had died compared with 22 patients with preserved SF. Absence of significant mitral or aortic regurgitation in this study excluded the possibility that valvular regurgitation contributed to a normal EF.

Another study undertaken at Yale University School of Medicine[16] examined the long-term outcome in patients with HF and "normal LV systolic function." Fifty-two patients were followed for 7 years. Average EF was 61%. At 7 years, cardiovascular mortality was 46% and morbidity, consisting of nonfatal recurrent HF, myocardial infarction, unstable angina, or other cardiovascular events was 29%. Combined cardiovascular mortality and morbidity was 75%. These researchers concluded that in patients with HF, intact SF did not confer a favorable prognosis. Results suggested that the risk of future cardiovascular events was high.

Diastolic heart failure

Diastolic HF, also referred to as "lusitropic HF," is due to an inability of the myocardium to relax, leading to a defect in filling.[17] Causes include: (1) hypertrophic cardiomyopathy (ventricular muscle becomes very thick; (2) pericardial disease (due to constriction, myocardium cannot completely relax); (3) infiltrative disease such as sarcoidosis or amyloidosis; and (4) ventricular aging.[10]

Maximal myocardial filling is dependent on complete relaxation at the beginning of diastole. With diastolic relaxation dysfunction, filling becomes more dependent upon late diastole and the atrial contraction or "atrial kick." Therefore patients with diastolic HF and atrial fibrillation have very poor ventricular filling due to poor relaxation and loss of the atrial kick.[10]

A tight and rigid ventricle at the beginning of diastolic relaxation phase prolongs compression of the intramyocardial vessels, and thus further reduces blood flow to the subendocardial layers. Myocardial blood flow and oxygenation are therefore impaired secondary to diastolic HF.[6] Once the subendocardial layers become ischemic, intramyocardial vessels maximally dilate and blood is driven by the pressure gradient between coronary diastolic pressure and left ventricular filling pressure throughout diastole.[11] Elevated left ventricular diastolic pressure secondary to poor ventricular distensibility tends to reduce the pressure gradient and subendocardial blood flow.[11] Any excessive increase in heart rate can also be detrimental to subendocardial blood flow because of shortened diastole and therefore decreased duration of perfusion.

Conti[18] recently discussed diagnosis of diastolic HF. "If there is evidence of pulmonary congestion either on physical exam or on chest x-ray in the absence of systolic dysfunction of the ventricle or valvular heart disease (e.g., aortic stenosis or constrictive pericarditis), then the diagnosis is highly suspect. A fourth heart sound is usually audible if the patient is in sinus rhythm. Probably the simplest clinical tool for identifying such patients is cardiac ultrasound, by which one can demonstrate excellent systolic function of the ventricle despite the presence of pulmonary rales and/or chest x-ray evidence of venous congestion. In addition, valve function and ventricular thickness can be assessed. Ventricular thickness may be normal or increased in these patients. However, it is important to remember that diastolic stiffness is a relationship of pressure and volume, and no noninvasive technique will measure left ventricular diastolic pressure. Thus, to confirm the diagnosis, elevated ventricular diastolic pressure or pulmonary capillary wedge pressure should be present." Conti further warns that "diastolic heart failure is going to become an increasing problem as our population ages because stiff ventricles are related to aging. More and more of our octogenarians and nonagenarians are going to be experiencing breathlessness on exertion without any evidence of systolic dysfunction."

Acute heart failure

Infarction is the most common cause of acute HF. Intracellular acidosis within the cell decreases the contractile ability of the myocardium within the first 60 seconds after myocardial infarction. Lack of high energy phosphates may further decrease contraction some minutes later.[12]

Chronic heart failure

Ischemic heart disease and dilated cardiomyopathy are the most frequent causes of chronic congestive HF. In contrast to acute syndromes, mechanisms responsible for chronic HF are unclear. Abnormal sarcoplasmic reticulum function and altered myofibril properties are suggested biochemical causes, along with fibrosis and altered geometry.[13]

Backward vs. forward heart failure

Braunwald[6] states "the clinical manifestations of HF arise as a consequence of inadequate cardiac output and/or damming up of blood behind one or both ventricles. These two principal mechanisms are the basis of the so-called forward and backward pressure theories of heart failure. It no longer seems fruitful to make a rigid distinction between backward and forward heart failure because both mechanisms appear to operate in the majority of patients with chronic heart failure. Some patients, particularly those with acute decompensation, develop relatively pure forms of forward or backward failure." Forward and backward conceptualizations of

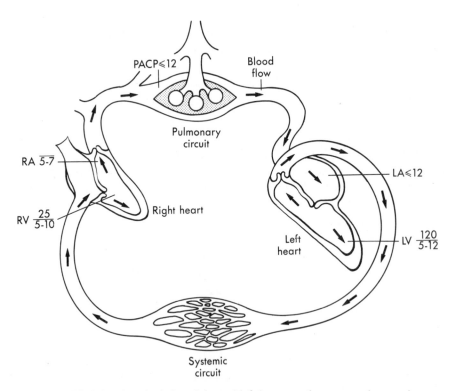

Fig. 4-4. Simplified drawing depicting right and left hearts, pulmonary and systemic systems arranged in a series circuit. Failure in one component affects the entire series circuit.

HF are oversimplified because the right and left ventricles are arranged within a series circuit (Fig. 4-4). Failure in one component of the circuit affects other components as well (see the box below).

Backward heart failure. The backward failure, first proposed in 1832 by James Hope,[20] proposes that as the left ventricle fails to fully empty during systole, blood accumulates and pressure rises in the ventricles, atria, and venous systems that empty into them. Elevation of left ventricular diastolic and atrial pressures, and pulmonary venous pressure, results in "backward" transmission pressure, causing increased volume and pressure in the pulmonic and systemic venous systems (Fig. 4-5). The rise in venous pressure may lead to an efflux of fluid across the capillary membranes into the extracellular spaces, which manifests as the clinical picture of edema. While increased blood volume shifts to the pulmonary circulation, pulmonary vessels enlarge. If the pulmonary capillary wedge pressure (PCWP) rises above plasma colloid osmotic pressure, fluid transudates out of the capillaries into the interstitial spaces and alveoli, resulting in pulmonary edema (Fig. 4-6).

Forward heart failure. Eighty years after Hope's theory was published, Macken-

---

EVENTS RESULTING FROM BACKWARD AND FORWARD HEART FAILURE

Backward effects

Failure of left ventricle to empty its stroke volume in systole
↓
Increased volume and pressure in left ventricle (end-diastolic pressure rises)
↓
Increased volume (pressure) in left atrium
↓
Increased volume (pressure) in pulmonary veins
↓
Increased volume (pressure) in pulmonary capillary bed
↓
Transudation of fluid from capillaries to alveoli
↓
Pulmonary edema
↓
Right ventricle may fail secondarily to elevated pulmonary pressures

Forward effects

Decreased cardiac output
↓
Decreased perfusion of body tissues
↓
Decreased blood flow to body organs
↓
Increased reabsorption of sodium and water via stimulation of renin-angiotensin aldosterone mechanism
↓
Increased extracellular fluid volume and blood volume

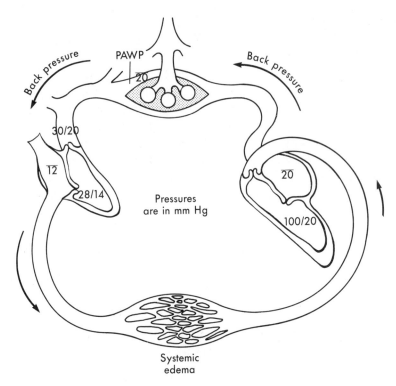

Fig. 4-5. Series circuit depicting pressure changes observed in left ventricular failure. Left ventricular end-diastolic pressures initially elevate with backwards transmission of elevated pressures to the left atrium, pulmonary capillaries, right ventricle, right atrium, and finally to the systemic circulation.

zie[21] proposed the "forward HF theory." According to this theory, clinical manifestations of HF are due to reduced cardiac output causing diminished perfusion of vital organs.

Relatively pure forward failure occurs in patients with acute right ventricular failure secondary to massive pulmonary embolism (Fig. 4-7).

Low and high output heart failure

Low output HF occurs in patients with valvular, coronary, hypertensive, and cardiomyopathic heart disease. Stroke volume decreases and body organs become symptomatic of hypoperfusion. Low output HF is commonly invoked by exercise; in severe HF it may manifest clinically, even at rest.

High output HF is caused by thyrotoxicosis, arteriovenous fistula, Paget's disease, anemia, beriberi, or pregnancy, which require an increased cardiac output and

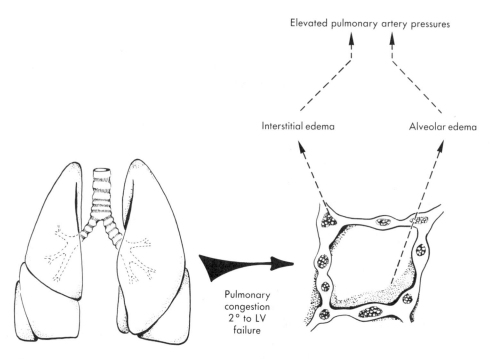

Fig. 4-6. Pathophysiology of pulmonary edema. Left ventricular failure causes volume over-load in the pulmonary capillaries. If pulmonary capillary pressure rises above the colloid os-motic pressure of plasma (approximately 28 mm Hg), fluid filters out of the capillaries into the interstitial spaces and alveoli, resulting in pulmonary edema.

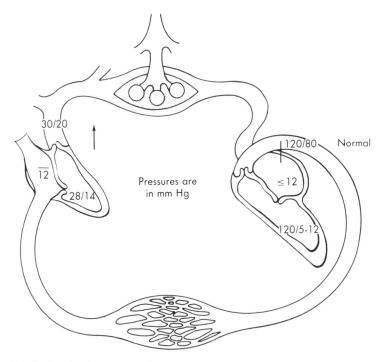

Fig. 4-7. Series circuit pressure changes, reflective of an acute pulmonary embolism.

oxygen delivery to the peripheral tissues. The heart may fail because it simply cannot keep up with increased tissue demands.[6]

COMPENSATORY MECHANISMS

When cardiac output decreases secondary to HF a chain of reflexes and compensatory mechanisms is activated in an attempt to restore normal hemodynamics. With severe HF, cardiac output is redistributed away from the cutaneous, renal, and splanchnic beds, with relative preservation of coronary and cerebral flow. Whatever the insult leading to development of HF, the heart and circulation have only limited means to adapt and compensate.

Starling regulation

The earliest mechanism responding to acute left ventricular failure, which regulates beat-to-beat variations in venous return, is the *Starling response*.[22] In early heart failure, increased end-diastolic volume maintains adequate stroke volume on the steep ascending portion of the Starling *curve* (Fig. 4-8). Small increments in preload (end-diastolic volume) produce substantial increases in stroke volume. At higher levels of preload the curve flattens, larger increases in preload are required to produce smaller increases in stroke volume, and the effectiveness of this compensatory mechanism becomes limited.

Two complications result from activation of the Starling compensatory mechanism in heart failure. First, increased ventricular diastolic pressure, which accompanies ventricular dilatation, is transmitted retrogradely into the pulmonary vasculature, where it causes pulmonary congestive symptoms. Second, increased ventricular preload increases ventricular wall tension, which, in turn, increases myocardial oxygen consumption.[22]

Compliance and the Starling curve. The original Starling curve was developed using a relationship between stroke volume and end-diastolic volume or pressure. This curve was based on the assumption that volume = pressure. However, the relationship between volume and pressure is curvilinear, rather than linear (Fig. 4-9, **A**). Volume therefore does not equal pressure.[22]

Compliance describes the relationship between end-diastolic volume and end-diastolic pressure. At a low preload a *large* change in volume will be reflected by a *small* change in pressure. At high preload a *small* change in volume will be reflected by a *large* change in pressure (Fig. 4-9, **B**). Many factors can alter compliance (see the box on p. 54). With an "increased compliance" a *large* change in volume may be reflected by a *small* change in pressure. With "decreased compliance" a *small* change in volume may be reflected by a *large* change in pressure.[24]

Fluid challenges may be administered in HF to maximize the Starling curve.

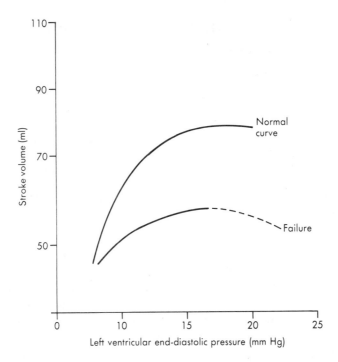

Fig. 4-8. Starling curve. Normally the left ventricle operates on a sharply rising Starling curve, where small changes in filling pressure yield appreciable changes in stroke volume. With ventricular failure additional pressure simply potentiates failure. The Starling mechanism does not represent the influence of compliance..

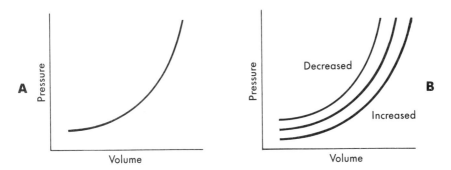

Fig. 4-9 A. Normal compliance representing the curvilinear relationship between volume and end-diastolic pressure. Because this relationship is curvilinear rather than linear, volume does not equal pressure. At low preload a large change in volume will be reflected by a small change in pressure. At high preload a small change in volume will be reflected by a large change in pressure. **B.** Increased and decreased compliance curves as compared to normal.

FACTORS THAT CAN ALTER COMPLIANCE[18]

Causes of increased compliance

Chronic ventricular dilatation
Congestive cardiomyopathy

Causes of decreased compliance

Myocardial ischemia
Myocardial fibrosis
Infiltrative cardiomyopathies
Ventricular hypertrophy

Classic end points of adequate fluid resuscitation have been pressure based parameters, which possess many inherent assumptions. Yet preload recruitability is not accurately measured by the pulmonary artery wedge pressure (PAWP) because changes in left and right ventricular compliance alter PAWP. Right ventricular volumetric measurements of end-diastolic volume index (RVEDI) and ejection fraction (EF) are a new entity, which affords a much more specific evaluation of right ventricular function.[26] If right ventricular ejection is subnormal (high RVEDVI and low EF), right ventricular stroke volume ejected is decreased; left ventricular stroke volume and cardiac output will also be diminished.

Sympathetic nervous system

Increased sympathetic activity is a reflexive response to depressed cardiac function. This results in an increased release of catecholamines by cardiac adrenergic nerves and adrenal glands. Increased levels of circulating catecholamines have been found in patients with HF. Increased norepinephrine increases contractility and heart rate to preserve cardiac output, elevate peripheral vascular resistance, increase venous tone, and redistribute cardiac output away from nonessential organs.[27,28]

Ventricular remodeling

Conti[29] described "ventricular remodeling" as a change in ventricular geometry. When myocardial infarction or any injury to the heart occurs, there is compensatory cardiac growth, referred to pathologically as "hypertrophy." Conti further described hypertrophy, referring to cellular oncogenic research. "Hypertrophy is a complex response that includes an increase in adult muscle proteins. It is also associated with a re-expression of genes that are active during the embryonic and fetal stages but have long since been suppressed. Studies of ventricles in intact animals, hypertrophied as a result of pressure overload, reveal an expression of several protoncogenes that clearly qualify as growth factors and may play a role in growth response."

In a clinical sense, ventricular remodeling consists of left ventricular wall thinning, thought to be due to cell slippage in the infarction area, ventricular chamber dilatation, and a compensatory hypertrophy of the uninfarcted portion of the myocardium. Thinning and chamber dilatation occur within 24 hours of the infarction and initially may be a physiological change to maintain myocardial pump function.[30] In essence, remodeling occurs analogous to a foot that develops a callus when a shoe doesn't fit.

Continuous pressure or volume load on the myocardium contributes to ventricular remodeling. Once ventricular symmetry is changed by hypertrophic growth of myocytes, inability to maintain blood flow to the increased muscle mass, and excess collagen formation, the actin-myosin ultrafilaments can no longer work as efficiently and HF typically ensues. The ideal sarcomere length for maximum effective contraction is 2.3 to 2.4 μm. As ventricular end-diastolic volume increases, sarcomere units become stretched. A stretch of the myocardial sarcomere unit beyond 2.3 to 2.4 μm produces an ineffective actin-myosin coupling, thereby reducing the force of contraction and stroke volume (Fig. 4-10).[31]

The remodeled ventricular wall fibers have to develop greater tension to produce a given pressure during isovolumetric contraction, which is explained by Laplace's law (Fig. 4-11). This equation states that ventricular wall tension is the product of pressure and radius ($T = P \times R$).[32]

Laplace's law explains functional limitations of the remodeled ventricle. The ventricle's radius may not sufficiently decrease during systole, which causes a rise in tension from the beginning of ejection, sustained to the point of peak systole. This tension invokes an additional type of afterload. Because of an increase in myocardial systolic wall tension resulting from the Laplace relationship, myocardial oxygen consumption may be significantly increased in patients with HF. This results in a greater amount of oxygen extracted from coronary blood flow and a widening of the arteriovenous oxygen difference.[33]

Francis and McDonald[34] recently further elucidated how the ventricular change in shape comes about. "The cardiac myocyte alters its sarcomere structure differently in response to varying mechanical loads. A pure pressure overload increases cell diameter and the number of sarcomeres in a parallel fashion (*concentric hypertrophy*). A volume-overloaded state increases cell diameter but also elongates cells by increasing the number of sarcomeres in a series (*eccentric hypertrophy*). It is possible that concentric hypertrophy is due solely to pressure load on the myocytes, whereas eccentric hypertrophy requires both alterations in loading conditions (i.e., myocyte stretch) and trophic factors, including input from the sympathetic nervous system and perhaps other peptides. Following myocardial injury caused by acute myocardial infarction, myocardial cells express both concentric and eccentric hypertrophy. Eccentric hypertrophy, however, appears to be more prominent, at least experimentally."

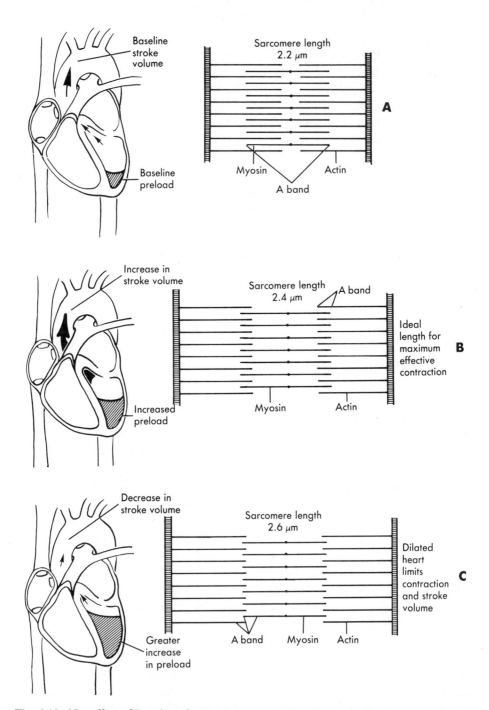

Fig. 4-10. Net effect of lengthened sarcomeres on stroke volume. **A,** Baseline preload, producing stretch on sarcomeres, lengthening to 2.2 μm. **B,** Ideal sarcomere stretch (2.4 μm for maximum contraction. **C,** Further stretch on the sarcomeres beyond 2.4 μm produces ineffective actin-myosin coupling. Actin filaments withdraw from the A band. Myosin overlap is decreased. Force of contraction and resultant stroke volume are reduced.

Laplace's law

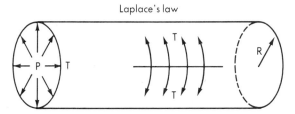

Fig. 4-11. Schematic illustration of Laplace's law. *T*, tension; *P*, pressure, *R*, radius. Tension on wall of chamber is the product of pressure within the chamber × radius.

The right ventricle is particularly sensitive to pressure overloading, with demonstrable decreases of contractility even before clinical failure ensues. These abnormalities are still reversible before the development of overt HF. Once failure ensues, it is not reversible.[35]

Renal compensation

HF activates the renin-angiotensin-aldosterone system by three mechanisms that trigger renin release: (1) hyponatremia; (2) increased sympathetic tone; and (3) renal hypoperfusion.[36,37] Increased secretion of the protein renin occurs from the kidney juxtaglomerular apparatus. Renin acts on a blood substrate to release the peptide angiotensin I, which is converted to angiotensin II by a converting enzyme, primarily found in the lungs and, to a lesser amount, in blood vessels and kidneys.[38] This peptide produces vasoconstriction of arteriolar smooth muscle; it is the most potent pressure substance released by the body—10 times more potent than norepinephrine. Angiotensin II is one of the most important stimuli for adrenal secretion of aldosterone, which causes distal tubular reabsorption of sodium, chloride, and water in exchange for potassium and hydrogen. Angiotensin II stimulates production of arginine vasopressin, which also causes vasoconstriction (Fig. 4-12). The net result is increased intravascular volume, thus increasing preload and afterload.[1]

In mild HF, retained fluid increases blood volume and venous return to the heart; cardiac output is increased, and arterial blood pressure and tissue perfusion are maintained. The resultant arterial pressure elevation deactivates renin secretion. Advanced heart failure does not lend itself to restoration of arterial pressure despite the sodium and water retention catalyzed by the renin-angiotensin-aldosterone mechanism because blood pressure is not restored to normal in the ventricles, atria, and great veins.[38]

There is new evidence suggesting the presence of angiotensin II receptors in cardiac tissue.[39] Dissected diseased hearts from patients undergoing transplantation and normal hearts from organ donors have revealed angiotensin II receptor sites in the midventricular portions of both left and right ventricles.[39] Although there is a

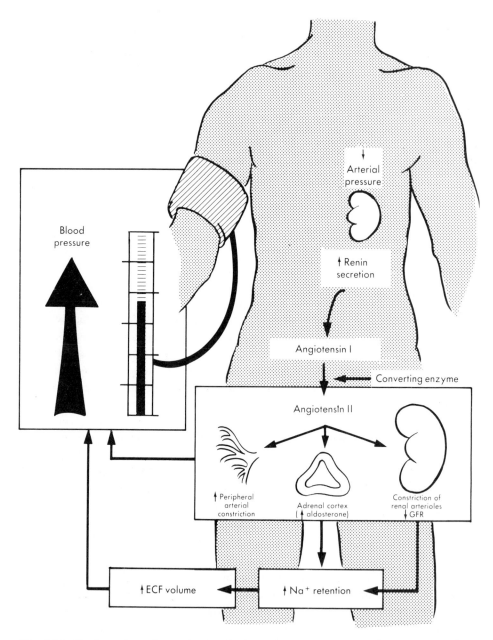

Fig. 4-12. Renin-angiotensin mechanism in heart failure. As the systemic pressure drops, blood flow to the kidney decreases and arterial constriction occurs. Renin is secreted by the kidney in response to renal arterial hypotension. Renin stimulates production of angiotensin I and is converted by angiotensin II, a potent vasoconstrictor, which promotes release of aldosterone from the adrenals. *ECF*, Extracellular fluid. *GFR*, Glomerular filtration rate.

recognized potential inotropic effect from cardiac angiotensin II, it may also have detrimental effects on cardiac function because it is a growth factor and may induce ventricular hypertrophy.

Atrial natriuretic factor

Specific granules have been found in the right atrial appendage, termed *atrial natriuretic factor* (ANF), which is a polypeptide suggested to have natriuretic (increased excretion of sodium), vasorelaxant, and aldosterone-inhibiting properties.[40] Atrial baroreceptors react to increased atrial filling pressures and release ANF, which regulates circulating fluid volume and lowers arterial blood pressure.[41] Assessment of plasma ANF levels in various blood vessels has demonstrated that ANF is secreted into the right atrial cavity through the coronary sinus and that a significant amount of ANF is extracted from the circulation by the kidney. It is also believed that ANF is extracted in the pulmonary circulation.[42]

Studies[42,43] suggest that patients with congestive heart failure have 5 to 20 times the normal circulating plasma concentrations of ANF. These patients have also exhibited peripheral vasoconstriction and oliguria, suggesting a lack of physiological response to the excess production of ANF. Other studies[44,45] have been undertaken to evaluate the hemodynamic efficacy of administering human ANP (anaritide) in HF patients. Decreased filling pressure and an increase in cardiac output were documented. Researchers have also demonstrated that preserving the right atrial appendage during cardiac operations significantly increases release of ANF, resulting in increased urinary sodium excretion and improved postoperative diuresis.[46]

Beta-adrenergic receptor down regulation

Subdivision of adrenergic receptors into subtypes of alpha and beta was originally postulated by Ahlquist.[47] Three adrenergic receptors, Beta$_1$, Beta$_2$, and Alpha$_1$ are found in the human heart. Nonfailing human ventricular myocardium contains 80% Beta$_1$ receptors and 20% Beta$_2$ receptors.[48] Stimulation of these receptors by an adrenergic compound such as norepinephrine causes increased production of adenylate cyclase and generation of cyclic adenosine monophosphate (cAMP), which is the carrier compound needed to move calcium from storage to the site of actin-myosin interaction. Calcium binds with troponin-C, the protein covering thin actin filaments. Thus the actin becomes "activated." Myosins then slide in place to align themselves with activated actin and form cross-bridges. This microcellular process of contraction is discussed in Chapter 3.

Beta$_1$ receptor density decreases in heart failure to about 60%, invoking a myocardial muscle subsensitivity to Beta$_1$ receptor stimulation. This process is referred to as "beta receptor down-regulation," presumably as a consequence of prolonged elevation of circulating norepinephrines.[49] Circulating norepinephrine concentrations have been measured at 2 to 3 times the norm in heart failure patients.[50,51]

Beta$_2$ receptor density appears to be unchanged in heart failure but responsiveness is also decreased, suggesting that these receptors are uncoupled from their pharmacological pathways.

G proteins

Cardiac cells contain two types of guanine nucleotide (G) proteins. G$_s$ mediates stimulation of adenylate cyclase causing a rise in intracellular cyclic AMP, needed to move calcium out of storage into the myocyte. G$_i$ mediates the inhibition of adenylate cyclase and has the opposite effect of calcium flux. Heart failure is associated with an increase in regulatory G$_i$ protein. This reduction in G$_s$ activity and the failing heart's ability to produce adenylate cyclase diminishes the inotropic effectiveness of beta adrenergic drugs such as dobutamine and phosphodiesterase inhibitors.[52]

Mitochondrial function

Considerable dispute exists regarding whether or not mitochondrial oxidative phosphorylation, i.e., energy production, is abnormal in HF. Chronic overloading causes each cell to sustain an increased level of work. Hypertrophy increases myocardial cell size and therefore reduces the load on each sarcomere. Compensation brought about by this increased muscle mass may not perfectly match the increased load. As a result the rate of energy expenditure by each sarcomere of the hypertrophied or remodeled heart remains elevated.[53]

Katz[54] also states that "there is abundant evidence, albeit mostly indirect, that the cells of the hypertrophied and failing heart are unable to generate sufficient energy to provide for this increased rate of energy expenditure; as a result, the failing heart is likely to be in an energy-starved state."

SIGNS/SYMPTOMS
Dyspnea

A cardinal manifestation of left ventricular failure is dyspnea, which presents with progressively increasing severity as (1) exertional dyspnea; (2) orthopnea; (3) paroxysmal nocturnal dyspnea; (4) dyspnea at rest; and (5) acute pulmonary edema.[6]

Exertional dyspnea differentiates normal subjects from HF subjects by the degree of activity required to produce the breathlessness.

Orthopnea is dyspnea that occurs in the recumbent position and alleviation may require several pillows. Orthopnea occurs rapidly, often within a minute or two of assuming recumbency. Braunwald[6] states "it is an important symptom of heart failure, but is far from specific and may occur in any condition in which vital capacity is low; dyspnea is exacerbated when recumbency elevates the diaphragm, reducing vital capacity even further. Patients frequently awaken short of breath if the head has slipped off the pillows, and they then often seek and find relief by sitting in front of an open window. In advanced left ventricular failure, orthopnea may be so severe that the patient cannot lie down and must spend the night in the sitting position. Often such patients are observed sitting at the side of the bed, slumped over a bedside table."

Paroxysmal nocturnal dyspnea typically occurs after prolonged recumbency. The patient falls asleep, awakens abruptly hours later, often with a feeling of severe anxiety and suffocation, gasping for breath. "Bronchospasm, which may be caused by congestion of the bronchial mucosa and by interstitial pulmonary edema compressing the small bronchi, increases ventilatory difficulty and the work of breathing, and is a common complicating factor of paroxysmal nocturnal dyspnea. The commonly associated wheezing is sometimes termed 'cardiac asthma.'"[6]

Dyspnea at rest can occur without the patient being aware of it. Patients may deny dyspnea but may then interrupt themselves in midsentence to take a breath. With increasing severity of heart failure, a patient may become extremely aware of not being able to carry out many activities because of breathlessness.

When hydrostatic pressure of pulmonary capillaries exceeds colloid osmotic blood pressure, transudation of fluid into the lungs occurs, producing *acute pulmonary edema*. Manifestations depend upon the extent to which the hydrostatic pressure is increased and the rapidity with which the condition develops. In milder cases, the patient may have moist rales and shortness of breath. In more severe cases, the alveoli may fill with so much fluid that adequate ventilation is difficult.

An often overlooked symptom of left ventricular failure is a cough, which is usually related to dyspnea. This is caused by pulmonary congestion that occurs during exertion or while the patient is recumbent.[55] Patients may complain of a dry hacking cough and may link it with stress, exercise, or sleep. A cough may severely interfere with a patient's sleep resulting in fatigue and insomnia.

Weakness and fatigue

Fatigue is an expected symptom associated with HF secondary to decreased cardiac output and disturbance in sleep patterns. Hypoperfusion of skeletal muscles may manifest as heaviness in arms and legs. Peripheral limb weakness may also be due to potassium depletion secondary to diuretic therapy. Fatigue usually worsens as the day's activities progress.

Exhaustion in a patient with HF most likely results from a disturbance in sleep and rest patterns, as well as a reduction in cardiac output. Patients may complain of chronic weakness, fatigability, or heaviness in arms or legs, generally because the reduction in cardiac output causes poor perfusion of skeletal muscles. Another common cause of these complaints is the use of diuretics, which can provoke sodium depletion, decreased potassium, and hypovolemia when given in improper dosages. Fatigue can result from the excessive work of breathing that occurs during activity or at rest, and generally worsens as the day progresses.

Urinary symptoms

Nocturia can be an early manifestation of myocardial pump failure. While the patient is upright and active, there is a redistribution of blood flow away from the kidneys to other organs; urine output is suppressed. At night, when the patient assumes a recumbent position, urine output increases because renal vasoconstriction diminishes.[53]

Edema and ascites

Systemic edema is a manifestation of right ventricular failure. Patients may become aware of dependent edema in their ankles, feet, and hands. They may observe impression marks from shoes, socks, or garters. Dependent edema is found over the sacrum in bedridden patients. If ascites is present, patients may notice their clothes tightening around the waist and may feel bloated. Massive ascites can affect breathing by forcing the diaphragm upward when the patient is recumbent. The most severe edema is *anasarca*, which involves the entire body.

Ventricular arrhythmias

Ventricular arrhythmias have been found in as many as 70% to 80% of HF patients. Although ventricular arrhythmias have been considered to be a cause of sudden death, they may be a sign of the severity of the underlying disease, rather than a causative factor. The mechanisms underlying sudden death have not been definitively established.[56]

BALLOON PUMPING IN HEART FAILURE

Intraaortic balloon counterpulsation has been extensively utilized to aid the failing heart. Its therapeutic benefits for the patient with HF are discussed in Chapter 7.

REFERENCES

1. Rutan P, Gavin E: Adult and pediatric heart failure, chap 1. In Quaal SJ: *Cardiac mechanical assistance beyond balloon pumping,* St Louis, 1993, Mosby–Year Book.
2. Chung TO: Congestive heart failure in coronary artery disease, *Am J Med* 91:409, 1991.
3. Ghali JK, Cooper R, Ford E: Trends in hospitalization rates for heart failure in the United States, 1973-1986. Evidence for increasing population prevalence, *Arch Intern Med* 150:769, 1990.
4. Kannel WB, Belanger AJ: Epidemiology of heart failure, *Am Heart J* 121:951, 1991.
5. Packer M: Survival in patients with chronic heart failure and its potential modification by drug therapy. In Cohn JN, ed: *Drug treatment of heart failure,* ed 2, Secaucus, NJ, 1988, ATC International.
6. Braunwald E, Grossman W: Clinical aspects of heart failure, chap 16. In Braunwald E, ed: *Heart disease,* ed 4, Philadelphia, 1992, WB Saunders.
7. Braunwald E: Pathophysiology of heart failure, chap 14. In Braunwald E, ed: *Heart disease: a textbook of cardiovascular medicine.* Philadelphia, 1988, WB Saunders.
8. Quaal SJ: The person with heart failure and cardiogenic shock, chap 11. In Guzzetta CE, Dossey BM: *Cardiovascular nursing holistic practice,* St. Louis, 1992, Mosby–Year Book.

9. Covinsky JO, Willett MS: Congestive heart failure. In Dipiro JT, Talbert RL, Hayes PE et al, eds: *Pharmacotherapy: a pathophysiologic approach,* New York, 1989, Elsevier Science Publishing.
10. Whitman G: Management of heart failure. Proceedings of the National Teaching Institute, 1992, Aliso Viejo, Calif, American Association of Critical Care Nurses.
11. Sonnenblick EH, Yellin E, LeJemtel TH: Congestive heart failure and intact systolic ventricular performance, *Heart Failure* 4:164, 1988.
12. Feldman MD, Copelas L, Gwathmey JK et al: Deficient production of cyclic AMP: pharmacologic evidence of an important cause of contractile dysfunction in patients with end-stage heart failure, *Circulation* 75:331, 1987.
13. Factor SM, Sonnenblick EH: The pathogenesis of clinical and experimental congestive cardiomyopathies: recent concepts, *Prog Cardiovasc Dis* 27:395, 1985.
14. Cohn JN, Johnson G, Veterans Administration Cooperative Study Group: Heart failure with normal ejection fraction. The V-Heft study, *Circulation* 82 (suppl III): III-48, 1990.
15. Ghali JK, Kadakia MD, Bhatt A et al: Survival of heart failure patients with preserved versus impaired systolic function: the prognostic implication of blood pressure, *Am Heart J* 123:993, 1992.
16. Selaro JF, Saufer R, Remetz MS: Long term outcome in patients with congestive heart failure and intact systolic left ventricular performance, *Am J Cardiol* 69:1212, 1992.
17. Schwinger R, Bohm M, Erdman E: Inotropic and lusitropic dysfunction in myocardium from patients with dilated cardiomyopathy, *Am Heart J* 123:116, 1992.
18. Conti CR: Ventricular diastolic function: clinical relevance, *Clin Cardiol* 15:399, 1992.
19. Conti CR: Personal communication, August 20, 1992.
20. Hope JA: *Treatise on the disease of the heart and great vessels,* London, 1932, Williams-Kidd.
21. Mackenzie J: *Disease of the heart,* ed 3, London, 1913, Oxford University Press.
22. Starling EH: *The Linacre lecture on the law of the heart,* London, 1918, Longmans, Green.
23. Waters DD, Forrester JS: Diagnosis and management of congestive heart failure and pulmonary edema. In Elliot RS, Forker AD, Saenz A: *Cardiac emergencies.* Mt Kisco, New York, 1983, Futura Publishers.
24. Tuman KJ, Carroll CG, Ivankovich AD: Pitfalls in interpretation of pulmonary catheter data, *J Cardiovasc Anesth* 3:625, 1989.
25. Raper R, Sibbald WJ: Misled by the wedge? The Swan-Ganz catheter and left ventricular preload, *Chest* 89:427, 1986.
26. Headley JM, Diethron ML: Right ventricular volumetric monitoring, *AACN's Clinical Issues in Critical Care Nursing:* 4:(120), 1993.
27. Chidsey CA, Braunwald E, Morrow AG: Catecholamine excretion and cardiac stores of norepinephrine in congestive heart failure, *Am J Med* 39:442, 1965.
28. Pierpont GL, Francis GS, DeMaster EG et al: Heterogeneous myocardial catecholamine concentrations in patients with congestive heart failure, *Am J Cardiol* 60:316, 1983.
29. Conti CR: Ventricular remodeling and prognosis after myocardial infarction, *Clin Cardiol* 15:141, 1992.
30. Mares A, Towbin J, Bies RD et al: Molecular biology for the cardiologist, *Curr Probl Cardiol* 12:21, 1992.
31. Ross J Jr: Diastolic geometry and sarcomere lengths in the chronically dilated left ventricle, *Circ Res* 28:49, 1971.
32. Grossman W, Braunwald E: Contractile state of the left ventricle in man as evaluated from end-systolic pressure-volume relations, *Circulation* 56:845, 1977.
33. Levine HJ, Wagman RJ: Energetics of the human heart, *Am J Cardiol* 9:372, 1968.
34. Francis GS, McDonald KM: Left ventricular hypertrophy: an initial response to myocardial injury, *Am J Cardiol* 69:3G, 1992.
35. Burkart F, Kiowski W: Circulatory abnormalities and compensatory mechanisms in heart failure, *Am J Med* 90:5B-19S, 1991.
36. Brozena S, Jessup M: Pathophysiologic strategies in the management of congestive heart failure, *Annu Rev Med* 41:65, 1990.

37. Leibovitch ER: Congestive heart failure: a current overview, *Geriatrics* 46:43, 1991.
38. Schlant RC, Sonnenblick EH: Pathophysiology of heart failure. In Hurst JW, ed: *The heart*, ed 7, New York, 1990, McGraw-Hill.
39. Grimstead VC, Young JB: The myocardial renin-angiotensin system: existence, importance and clinical implications, *Am Heart J* 123:1039, 1992.
40. Genest J, Cantin M: Atrial natriuretic factor, *Circulation* 75:118, 1987.
41. Cosgrove JA: Atrial natriuretic peptide: a new cardiac hormone, *Heart Lung* 18:461, 1989.
42. Fife MA, Cesar R, Molina MD et al: Hemodynamic and renal effects of atrial natriuretic peptide in congestive heart failure, *Am J Cardiol* 65:211, 1990.
43. Crozier IG, Nicholls MG, Ikram H et al: Hemodynamic effects of atrial natriuretic peptide infusion in heart failure, *Lancet* 2:1242, 1986.
44. Saito Y, Nakao K, Nishimura K et al: Clinical application of atrial natriuretic polypeptide in patients with congestive heart failure: beneficial effects on left ventricular function, *Circulation* 76:115, 1987.
45. Fife MA, Molina CR, Quiroz AC et al: Hemodynamic and renal effects of atrial natriuretic peptide in congestive heart failure, *Am J Cardiol* 65:211, 1990.
46. Omari BO, Nelson RJ, Robertson JM: Effect of right atrial appendectomy on the release of atrial natriuretic hormone, *J Thorac Cardiovasc Surg* 102:272, 1991.
47. Alquist RP: A study of the adrenotropic receptors, *Am J Physiol* 53:586, 1948.
48. Brodde OE: Molecular pharmacology of beta-adrenoceptors, *J Cardiovasc Pharmacol* (suppl 5): S16, 1986.
49. Bristow MR, Ginsburg R, Fowler M: Beta$_1$ and Beta$_2$ adrenergic receptor pathways in the failing human heart, *Heart Failure* 5:77, 1989.
50. Hasking GJ, Eglu MD, Jennings GL et al: Norepinephrine spillover to plasma in patients with congestive heart failure: evidence of increased overall and cardiorenal sympathetic nervous activity, *Circulation* 73:615, 1986.
51. Bristow MR, Ginsburg R, Minobe W et al: Decreased catecholamine sensitivity and beta-adrenergic receptor density in failing human hearts, *N Eng J Med* 307:205, 1982.
52. Neumann J, Schmitz W, Scholtz H et al: Increase in myocardial proteins in heart failure, *Lancet* 22:936, 1988.
53. Katz AM: Future prospectives in basic science understanding of congestive heart failure, *Am J Cardiol* 66:468, 1990.
54. Katz AM: Changing strategies in the management of heart failure, *J Am Coll Cardiol* 13:513, 1989.
55. Glover DR, Littler WA: Factors influencing survival and mode of death in severe chronic ischemic cardiac failure, *Br Heart J* 57:125, 1987.

CHAPTER 5

Pharmacological management of myocardial pump failure

Susan J. Quaal

During the past 20 years, numerous pharmacological therapies have been used in treatment of heart failure (HF). Many drugs have demonstrated their effectiveness in improving ventricular function and clinical symptoms. Heart failure is associated with a high rate of mortality[1]; treatment is therefore directed toward reducing mortality, as well as relieving symptoms. In recent years large-scale studies have examined the impact of various pharmacological regimes on mortality. Current practice is, in part, guided by results of these trials. Credible evidence has resulted from trials suggesting that vasodilators and angiotensin-converting enzyme (ACE) inhibitors are associated with symptomatic improvement and reduced mortality.[2]

Pharmacological therapy is used before and concomitant with balloon pump therapy. Therefore this chapter offers a literature based review of existing pharmacological therapy options.

DIURETICS

Retention of sodium and water and expansion of extracellular volume are most important adverse physiological responses to HF. Thus diuretic therapy is one of the basic components of treatment. Although diuretics may not influence the natural history of HF, they improve symptoms by acting directly on nephrite solute and water resorption and may slow progression of cardiac chamber dilation by reducing ventricular filling pressure.[3]

Therapeutic mechanisms of diuretics are best appreciated by reviewing normal nephron function (Fig. 5-1). Each nephron consists of a (1) *glomerular capillary tuft*, surrounded by Bowman's capsule; (2) *proximal convoluted tubule*; (3) *loop of Henle*; and (4) *distal convoluted tubule*. There are about 1 million nephrons in each kidney. Primary kidney function is to maintain normal extracellular fluid volume and com-

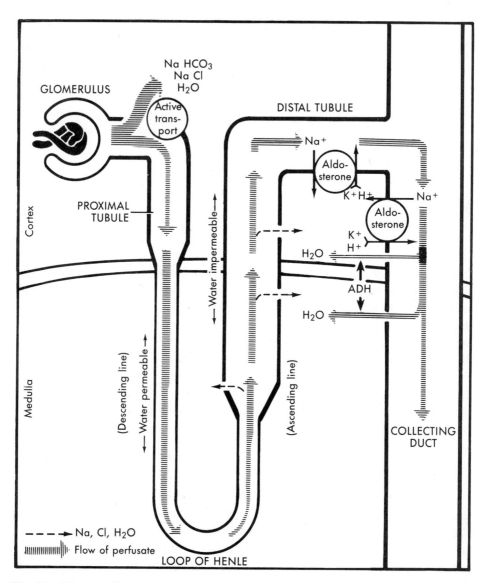

Fig. 5-1. Schematic illustrating normal nephron anatomy and filtration, reabsorption, and secretion processes through the glomerulus, proximal tubule, ascending and descending loop of Henle, distal tubule, and collecting duct (see text for discussion).

position. Regulation is controlled by glomerular filtration, tubular reabsorption, and secretion.[4] Each of these processes is further discussed.

Glomerular filtration

The process of urine formation begins with glomerular plasma filtration. Renal blood flow equals about 25% of cardiac output or 1200 ml/min. Glomerular filtration consists of "restraining" blood cells and large molecules such as proteins by membrane pores. Water and small molecular substances such as crystalloids are filtered. Approximately 173 liters of fluid are filtered through the glomerulus each day. Glomerular filtration is entirely passive; the kidney does not expend any energy.[4]

Resorption and secretion

These processes take place by active and passive transport mechanisms. Along the proximal tubule, glucose and amino acids, potassium, calcium, and phosphate are completely resorbed by "active transport," which means that energy is expended as substances are transported against an electrochemical gradient. Approximately two thirds of sodium entering the nephron is actively resorbed in the proximal tubule. Sodium resorption continues in the ascending loop of Henle, distal tubule, and collecting ducts, so that less than 1% is actually excreted in urine. Water, chloride, and urea are resorbed in the proximal tubule by "passive transport," which means they move down an electrochemical gradient that does not require any energy expenditure. Approximately 90% of bicarbonate is resorbed in the proximal tubule indirectly by Na^+ and H^+ exchange. Chloride is actively transported out of the loop of Henle ascending limb, followed passively by Na^+; approximately 35% of NaCl is therefore resorbed.

Resorption is complete in the distal tubule and collecting duct. The distal tubule is responsible for final regulation of water and acid-base balance. The distal tubule contains the active Na^+ pump, which is under the control of aldosterone. Potassium and H^+ are exchanged for Na^+; for every molecule of Na^+ resorbed, one molecule of K^+ is excreted. Consequently, the more Na^+ delivered to the distal tubule, the greater the exchange of Na^+ with K^+. As the aldosterone level increases, Na^+ resorption increases and a greater K^+ loss occurs. Potassium-sparing diuretics antagonize aldosterone and depress this resorption mechanism. Specific diuretic drugs are categorized below as weak, moderate, and potent. Their function is related to nephron anatomy and physiology as described above. Recommended dosages are listed in Table 5-1.

Weak diuretics

Mannitol, acetazolamide, and potassium-sparing agents are relatively weak natriuretic (drugs increasing sodium excretion) agents. Osmotic diuretics such as manni-

Text continued on p. 72.

Table 5-1.   Diuretics

Agent	Onset of action	Dosage/administration	Plasma concentration time (Hours)		Plasma half-life (Hours)
			Peak	Plateau	
Sulfonamide and Indolamine derivatives					
Chlorothiazide sodium (Diuril)		PO: 125-1000 mg qd★ max: 2000 mg qd★ IV:500-2000 mg qd★			14
Chlorthalidone (Hygroton, Thalitone)		PO: 12.5-50 mg qd Max: 200 mg qd action prolonged up to 48 hr			
Cyclothiazide (Anhydron)		PO: 1.0-2.0 mg qd			
Hydrochlorothiazide (Esidrex, Hydrodiuril, Oretic)		PO: 12.5-50 mg qd max: 200 mg qd★			
Hydroflumethiazide (Diucardin, Saluron)		PO: 12.5-50 mg qd max: 200 mg qd★			
Indapamide (Lozol)		PO: 2.5-5.0 mg qd			
Methyclothiazide (Aquatensen, Enduron)		po: 2.5-5.0 mg qd max: 10 mg qd			
Metolazone (Zaroxolyn)		PO: 2.5-10 mg qd max: 20 mg qd			
Polythiazide (Renese)		po: 2.0-4.0 mg qd			
Quinethazone (Hydromox)		PO: 25-100 mg qd max: 200 mg qd★			
Loop diuretics					
Bumetanide (Bumex)	PO: 30 min	PO: 0.5-2.0 mg qd★ max: 10 mg qd★	PO: 0.5-2.0	PO: 0.5	PO: 1.5
	IV: 10 min	IV or IM: 0.5-1.0 mg, may repeat every 2-3 hr to max dose of 10 mg	IV: 0.5		IV: 1.5

Metabolism and excretion	Drug interactions and incompatibilities	Side and toxic effects
70% renal, 23% GI (bile)	Potentiates: other antihypertensive drugs, lithium Potentiated by: hypercalcemic effect enhanced by vitamin D and calcium products; hypokalemic effect increased by adrenal corticosteroids Inhibited by: NSAIDs Inhibits: arterial response to norepinephrine, oral anticoagulants	CNS: headache, dizziness, fatigue, weakness, lethargy, nervousness, tension, anxiety, irritability, agitation, depression, blurred vision GI: anorexia, nausea, vomiting, constipation, diarrhea, gastric irritation, abdominal pain or cramps, dry mouth, bad taste, pancreatitis MS: muscle cramps or spasm, rhabdomyolysis from severe hypokalemia (more common with chlorthalidone) CV: orthostatic hypotension, premature ventricular contractions, irregular heart beat, palpitations Derm: rash, hives, pruritis, flushing Met: hyperuricemia, increased BUN, hyperglycemia, hyperlipidemia, hyponatremia, hypochloremia, fever, hypercalcemia GU: frequent urination, nocturia, polyuria, oliguria Hypersensitivity: vasculitis, photosensitivity
80% renal, 15% GI	Inhibited by: probenecid	CNS: headache, dizziness, weakness, hearing loss, encephalopathy GI: nausea, vomiting, abdominal pain MS: muscle cramps, arthritic or musculoskeletal pain CV: hypotension, ECG changes Derm: pruritus, hives, rash

Continued.

Table 5-1.   Diuretics—cont'd

Agent	Onset of action	Dosage/ administration	Plasma concentration time (Hours)		Plasma half-life (Hours)
			Peak	Plateau	
Furosemide (Lasix)	PO: 60 min IV: 2-10 min	PO: 20-480 mg qd* max: 600 mg qd* IV: 20-40 mg over 1-2 min, repeat in 20 mg increments every 2 hr if needed 100-200 mg IV in 1-2 min for hypertensive emergencies. Do not use if solution has a yellow color	PO: 1 IV: 0.5		1.5
Ethacrinic Acid (Edecrin)	PO: 30 min IV: 2-10 min	PO: 25-200 mg qd* after meals; preferably on alternate days IV: 0.5-1.0 mg/kg or 50 mg for the average adult	PO: 1.0-2.0 IV:0.5	po: 6-8	0.5-1.0
Potassium-sparing diuretics					
Spironolactone (Aldactone)	2 hr	PO: 25-200 mg qd* max: 400 mg qd*	2.0-4.0	Up to 2 weeks to achieve maximum effect	2 phases: 4 hr; 10-35 hr

Metabolism and excretion	Drug interactions and incompatibilities	Side and toxic effects
66% renal, 33% GI (bile)	Potentiates: digitalis toxicity if excessive K^+ loss; antihypertensive drugs; ganglionic or peripheral adrenergic blocking drugs; ototoxic potential of aminoglycoside antibiotics; salicylate toxicity; tubocurarine and succinylcholine; nephrotoxicity of cephaloridine; lithium toxicity; cisplatinum; hypokalemia from adrenal corticosteroids Inhibited by NSAIDs; steroids and amphotericin increase K^+ loss; patients allergic to sulfonamides may be allergic to loop diuretics Potentiated by: clofibrate	CNS: dizziness, vertigo, paresthesias, headache, blurred vision, tinnitus, weakness, restlessness, hearing loss MS: muscle spasms GI: anorexia, oral and gastric irritation, nausea, vomiting, cramping, diarrhea CV: orthostatic hypotension, potentiated by alcohol; barbiturates or narcotics; thrombophlebitis Derm: pruritus, purpura, rash, photosensitivity Hemat: anemia, leukopenia, thrombocytopenia Met: increased BUN, serum uric acid, glucose; hypokalemia; systemic alkalosis due to loss of sodium chloride, potassium, and water GU: bladder spasm
66% renal, 33% GI	See furosemide In addition: potentiates warfarin	See furosemide In addition: CNS: fatigue; apprehension; mental confusion; deafness more common than with furosemide GI: dysphagia, liver dysfunction, GI bleeding, profuse watery diarrhea Hemat: severe neutropenia, agranulocytosis Met: chills, fever, hypoglycemia with convulsion in persons with uremia
25-50% urine, 50-75% GI (bile)	Potentiates: other diuretics, increases half-life of digoxin Inhibits: vascular response to norepinephrine Inhibited by: NSAIDs Potentiates: lithium	CNS: ataxia GI: cramping, diarrhea Derm: skin eruptions Met: hyperkalemia that can lead to fatal arrhythmias, drug fever, increased BUN, hyperchloremic metabolic acidosis GU: irregular menses or amenorrhea, postmenopausal bleeding, hirsutism, deepening of voice, interference with sexual function, breast enlargement, conflicting data on potential relationship with incidence of breast cancer

Continued.

Table 5-1. Diuretics—cont'd

Agent	Onset of action	Dosage/ administration	Plasma concentration time (Hours)		Plasma half-life (Hours)
			Peak	Plateau	
Amiloride (Mida-mor)	2 hr	PO: 5-10 mg qd* max: 20 mg qd*	6-10 Duration of action 24		6-9
Triamterene (Dyre-nium)	2-4 hr	PO: 100-200 mg qd max: 300 mg qd*	3 Duration of action: 7-9		1.5- 2.5

PO, orally; IV, intravenously; IM, intramuscularly; qd, every day
*divided doses; CNS, central nervous system; MS, musculoskeletal; GI, gastrointestinal; CV, cardiovascular; Derm, dermatologic; Hemat, hematologic; Met, metabolic; GU, genitourinary; NSAID, nonsteroidal antiin-flammatory drugs; BUN, blood urea nitrogen.
(Modified from Underhill SL, Woods SL, Froelicher ESS et al: *Cardiovascular medication for cardiac nursing*, Philadelphia, 1990 JB Lippincott.)

tol promote a modest natriuresis, but if not eliminated, they can cause dilutional hyponatremia and/or extracellular fluid volume expansion.[5]

Spironolactone, triamterene, and *amiloride* are potassium-sparing and often are used in combination with the more potent loop diuretics. Potassium sparing diuretics subdivide into two classes of agents: (1) aldosterone agonists and (2) direct inhibitors of Na^+ in the collecting duct. Normally, aldosterone facilitates distal tubule Na^+ reabsorption in exchange for K^+, thus retaining extracellular fluid Na^+ concentration. When this action is blocked by spironolactone, Na^+ is excreted, while K^+ is retained or "spared." Spironolactone is extensively metabolized in the liver and bound to plasma proteins. Maximal effects may not be seen for at least 5 days, and up to weeks after initiating therapy.[6,7]

Amiloride inhibits Na^+ uptake in the distal tubule's latter two-thirds and in the

Metabolism and excretion	Drug interactions and incompatibilities	Side and toxic effects
52% renal, 40% GI	Inhibited by: NSAIDs Potentiates: lithium	CNS: dizziness, headache, weakness, fatigue, encephalopathy GI: anorexia, nausea, vomiting, diarrhea, flatulence, constipation, abdominal pain MS: muscle cramps Met: hyperkalemia
45-70% renal, 30-55% GI (bile)	Potentiates: antihypertensive drugs, other diuretics, preanesthetic and anesthetic agents, skeletal muscle relaxants, lithium Potential for hyperkalemia increased by: stored blood; K^+-containing drugs such as penicillin G, salt substitutes, and low-salt milk	CNS: weakness, fatigue, dizziness, headache, dry mouth GI: nausea, vomiting, diarrhea, liver enzyme abnormalities, jaundice MS: muscle cramps Derm: rash Hemat: thrombocytopenia, megaloblastic anemia Met: hyperkalemia, hyperglycemia, hypokalemia GU: renal colic, renal calculi Hypersensitivity: anaphylaxis, photosensitivity

collecting duct. Secondary to the effect on sodium, amiloride also inhibits urinary loss of potassium, hydrogen ions, magnesium, and calcium.[7] The exact mechanism of *triamterene* is uncertain. It is thought to inhibit distal tubule K^+ secretion.[7] Efficacy of these K^+ sparing diuretics is enhanced in conditions characterized by high aldosterone levels such as ascites due to cirrhosis. They are relatively ineffective in the therapy of HF, unless combined with a second diuretic.[3]

Moderate diuretics

The sulfonamide derivatives are the oldest orally effective diuretics in use; their fundamental cellular mechanism of action remains unclear. They increase excretion of Na^+ and Cl^- in the distal tubule's proximal portion. These thiazide diuretics include a number of agents that are chemically and pharmacologically similar, and are the prototypes of chlorothiazide: *chlorthalidone, hydrochlorothiazide, indapamide, metolazone,* and *quinethazone.*[7] With the exception of metolazone, thiazide diuretics become ineffective as the glomerular filtration rate falls below about 30 ml/min. The thiazides are useful in the initial management of HF.[4]

Potent diuretics

Loop diuretics *furosemide, bumetanide,* and *ethacrynic acid* exert their major effect on the thick ascending loop of Henle limb. They inhibit sodium, chloride, and potassium absorption. "Since the thick ascending limb of the loop of Henle is relatively impermeable to water, this inhibition results in delivery to the distal tubule of an increased volume of tubular fluid. The increased volume of fluid delivered to the distal tubule results in even further potassium secretion at that site. Inhibition of NA^+, Cl^+, and K^+ absorption in the ascending limb also results in a decrease in the osmolality of the renal medulla, which impairs reabsorption of free water in the cortical collecting duct. In addition, reabsorption of calcium and magnesium in the ascending limb is inhibited, resulting in an increased excretion of these two electrolytes."[7]

Loop diuretics have a rapid onset when given intravenously. These agents may inhibit as much as 25% of the filtered sodium from reabsorption in the ascending loop of Henle limb. They all cause an increase in systemic resistance due to stimulation of the renin-angiotensin-aldosterone, catecholamine, and antidiuretic hormones. The resulting increase in afterload is transient and offset by vasodilator prostaglandins, which are then secreted in increased quantities, stimulated by the increased natriuresis.[8]

INOTROPIC AGENTS

An early theory of HF was thought to be a weakening of systolic heart muscle function. A seemingly obvious early corollary to depressed myocardial contractility was a belief that more powerful inotropics produced a greater effect in treating HF patients. However, a number of theoretical concerns suggested that positive inotropic drugs might exert significant detrimental long-term effects in HF patients. These include worsening of the deficit between energy production and utilization, exacerbation of relaxation abnormalities, arrhythmogenic effects, and lack of any effect due to down regulation of beta receptors.[9,10]

Theoretically, cardiotonic agents may decrease systemic vascular resistance, left ventricular filling pressure, and chamber size, thereby decreasing myocardial wall tension. The net result is a decrease in myocardial oxygen demands and an increase in the coronary perfusion pressure gradient, with increased oxygen delivery to ischemic tissues. However, in mild HF the increased myocardial energy expenditure required to support an increase in inotropy may not be compensated for by a fall in wall tension and enhanced subendocardial perfusion. Thus potent inotropes are used cautiously in patients with HF.[11]

Inotropic therapy is predicated on the supposition that residual myocardial function, or a contractile reserve, can be elicited from the failing heart. Residual contractile activity in failing hearts has been demonstrated by post-extrasystolic potentiation of myocardial contractility and paired electrical stimulation.[12] Positive inotropic agents presumably elicit this contractile reserve by increasing the amount of calcium available to the contractile apparatus.[11]

In the failing heart there is an impaired ability to deliver calcium ions to myofibrilar elements, a process that is critical to contraction. Katz[9] hypothesized that this decrease in contractile state was an important compensatory mechanism to conserve energy utilization and improve long-term myocardial function. Consequently augmentation of the heart's inotropic state could provide a temporary improvement in cardiac contractility at the expense of increasing myocardial energy consumption and accelerating myocardial cell death.

Long-term inotropic therapy may exacerbate ventricular tachyarrhythmias through a number of interrelated mechanisms. Nearly all inotropic agents increase intracellular calcium, which may precipitate arrhythmias. Beta receptor agonists may promote transmembrane transport of extracellular potassium into cells, which may also precipitate arrhythmias.[13]

Isoproterenol has recently been used to evaluate prognosis in HF patients.[14] Sinus cycle length measured during infusion of 4 μg/min of isoproterenol is suggestive of patient prognosis. Between 89% to 93% of patients whose sinus cycle length was ≤15% died within 28 months. Researchers suggest that infusion of low dose isoproterenol be used as a prognostic indicator. It is recommended that patients exhibiting a weak increase in heart rate undergo evaluation for cardiac transplantation.

Dobutamine

Dobutamine is a synthetic sympathomimetic amine that increases myocardial contractility through stimulation of the beta-adrenergic receptors. Beta receptor stimulation activates production of adenyl cyclase, a precursor to cyclic AMP, which mobilizes calcium from its stores to the sight of actin/myosin interaction. More cross-bridges can then be formed through actin/myosin coupling, hence a greater force of contraction occurs.

A series of landmark studies by Leier et al.[15,16] first established a role for dobutamine as an acute short-term therapy for severe HF. The most obvious affect of dobutamine was that it could temporarily improve cardiac output and decrease left ventricular filling pressure without promoting peripheral vasoconstriction or an excessive increase in heart rate.

"Dobutamine does not activate dopaminergic receptors and does not release norepinephrine from adrenergic nerve endings. At equivalent inotropic responses, dobutamine exerts a much weaker beta$_2$-adrenergic action than does isoproterenol and a much weaker alpha$_1$-adrenergic action than do either norepinephrine or dopamine. When administered to patients with heart failure, dobutamine results in a reduction in systemic vascular resistance as cardiac output rises and arterial pressure remains relatively constant."[3]

"In contrast to dopamine, dobutamine is not a renal vasodilator. Also, it causes a redistribution of cardiac output in favor of the coronary and limb beds over the mesenteric and renal vascular beds. However, it has been reported not to increase oxygen delivery to working skeletal muscles of patients with heart failure. A low-dose infusion of dopamine may be added to dobutamine to obtain a renal vasodilator effect from the former and a positive inotropic effect from the latter."[3]

Dobutamine should be administered via an intravenous infusion pump, since accurate delivery of the proper dosage is critical. Initial infusion is begun at 2.5 μg/kg/min and increased by 2.5 μg/kg/min no more frequently than every 30 minutes. The heart rate should not be allowed to increase more than 15% over baseline and the dosage should be reduced if left ventricular filling pressure increases or if ventricular ectopic rhythms develop. Maximum dosage is 15 to 20 μg/kg/min up to 40 μg/kg/min in rare instances. In an ideal situation, cardiac output will be increased by 20% to 30%. To achieve this end, the dose must be highly individualized.[17]

Dopamine

Dopamine acts by stimulation of alpha-adrenergic, beta-adrenergic, and dopaminergic receptors. Effects of dopamine on vascular resistance and arterial pressure are dose dependent. With infusion rates < 2μg/kg/min, dopamine predominantely stimulates the dopamine receptors in renal, splanchnic, cerebral, and coronary vascular beds, thereby lowering resistance.[3] Other effects include improved renal perfusion, increased glomerular filtration rate, and natriuresis.[18,19]

Doses of 2 to 5 μg/kg/min exert a positive inotropic effect; cardiac contractility and cardiac output increase, with little change in heart rate, and either a reduction or no change in peripheral vascular resistance. With higher infusion rates (5 to 10 μg/kg/min), arterial pressure, peripheral resistance, and heart rate increase, and renal blood flow may decline.[3]

Comparison of dobutamine and dopamine in management of heart failure. Smith, Braunwald and Kelly[3] published a comprehensive summary of studies that compared the effects of dobutamine and dopamine in patients with severe HF. In one study,[20] dobutamine raised cardiac index while lowering left ventricular end-diastolic pressure with no effect on mean arterial pressure. Dopamine also improved cardiac index but with a greater increase in heart rate. Dopamine increased mean aortic pressure but was ineffective in lowering left ventricular end-diastolic pressure. Both dopamine and dobutamine increased myocardial contractility and thereby augmented myocardial oxygen consumption. Since dobutamine had little effect on heart rate, aortic pressure, and reduced ventricular filling pressure, it may perhaps be superior to dopamine in patients with low cardiac output states.[21]

Dobutamine in doses up to 10 μg/kg/min progressively increased cardiac output while decreasing systemic and pulmonary vascular resistance and filling pressure without a significant effect on heart rate and ventricular irritability. In contrast, dopamine also increased heart rate, and systemic and pulmonary vascular resistance.[22]

Norepinephrine

Norepinephrine is a naturally occurring catecholamine that is the neurotransmitter released at most sympathetic postganglionic fibers. It is a potent $Beta_1$ agonist. Its alpha agonist effects cause vasoconstriction, which reduces renal and mesenteric perfusion, while increasing left ventricular afterload. Increases in myocardial inotropy and peripheral vascular resistance increase myocardial oxygen consumption, which can exacerbate ischemia and compromise left ventricular function.[23]

Norepinephrine infusions are generally initiated at 2 to 4 µg/min and are increased until satisfactory blood pressure is achieved. Heart rate usually remains constant due to baroreceptor stimulation. Local subcutaneous necrosis may result from intravenous extravasation.[23]

Epinephrine

Epinephrine is an endogenous adrenal hormone with potent alpha and $beta_1$ agonist effects and moderate $beta_2$ agonist effects. At lower doses (0.04 to 0.1 µg/kg/min), beta effects predominate (increased heart rate, cardiac output, stroke volume, and peripheral resistance). With higher dosages, peripheral vasoconstriction due to alpha effects occurs, and venous return may be enhanced as a result of venoconstriction.[23]

"The alpha effects probably account for epinephrine's salutary effects during cardiac resuscitation, since increased arterial resistance is thought to augment coronary perfusion pressure."[23]

Digitalis

For more than 200 years, digitalis glycosides have been used in the management of congestive heart failure.[24] Forty years ago cardiac glycosides were the only useful positive inotropic agent for the treatment of heart failure. Katz[25] stated "I suspect, however, that the benefit of these agents was due, in large part, to their ability to slow ventricular rate in atrial fibrillation." Such a view had been expressed in 1918 by the British cardiology giant, Sir James MacKenzie, who wrote "In searching the records in literature for the evidence of the good effects of digitalis, I feel fairly certain that it is in patients with auricular fibrillation, particularly when it is subsequent to rheumatic fever, that the extraordinarily good results have been obtained. If one reads carefully the records given by Withering in the first valuable account of digitalis in 1785, though he used it as a diuretic, yet he noted its good effects in heart cases; and several of his successful cases had undoubtedly auricular fibrillation."[26]

While controversy exists regarding the mechanism of digitalis induced inotropy, it seems to exert a partial inhibition of the enzyme that activates adenosine triphosphate (ATP). This enzyme supplies energy for operation of the sodium-potassium membrane pump. Sodium transport out of the cell is impeded; intracellular sodium is therefore increased. Such a process creates an environment conducive to a calcium-sodium exchange. More calcium ions are retained in the cell, maximizing the actin-myosin coupling of contraction.[3] It has been demonstrated that an intact myocardial cell membrane (sarcolemma) is required for inotropic effects of digitalis to occur; no effect results after administration of digitalis in the skinned myocardial fiber.[27]

Digitalis glycosides exert a positive inotropic effect on cardiac muscle, but not on skeletal muscle. Marked positive inotropic effects persist in the presence of full beta blockade, suggesting that the inotropic effects of digitalis are not mediated by catecholamine release or increased sensitivity to catecholamines. Adenylate cyclase does not appear to be influenced by digitalis glycosides.[27]

In patients with very mild HF and a relatively well preserved left ventricular systolic function, with only slight impairment of exercise tolerance, digoxin therapy is less likely to produce any sustained benefit. Digitalis toxicity occurs in approximately 20% of digitalized patients.[28]

Only recently have double-blind, randomized placebo-controlled trials of digoxin therapy been conducted in patients with moderate HF and sinus rhythm.[29] These studies suggest that digoxin, alone or in combination with ACE inhibitors, is beneficial in patients with any signs or symptoms of HF due to systolic dysfunction.

Another study undertook an investigation to determine the effect of digitalis on norepinephrine uptake and beta receptor down regulation in right HF.[30] Results suggested that chronic digitalis therapy in HF may be deleterious because it reduces norepinephrine reuptake and decreases beta receptor density in the failing myocardium.

A controlled prospective mortality study in over 8000 patients is currently underway to evaluate the efficacy of digitalis in HF in patients who are also maintained on a diuretic and converting enzyme inhibitor.[31]

Oral beta agonists

Some oral beta agonist agents are relatively selective for Beta$_1$ receptors (*prenalterol, butopamine, denopamine,* and *xamoterol*), while others are selective for Beta$_2$ receptor activity (*salbutamol, terbutaline, pirbuterol,* and *albutamol*).[32-35] Several of these agents have demonstrated improvement in left ventricular hemodynamic performance, but sustained effectiveness has been difficult to demonstrate in HF patients. Pirbuterol has been demonstrated to increase cardiac output and decrease left ventricular filling pressure in patients with chronic and severe HF, refractory to digitalis therapy. Tolerance to the favorable effects occurs in 1 month, accompanied by a decrease in numbers of beta adrenoreceptors on the lymphocytes, suggesting a mechanism for decreased responsiveness.[35] A high incidence of ventricular arrhythmias has resulted in withdrawal of prenalterol, terbutaline, and pirbuterol from clinical trials.[36,37]

Ibopamine and *levodopa* are under investigation in clinical trials. Increased diuresis, peripheral vasodilation, and improved contractility have been demonstrated with these agents. Ibopamine is an orally active derivative of dopamine, which metabolizes to its active form, *epinine*. It increases cardiac output, reduces peripheral vascular resistance, and increases renal blood flow, exerting a lesser effect on preload parameters. This hemodynamic improvement has been sustained even after relatively long-term treatment. There is no evidence of pharmacological tolerance. Ibopamine modulates the neurohumoral consequence of HF with decreases in plasma renin activity and aldosterone and norepinephrine plasma levels.[38] Following a single oral dose of 100 or 200 mg, primary vasodilating action has been demonstrated in HF patients.[39] Levodopa, also a precursor of dopamine, exerts a similar salutary hemodynamic effect in HF.[40]

Xamoterol is a new partial beta$_1$ agonist that modulates cardiac response to variations in sympathetic tone in HF patients. It offers beta-receptor stimulatory effects at low levels of sympathetic tone and beta-receptor protective effects at higher levels of sympathetic tone. In a 6-month, double-blind, placebo-controlled cross-over study of chronic oral xamoterol therapy, at 200 mg twice daily, cardiac performance improved at rest and during exercise in mild to moderate HF. Furthermore, 24-hour ambulatory electrocardiographic monitoring showed no change in ventricular arrhythmias and no tachyphylaxis during oral treatment.[41]

PHOSPHODIESTERASE INHIBITORS

Phosphodiesterase inhibitors *(amrinone, milrinone, enoximone, imazodin, prioximon)* are potent inotropic and vasodilator agents that have undergone extensive investigation in the past few years. These agents increase intracellular calcium availability by increasing cyclic AMP levels. They improve cardiac performance by enhancing contractility, reducing left ventricular afterload, and improving left ventricular diastolic compliance. Cardiac index is increased by about 50% and is accompanied by marked decreases in pulmonary capillary wedge pressure (PCWP) and systemic vascular resistance. Systemic venous pressure and, in some cases, mean arterial pressure also decrease while heart rate increases slightly. Increased cardiac work leads to an increase in myocardial oxygen consumption, but increased coronary flow prevents an imbalance of myocardial oxygen supply and demand. Renal perfusion may increase as a result of the increase in cardiac output. Hemodynamic improvements associated with these agents are well documented, but whether they impact the prognosis of HF patients is yet to be determined.[42-46] Some concerns have been raised about the adverse effects on myocardial energetics. Increase of cyclic AMP and intracellular calcium may produce toxic effects on the myocardium.[23]

Amrinone

Amrinone has slight positive inotropic and marked vasodilating properties. Because of its pronounced vasodilating properties, a dose-dependent decline in blood pressure occurs, which may limit its use in severe HF and hypotension. The relatively long plasma half-life (6 hours in HF) may hamper dose titration and control of plasma levels and clinical effects. Amrinone is indicated for short-term therapy of cardiac failure not responding to conventional treatment with digitalis, diuretics, and vasodilators and for patients not responding to dobutamine because of beta receptor down regulation.[23]

Milrinone

Milrinone is a second-generation congener of amrinone, therefore it is similar to amrinone, but the positive inotropic effect is about 15 times more potent than with amrinone. Milrinone has also been demonstrated to improve myocardial relaxation and increase coronary perfusion.[23]

Enoximone

Enoximone is similar to amrinone and milrinone. In chronic HF, symptomatic improvement was demonstrated in a controlled cross-over trial; however, gastrointestinal side effects may limit its use.[47]

CALCIUM-SENSITIZING AGENTS

Cardiac sensitizers are a new class of drugs that increase the affinity of troponin C for calcium. As a result, more calcium binds to troponin C in the presence of the drug. Therefore the potentially deleterious effects of inotropic drugs that increase cycle AMP levels or cellular calcium are circumvented.[48]

Pimobendan and *sulmazole* are calcium-sensitizing agents. Both also inhibit cyclic AMP.[49] Sulmazole was withdrawn from clinical trials because it produced severe gastrointestinal side effects and hepatic neoplasms.[50]

Oral pimobendan has been observed to significantly improve myocardial contractility and relaxation with immediate and prolonged vasodilatory effects. Pimobendan also had favorable effects on myocardial energetics and did not induce rhythm disturbances.[51] Its long-term efficacy, effect on exercise tolerance, and influence on patient survival has yet to be determined.

VASODILATOR THERAPY

Vasodilators have achieved widespread acceptance in the management of heart failure.[52,53] Nitrates act to attenuate the peripheral vasoconstriction that contributes to hemodynamic derangements associated with HF. Because the capacity of venous beds is large, a relatively small reduction in venous tone can result in pooling of substantial quantities of blood and its redistribution from pulmonary to systemic circuits.[3] Cardiac performance can be affected profoundly by alterations in the resistance and capacitance of peripheral vascular beds. When contractility is normal, an increase in afterload results in stroke volume improvement, with little elevation of ventricular end-diastolic volume or pressure. In patients with left ventricular dysfunction, increasing afterload decreases stroke volume and elevates left ventricular end-diastolic pressure and volume.[3]

Nitrates may exhibit coronary artery vasodilating properties and therefore improve myocardial blood flow, which may be particularly important in HF because ischemia contributes to left ventricular dysfunction. Even without an antiischemic effect, nitrates might reduce the long-term morbidity and mortality associated with HF because they can potentially minimize progressive ventricular failure.[54]

Vasodilators that act equally on arterial and venous beds are referred to as "balanced vasodilators" (nitroprusside and prazosin). Their actions are intermediate between those of pure arterial dilators (hydralazine, minoxidil, and phenoxybenzamine) and pure venous dilators (nitroglycerin and isorbide dinitrate).[54]

Packer[55] published a literature review and commentary addressing the issue of nitrate effectiveness in the treatment of HF. He concluded that "few data are available to support the widespread belief that nitrates are effective drugs in the treatment of chronic HF. At least in the doses and dosing regimens that have been utilized in controlled trials, therapy with nitrates does not produce predictable long-term hemodynamic or clinical benefits. Although mortality may be favorably affected when nitrates are combined with hydralazine, this benefit appears to be more closely related to the use of hydralazine than to the use of nitrates." In response to the question, "Are nitrates worthless drugs in the treatment of HF?" he responded, "No. Current studies are plagued by inherent flaws in design and interpretation; future trials (if better executed) may demonstrate a favorable effect of nitrates in these patients. Yet the problem with nitrates lies not only in the design of studies but also with the drugs themselves. Tolerance is the inevitable result of any attempt to use nitrates to produce round-the-clock hemodynamic improvement. To the extent that such a goal is important in improving the clinical status of patients with CHF, we will almost certainly need to look to other vasodilator drugs."

Sodium nitroprusside

Intravenous sodium nitroprusside produces a balanced and potent vasodilator effect. Intended therapeutic effects are to reduce (1) pulmonary congestion by increasing venous capacitance and (2) pulmonary artery wedge pressure. Impedance to left ventricular ejection should be reduced because of arterial tone relaxation and the lowering of systemic vascular resistance. Recommended starting dosage is 3 μg/kg/min for both adults and children (range 0.5-10 μg/kg/min). At 3 μg/kg/min, blood pressure can be lowered to about 30% to 40% below the pretreatment diastolic levels. To avoid possible thiocynate overdosage and the possibility of precipitous drops in blood pressure, dosage should not exceed 10 μg/kg/min.[56]

Effect of nitroprusside on radial artery pressure measurements. Effects of nitroprusside on pressure wave transmission from ascending aorta to radial artery were studied in 10 patients with severe HF.[57] In six patients with an identified late systolic peak of aortic pressure, nitroprusside reduced aortic systolic pressure more than radial systolic pressure, resulting in up to a 20 mm Hg difference between aortic and radial artery systolic pressures. In four patients in whom no aortic late systolic pressure wave was apparent, nitroprusside did not alter the difference between aortic and radial systolic pressures. These results suggest that a reduction of radial systolic pressure induced by nitroprusside may underestimate the true reduction of aortic systolic pressure and thus the vasodilator effect on left ventricle arterial load.

Nitroglycerin

Intravenous sodium nitroglycerin has a potent effect on venous tone even at low dosages. Arterial dilatation occurs at dosages of approximately 200 μg/min.[58] Its effect on systemic vascular resistance is less than that of sodium nitroprusside. Nitroglycerin also has been demonstrated to increase flow through collateral coronary beds by a greater magnitude than nitroprusside.[59]

The initial dosage is 5 μg/min, increasing by 5 μg/min every 10 minutes. After a dosage of 20 μg/min is reached, infusion can be increased by increments of 10 μg/min until a hemodynamic response is achieved.[60] Adherence of nitroglycerin to polyvinyl chloride has been demonstrated. One study[61] reported that the relative absorption of nitroglycerin from PVC infusion sets was 41.5%, 62.9%, and 76.0% for the 6, 12, and 24 ml/hr infusion rates. Loss of nitroglycerin was related to the rate of infusion, with slower infusion rates resulting in more nitroglycerin loss. Only minimal loss of nitroglycerin occurred with non-PVC or polyethylene administration sets.

Hydralazine

Hydralazine is an oral vasodilator that acts directly on arteriolar smooth muscle. Usual dosage ranges from 25 to 100 mg 3 to 4 times daily. The degree of left ventricular enlargement and level of peripheral vascular resistance appear to be important determinants of hydralazine responsiveness. Patients with marked cardiomegaly and markedly elevated systemic vascular resistance exhibit the most salutary responses. A lupus-like syndrome manifests in approximately 15% of patients receiving 400 mg daily. Some patients also develop circulating antinuclear antibodies.[3]

Nitroglycerin tolerance in heart failure

Development of nitrate tolerance may negate the beneficial effect of nitrate therapy in the management of patients with HF. At constant doses of nitrates, ventricular filling pressures and cardiac output return to baseline values in many patients within 24 to 48 hours.[62] A study was therefore undertaken to characterize in more detail the magnitude, hemodynamic spectrum, and temporal course of tolerance developed during intravenous nitroglycerin therapy.[63] The extent of nitrate tolerance at 24 hours was calculated as the percentage loss of benefit achieved at time of peak nitroglycerin effect. Tolerance had a different time course and magnitude in the venous, arterial, and pulmonary circulations. At 24 hours, right atrial pressure and pulmonary vascular resistance returned to control values in most patients, while 40% to 50% of the effect on systemic vascular resistance, cardiac index, and pulmonary wedge pressure was maintained.

Clinical trial of vasodilatory therapy in heart failure

The Veterans Administration Cooperative Study on Vasodilator Therapy of Heart Failure (V-HeFT trial)[64] was designed to determine whether vasodilator drugs could alter the survival of patients with chronic congestive HF treated with digitalis and diuretics. Among the 642 patients entered into the study, 273 were randomly assigned to placebo, 186 were randomly assigned to prazosin; all patients were followed for periods ranging from 6 months to 5.7 years. Patients were stratified by the presence of coronary artery disease.

The vasodilator regime of hydralazine and isosorbide dinitrate was shown to reduce the risk of mortality in comparison with placebo by 28%. No mortality reduction was obtained with the vasodilator prazosin in comparison with placebo.[64]

Reduction of atrial overload during vasodilator therapy

The effect of vasodilator therapy on atrial overload contributing to HF symptoms was also studied.[65] Right atrial pressure decreased by 45%. Echocardiography showed simultaneous reductions in left and right atrial volumes. Mitral and tricuspid regurgitation measured by color flow fraction both decreased by a mean of 44%.

Future of nitrate therapy for heart failure

Cohn[53] described one of the most exciting developments in the nitrate field, which was evidence that nitric oxide, the active product of a nitrodilator drug, is also the active substance released from the endothelium in response to a variety of physiological and pharmacological stimuli. Cohn stated "Evidence has accumulated that this endothelial derived relaxing factor is deficient in atherosclerotic coronary arteries and in the peripheral vasculature in other disease states. Nitrates may therefore now be viewed as endogenous vasodilators and their administration may actually be restoring deficient endogenous nitric oxide."

With parenteral vasodilation, arterial blood pressure may fall unless there is a concomitant increase in cardiac output. For this reason, it is imperative that arterial blood pressure, intracardiac pressures, and cardiac output measurements be carefully monitored and evaluated. An arterial pressure monitoring line and pulmonary artery catheter should be in place before beginning intravenous vasodilator therapy.

ANGIOTENSIN-CONVERTING ENZYME (ACE) INHIBITORS

The renin-angiotensin system response in HF was described in Chapter 4. During the early compensatory phase, this mechanism contributes to sodium and water retention. With expansion of extracellular fluid volume and restoration of blood pressure, the renin-angiotensin system is deactivated. During profound cardiac failure, such stabilization may not occur and the renin-angiotensin remains activated. Resultant sodium retention and expansion of extracellular fluid volume contribute to increased preload and subsequent edema. Angiotensin is also a powerful renal vasoconstrictor.[66]

The principle action of an ACE inhibitor is blocking conversion of angiotensin I to angiotensin II. ACE inhibitors also degrade the potent vasodilator bradykinin to inactive metabolites. Tissue accumulation of bradykinin has been postulated to be responsible, in part, for the vasodilator effect.

There is an inverse relationship between plasma renin levels and serum sodium concentration in patients with HF. Patients with serum sodium less than 130 mg/L are 30 times more likely to develop symptomatic hypotension during initiation of captopril therapy.[67] Three ACE inhibitors are currently FDA approved for use in the United States.

Captopril

The first ACE inhibitor to be approved has demonstrated an improvement in pump efficiency by reducing MVO_2. *Captopril* dosage suggested for heart failure is 6.25 mg to 25 mg three times/day. Captopril is rapidly absorbed after oral administration. In the fasting state, 60% to 75% of the orally administered dose is bioavailable. Only 30% to 40% of each dose is absorbed when ingested with food. Serum levels can be detected 15 minutes following ingestion. Peak levels are reached in 30 to 90 minutes. Approximately 25% to 30% of captopril is protein bound. Captopril is excreted during the first 4 hours and 95% of the dose is eliminated over a 24-hour period.[68]

Enalapril

Enalapril is a relatively weak ACE inhibitor. Recommended initial dosage is 2.5 to 5.0 mg. Maintenance doses range from 5.0 mg to 40 mg daily. Following oral ingestion, approximately 60% to 70% of enalapril is absorbed and bioavailable; absorption is not influenced by food in the gastrointestinal tract. Onset of action is approximately 1 hour after ingestion, and peak ACE inhibition occurs 4 to 6 hours after dosing. Over 90% of enalapril is eliminated in the urine; half-life is approximately 11 hours.[69]

Clinical trials with ACE inhibitors

Captopril (25 to 100 mg 3 times daily after a lower initial dose) demonstrated sustained benefit in the therapy of severe HF during double-blind randomized trials.[70] Onset of action with captopril is rapid. Patients may experience a reactive hypotension. Therefore a test dose of 6.25 mg is usually administered while avoiding diuresis and maintaining circulating volume.[70]

Enalapril (5 mg 2 times daily after a test dose of 2.5 mg; range 2.5 to 20 mg 2 times daily) demonstrated equal effectiveness in a double-blind randomized trial.[70] Onset of action is slower, so reactive hypotension may be less of a problem than with captopril.

The CONSENSUS trial[71] was designed to study the effect of enalapril on 6-month mortality in patients with severe HF (New York Heart Association Class IV). Thirty-five Scandinavian centers participated in this double-blind study in which 253 patients were randomly assigned to receive enalapril or placebo in addition to conventional therapy with digitalis, diuretics, and vasodilators other than ACE inhibitors. At the end of 6 months, mortality was 26% in the enalapril group and 44% in the placebo group.

A metaanalysis of 28 placebo-controlled trials of various vasodilators suggested that ACE inhibitors were the only drug class with a consistent positive effect on mortality and functional symptoms of HF.[72]

SOLVD is a randomized, double-blind, placebo-controlled study[73] designed to determine the effect of treatment with enalapril on mortality of patients with left ventricular ejection fraction ≤35%. This study, with 23 participating centers, was designed to include 2500 patients in a treatment trial and 4600 patients in a prevention trial. Patients with symptoms of HF, who required digitalis, diuretics, or non-ACE inhibitor vasodilators, were admitted to the treatment trial. Those who did not require therapy were assigned to the prevention trial. Within each trial, patients were randomized to receive either placebo or enalapril, starting at 2.5 mg bid and increasing to 5 to 10 mg bid, if tolerated. The results showed that enalapril reduced mortality by 16% and reduced deaths or hospitalizations for HF by 25% in patients with mild-to-moderate HF.

The V-HeFT II trial was designed to compare double-blind treatment with hydralazine-isorbide dinitrate with enalapril titrated to a maximum dose of 20 mg daily. Data from V-HeFT II in 804 men showed that patients randomized to enalapril had a survival rate of 82% compared with those receiving hydralazine and isorbide dinitrate (75%).[74]

As part of the V-HeFT II trial, the relationship of arrhythmia to mortality was evaluated in HF patients. Ventricular tachycardia persisted less at 3 months in the enalapril group. New ventricular tachycardia was also less frequent in the enalapril group.[75]

BETA-ADRENERGIC BLOCKADE THERAPY

Conventionally, beta-adrenergic blockers have been contraindicated in HF because it was believed that high reflex sympathetic tone was necessary to maintain cardiac output.[76] The consequence of catecholamine stimulation is an increase in heart rate and contractility; continued sympathetic stimulation results in beta-adrenergic receptor down regulation and possibly a direct toxic effect on the myocardium.[77] Vasoconstriction and release of vasopressin with activation of the renin-angiotensin system, along with an increase in systemic vascular resistances, are all untoward side effects of sympathetic overstimulation.

Clinical trials

A large, multicenter, randomized double-blind investigation, "Metoprolol in Dilated Cardiomyopathy," was organized by a Goteborg, Sweden, group and initiated in 1986 to assess the efficacy of metoprolol in management of HF.[78] Recommendations from that study include beginning metoprolol orally at 5 mg bid; observing patients in the inpatient setting overnight; and performing dosage titration weekly, increasing up to 50 mg tid. Metoprolol doses are not increased if the heart rate is below 60 beats per minute or systolic pressure is less than 90 mm Hg. Contraindications include a history of asthma, significant atrioventricular block, and insulin-dependent diabetes. Fatigue, lightheadedness, and dizziness have been reported, but most patients have tolerated the drug well.

The Beta Blocker Heart Attack Trial (BHAT)[79] evaluated the effect of long-term therapy with propranolol after an acute myocardial infarction with congestive heart failure. This retrospective analysis indicated that the use of propranolol is generally safe in survivors of acute myocardial infarction, including those with a history of HF. During the average follow-up of 25 months, BHAT with prior HF, who were assigned to receive propranolol, experienced a relatively greater reduction in total mortality rate and all coronary events without incurring an overall increased rate of HF. An increased incidence of HF (14.8%) compared with placebo (12.6%) was observed in the propranolol group who had a history of prior HF.

A randomized trial was conducted to evaluate the beneficial effects of metoprolol in HF associated with coronary artery disease.[80] The study suggested that HF associated with ischemic heart disease can be safely and effectively treated with beta blockers. Patients with high plasma norepinephrine (PANE) are more likely to benefit from metroprolol compared with those having low PANE, who rarely respond.

REFERENCES

1. Chung TO: Congestive heart failure in coronary artery disease, *Am J Med* 91:409, 1991.
2. Pitt B, Cohn JN, Francis GS et al: The effect of treatment on survival in congestive heart failure, *Clin Cardiol* 15:323, 1992.
3. Smith TW, Braunwald E, Kelly RA: The management of heart failure. In Braunwald E, ed: *Heart disease*, ed 4, Philadelphia, 1992, WB Saunders.
4. Rose BD: Clinical assessment of renal function (chap 1). In Rose BD, ed: *Pathophysiology of renal disease*, ed 2, New York, 1987, McGraw-Hill.
5. Sica DA, Gehr T: Diuretics in congestive heart failure, *Cardiol Clin* 7:87, 1989.
6. Muller J: Spirolactone in the management of congestive heart failure, *Am J Cardiol* 65: 51K, 1990.
7. Cunningham SG: Diuretics (chap 8). In Underhill SL, Woods SL, Froelicher ESS et al: *Cardiovascular medications for cardiac nursing*, Philadelphia, 1990, Lippincott.
8. Francis GS, Siegel RM, Goldsmith SR et al: Acute vasoconstrictor response to intravenous furosemide in patients with chronic congestive heart failure, *Ann Intern Med* 103:1, 1985.
9. Katz AM: Future perspectives in basic science understanding of congestive heart failure, *Am J Cardiol* 66:468, 1990.
10. Poole-Wilson PA: Future perspectives in the management of congestive heart failure, *Am J Cardiol* 66:462, 1990.
11. Zelcer AA, LeJemtel TH, Sonnenblick EH: Inotropic therapy in heart failure, *Heart Failure* 10:7, 1985.
12. Packer M, Leier CV: Survival in congestive heart failure during treatment with drugs with positive inotropic action, *Circulation* 75 (suppl IV):IV-55, 1987.
13. Helfant RH: Short and long term mechanism of sudden cardiac death in congestive heart failure, *Am J Cardiol* 65:41K, 1990.
14. Brembilla-Perrot B: Heart rate variations during isoproterenol infusion in congestive heart failure: relationships to cardiac mortality, *Am Heart J* 12:989, 1992.
15. Leier CV, Webel J, Bush CA: The cardiac output effects of dobutamine in patients with severe cardiac failure, *Circulation* 56:468, 1977.
16. Unverferth DV, Leier CV, Magorien RD et al: Improvement of human mitochondria after dobutamine: a quantitative ultrastructural study, *J Pharmacol Exp Ther* 215:527, 1980.
17. Francis GS: Dobutamine in chronic CHF (chap 6). In Chatterjee K, ed: *Dobutamine: a ten year review*, New York, 1989, NCM Publisher.
18. Goldberg IF, Olivari MT, Levine B et al: Effect of dobutamine on plasma potassium in congestive heart failure secondary to idiopathic or ischemic cardiomyopathy, *Am J Cardiol* 63:843, 1989.
19. Goldberg LI, Rajfer WI: Dopamine receptors: application in clinical cardiology, *Circulation* 72:245, 1985.
20. Stoner JD III, Bolen JL, Harrison DC: Comparison of dobutamine and dopamine in treatment of severe heart failure, *Br Heart J* 39:536, 1977.
21. Loeb HS, Bredalos K, Gimmar RM: Superiority of dobutamine over dopamine for augmentation of cardiac output in patients with chronic low output heart failure, *Circulation* 55:375, 1977.
22. Leier CV, Heban PT, Huss P et al: Comparative systemic and regional hemodynamic effects of dopamine and dobutamine in patients with cardiomyopathic heart failure, *Circulation* 58:486, 1978.
23. Lologen H, Drexler H: Use of inotropes in the critical care setting, *Crit Care Med* 18:S56, 1990.
24. Withering, W: An account of the foxglove and some of its medical uses with practical remarks on dropsy and other disease. In Willis FA and Keys TE, eds: *Classics of cardiology*, New York, 1941, Henry Schuman.
25. Katz AM: Changing strategies in the management of heart failure, *JCC* 13:513, 1989.
26. MacKenzie J: *Diseases of the heart*, ed 3, Oxford, 1918, Oxford University Press.
27. Marsh JD and Smith TW: Clinical use of cardiac glycosides in congestive heart failure. In Smith TW, ed: *Digitalis glycosides*, Orlando, Fla, 1985, Grune and Stratton.
28. Smith TW, Antman EM, Friedman PL et al: Digitalis glycosides: mechanisms and manifestations of toxicity, *Prog Cardiovas Dis* 26:413, 1984.

29. Gheorghiade M, Zarowitz BJ: Review of randomized trials of digoixin therapy in patients with chronic heart failure, *Am J Cardiol* 69:48G, 1992.
30. Imai N, Kashiki M, Masakuni S et al: Chronic digoxin administration decreased beta-adrenocepter density in right heart failure, *Circulation* (suppl II)84:II-259, 1991.
31. Pitt B, Cohn JN, Francis GS: The effect of treatment on survival in congestive heart failure, *Clin Cardiol* 15:323, 1992.
32. Colucci WS, Wright RF, Braunwald E: New positive inotropic agents in the treatment of congestive heart failure. Mechanisms of action and recent clinical developments, *N Engl J Med* 314:290, 1986.
33. Wahr DW, Swedberg K, Rabbino M et al: Intravenous and oral prenaterol in congestive heart failure: effects on systemic and coronary hemodynamics and myocardial catecholamine balance, *Am J Med* 76:999, 1984.
34. Sharma B, Goodwin JF: Beneficial effects of salbutamol on cardiac function in severe congestive cardiomyopathy. Effects on systolic and diastolic function of the left ventricle, *Circulation* 58:449, 1978.
35. Awan NA, Evenson MK, Needham KE et al: Hemodynamic effects of oral pirbuterol in chronic severe congestive heart failure, *Circulation* 6:96, 1981.
36. Colucci WS, Alexander RW, Williams GH et al: Decreased lymphocyte beta-adrenergic receptor density in patients with heart failure and tolerance to the beta-adrenergic agonist pirbuterol, *N Engl J Med* 305:185, 1981.
37. Chatterjee K: Newer oral inotropic agents, *Crit Care Med* 18:S34, 1990.
38. Lopez-Sendon J: Ibopamine in chronic congestive heart failure: hemodynamic and neurohumoral effects, *Am J Med* 90(suppl 5B):43S, 1991.
39. Itoh H: Clinical pharmacology of ibopamine, *Am J Med* 90(suppl 5B):36S, 1991.
40. Fajfer WI, Anton AH, Rosen JD et al: Beneficial hemodynamic effects of oral levodopa in heart failure. Relations to the generation of dopamine, *N Engl J Med* 30:1357, 1984.
41. Surinder JS, Virk MRCP, Qiang F et al: Acute and hemodynamic effects of xamoterol in mild to moderate congestive heart failure, *Am J Cardiol* 67:48C, 1991.
42. Massie B, Bourassa M, DeiBianco R et al: Long-term oral administration of amrinone for congestive heart failure: lack of efficacy in multicenter controlled trial, *Circulation* 72:963, 1985.
43. Packer M, Carver JR, Rodeheffer RJ: Effect of oral milrinone on mortality in severe chronic heart failure, *N Engl J Med* 325:1468, 1991.
44. Ferrick KJ, Fein SA, Ferrick AM et al: Effect of milrinone on ventricular arrhythmias in congestive heart failure, *Am J Cardiol* 66:431, 1990.
45. Weber KT, Janicki JS, Jain MC: Enoximone (MDL 17,043) a phosphodiesterase inhibitor in the treatment of advanced unstable chronic heart failure, *J Heart Transplant* 5:105, 1986.
46. Jessup M, Ulrich S, Samaha S et al: Effects of low dose enoximone for chronic congestive heart failure, *Am J Cardiol* 60:80C, 1987.
47. Uretsky B, Jessup M, Konstam MA et al: Multicenter trial of oral enoximone in patients with moderate to moderately severe congestive heart failure, *Circulation* 82:774, 1990.
48. Schwertz DW, Piano MR: New inotropic drugs for treatment of congestive heart failure, *Cardiovasc Nurs* 26:7, 1990.
49. Endoh M, Yanagisawa T, Taira N et al: Effects of new inotropic agents on cyclic nucleotide metabolism and calcium transients in canine ventricular muscle, *Circulation* 73 (suppl III):III-117, 1986.
50. Diederen W, Kadatz R: Effects of Ar-L 115 BS, a new cardiotonic compound, on cardiac contractility, heart rate and blood pressure in anesthetized and conscious animals, *Arneimittelforschung* 31:146, 1981.
51. Baumann G, Ningel K, Permanetter B: Clinical efficacy of pimobendan (UDCG 115 BS) in patients with chronic congestive heart failure, *J Cardiovasc Pharmacol* 14 (suppl II):S 23, 1989.
52. Giles D: Principles of vasodilator therapy for left ventricular congestive heart failure, *Heart Lung* 9:2, 1980.
53. Cohn JN: Nitrates are effective in the treatment of chronic congestive heart failure: the protagonist's view, *Am J Cardiol* 66:444, 1990.
54. Packer M: Do vasodilators prolong life in heart failure? *N Engl J Med* 316:1471, 1987.

55. Packer M: Are nitrates effective in the treatment of chronic heart failure? Antagonist's viewpoint, *Am J Cardiol* 66:458, 1990.
56. Nitropress: Sodium Nitroprusside, USP package insert, North Chicago, March 1987, Abbott Laboratories.
57. Simkus GJ, Fitchett DH: Radial arterial pressure measurements may be a poor guide to the beneficial effects of nitroprusside on left ventricular systolic pressure in congestive heart failure, *Am J Cardiol* 66:323, 1990.
58. Saxon SA, Silverman ME: Effects of continuous infusion of intravenous nitroglycerin on methemoglobin levels, *Am J Cardiol* 56:461, 1985.
59. Flaherty JT: Comparison of intravenous nitroglycerin and sodium nitroprusside on ischemic injury during acute myocardial infarction, *Circulation* 65:1072, 1982.
60. Underhill SL, Woods SL, Froelicher ESS et al: *Cardiovascular medications for cardiac nursing*, Philadelphia, 1990, JB Lippincott.
61. Nix DE, Tharpe WN, Francisco GE: Intravenous nitroglycerin delivery: dynamics and cost considerations, *Hosp Pharm* 20:230, 1985.
62. Abrams J: Tolerance to organic nitrates, *Circulation* 74:1181, 1986.
63. Makhoul N, Dakak N, Flugelman MY et al: Nitrate tolerance in heart failure: differential venous, pulmonary and systemic arterial effects, *Am J Cardiol* 65:28J, 1991.
64. Cohn JN, Archibald DG, Phil NW et al: Effect of vasodilator therapy on mortality in chronic congestive heart failure: results of a Veterans Administration Cooperative Study, *N Eng J Med* 314:1547, 1986.
65. Hamilton MA, Stevenson LW, Child JS et al: Acute reduction of atrial overload during vasodilator and diuretic therapy in advanced congestive heart failure, *Am J Cardiol* 65:1209, 1990.
66. Swartz SL, Williams GH: Angio-converting enzyme inhibition and prostaglandins, *Am J Cardiol* 49:1405, 1982.
67. Packer M, Medina N, Yushak M: Relations between serum sodium concentration and hemodynamic and clinical response to converting enzyme inhibition with captopril in severe heart failure, *J Am Coll Cardiol* 3:1035, 1984.
68. Dzau VJ, Creager MA: Progress in angiotensin-converting enzyme inhibition in heart failure: rationale, mechanisms, and clinical responses, *Cardiol Clin* 7:119, 1989.
69. Sharpe DN, Murphy J, Connon R et al: Enalapril in patients with chronic heart failure: a placebo-controlled, randomized double blind study, *Circulation* 70:271, 1989.
70. Opie LH: *Drugs for the heart*, ed 2, New York, 1987, Grune and Stratton.
71. Swedberg K, Kjekshus J: Effects of enalapril on mortality in severe congestive heart failure: results of the Cooperative North Scandinavian Enalapril Survival Study (CONSENSUS), *Am J Cardiol* 62:60A, 1988.
72. Mulrow CD, Mulrow JP, Linn WD et al: Relative efficacy of vasodilator therapy in chronic congestive heart failure. Implications of randomized trials, *JAMA* 259:3422, 1988.
73. The SOLVD investigators: effect of enalapril on survival of patients with reduced left ventricular ejection fraction and congestive heart failure, *N Engl J Med* 325: 293, 1991.
74. Cohn JN, Johnson G, Xiesche S et al: A comparison of enalapril with hydralazine-isosorbide dinitrate in the treatment of chronic congestive heart failure, *N Engl J Med* 325:303, 1991.
75. Fletcher R, Cinton G, Johnson G: Enalapril decreases ventricular tachycardia in heart failure:V-HeFT II, *Circulation* 84(suppl II):II-310, 1991.
76. Gerber JG, Niew AS: Beta-adrenergic blocking drugs, *An Rev Med* 36:145, 1985.
77. Fowler MB, Bristow MR: Rationale for beta-adrenergic blocking drugs in cardiomyopathy, *Am J Cardiol* 55:120D, 1985.
78. Swedberg K, Hjalmarson A, Waagstein F et al: Beneficial effects of long-term beta-blockage in congestive cardiomyopathy, *Br Heart J* 44:117, 1980.
79. Chadda K, Goldstein S, Byington R et al: Effect of propranolol after acute myocardial infarction in patients with congestive heart failure, *Circulation* 73:503, 1986.
80. Fisher ML, Gottlieb SS, Hamilton B et al: Beneficial effects of metoprolol in CHF associated with coronary artery disease: a randomized trial, *Circulation* 84(suppl II):II-312, 1991.

PART TWO

CLINICAL APPLICATION OF INTRAAORTIC BALLOON COUNTERPULSATION (IABC)

CHAPTER 6

Basic principles of IABC

Susan J. Quaal

Intraaortic balloon counterpulsation (IABC) is instituted by insertion of a distensible polyurethane, nonthrombogenic balloon (usually 40 cc) in the patient's descending thoracic aorta. The balloon is passed retrogradely to a position in situ just below the left subclavian artery, but above the renal arteries (Fig. 6-1).

An instructional paper on proper intraaortic balloon (IAB) placement was published by Chiles et al. from the Department of Radiology, McMaster University Medical Center in Hamilton, Ontario.[1] The tip of the catheter is visible radiographically as an opaque rectangle, 3 × 4 mm, paralleling the walls of the descending aorta. An IAB is correctly positioned with this tip in the proximal descending aorta, just below the left subclavian artery (Fig. 6-2). The distance from the top of the aortic arch to the more cephalad renal artery ranged from 19.0 to 27.8 cm (mean 23.2 cm) in 28 chest IABC radiographs reviewed by this group. They found that the balloon crossed the renal artery ostia, even when it was properly positioned in the descending thoracic aorta. When the catheter is overadvanced in the aortic arch, the normally rectangular tip is foreshortened and may even be visible end-on as a radiopaque ring (Fig. 6-3).

This balloon is mounted on a vascular catheter, which has multiple pores (Fig. 6-4). Helium gas is shuttled from the balloon pump console into the balloon catheter, escapes through the pores, and inflates the balloon. Helium is a molecularly light gas, which minimizes shuttle transfer time and thus increases efficiency.

Inflation occurs immediately upon onset of diastole. Deflation occurs during isometric contraction or early systole. Thus the balloon is phasically pulsed in counterpulsation to the patient's cardiac cycle. Catheter attachment is made externally to a balloon pump console equipped with R-wave detector circuitry.

Arterial entry is usually through a femoral artery; axial artery[2] or open chest proximal aorta[3,4] insertions are alternative options. Femoral insertion is accomplished via an arterial cutdown[5] or percutaneously,[6] the latter being most commonly used. The femorally inserted IAB is then passed retrogradely up the descending thoracic aorta to a position in situ, just distal to the left subclavian artery.

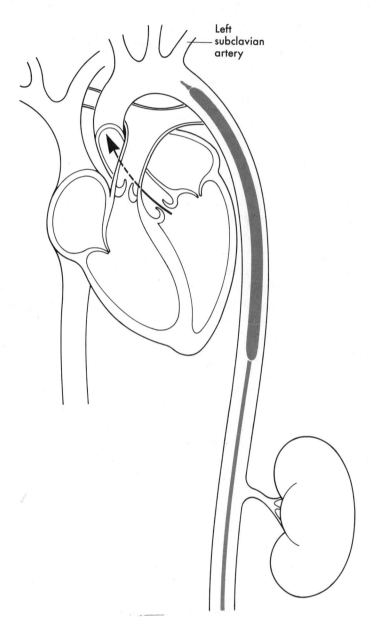

Left subclavian artery

Fig. 6-1. Schematic illustration of the intraaortic balloon (IAB) positioned in the descending thoracic aorta, just below the left subclavian artery, but above the renal artery.

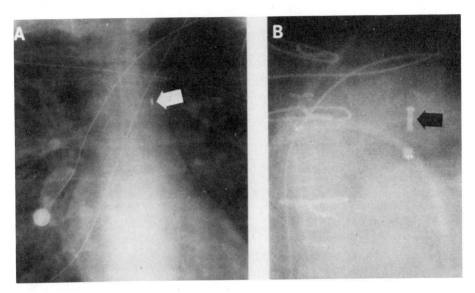

Fig. 6-2. Chest radiographies illustrating correct positioning of IAB. **A,** Datascope Percor IAB catheter; **B,** Kontron percutaneous catheter. The tip of each catheter is identifiable as a 3 × 4 mm rectangular opacity *(arrows)* in the proximal descending thoracic aorta. (From Chiles C, Vail CM, Coblentz CL et al: *Can Assoc Radiol J* 42:257, 1991.)

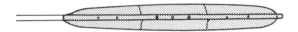

Fig. 6-3. The intraaortic balloon is mounted on a vascular catheter, which contains multiple pores. Helium gas escapes through these pores and inflates the balloon.

PRINCIPLES OF COUNTERPULSATION

Counterpulsation is the term that describes balloon inflation in diastole and deflation during isometric contraction or early systole[7] (Fig. 6-5). In a mechanical sense, balloon inflation causes "volume displacement." Blood volume within the intraaortic balloon is displaced both proximally and distally, concomitant with balloon inflation. Balloon inflation can be conceptualized as "compartmentalizing" the aorta (Fig. 6-6). The *proximal compartment* includes aortic root and coronary arteries. The aortic segment extending beyond the distal balloon tip together with the systemic circulation comprise the *distal compartment*.[8]

Total or regional blood flow is potentially improved by balloon inflation. Collat-

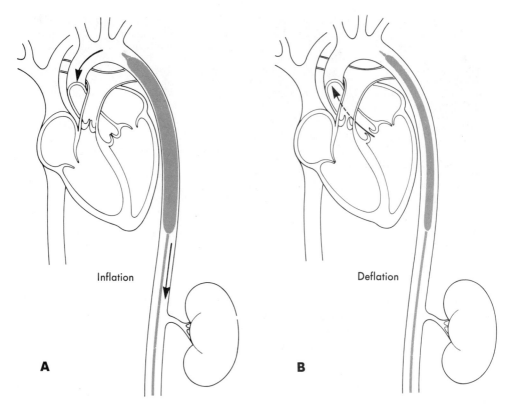

Fig. 6-4. The intraaortic balloon is inflated in diastole (**A**) and deflated during systole (**B**).

eral coronary circulation is also enhanced. Perfusion to aortic arch trifurcated vessels is potentially increased and systemic perfusion improves because balloon inflation facilitates peripheral runoff. Although the exact physiological mechanisms have not been conclusively clarified, the hypothesis is that balloon inflation augments the intrinsic "Windkessel" effect, which augments peripheral perfusion (see discussion in Chapter 1).[9]

Balloon deflation conventionally occurs during isovolumetric contraction. However, more recent research findings suggest that later deflation in early systole may actually be therapeutic in certain hemodynamic states.[10] Recall that during inflation blood volume is displaced. Therefore at the time of deflation, intraaortic blood volume is decreased with concomitant lowering of pressure. This process occurs at the end of diastole (AoEDP), just as isovolumetric contraction is commencing. A de-

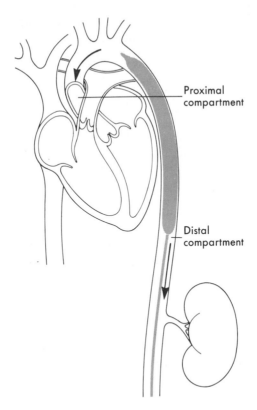

Fig. 6-5. Balloon inflation "compartmentalizes" the aorta. The proximal compartment includes aortic root and coronary arteries. The distal compartment contains the aortic segment extending beyond the IAB's distal tip.

crease in AoEDP "reduces the impedance" against which the left ventricle (LV) must eject. Balloon deflation during isovolumetric contraction therefore potentially lowers the afterload component of cardiac work.[11]

POSITIONING OF THE BALLOON

If the balloon was positioned at the aortic root, inflation would compromise flow to the aortic arch and its trifurcated vessels, which would invoke a risk of neurological insult. Placement of the IAB's proximal tip just distal to the left subclavian artery expands the proximal compartment to include subclavian and carotid arterial systems.

Positioning of the IAB remotely from the aortic root imposes a time delay between actual balloon inflation and its physiological impact on aortic root pressure, which must be taken into account when "timing" of inflation via a radial or even more peripheral arterial line. This situation is discussed more completely in Chapter 16.

A debate over what happens to renal blood flow when IABs are adjacent to renal arteries prompted a study undertaken by the Department of Surgery at St. Louis University.[12] Balloon positioning in 14 dogs was randomized so that it was positioned (1) above the renals in the descending thoracic aorta (control) or (2) at the level of the renal arteries (experimental position). Intraaortic balloon counterpulsation was performed for 4 hours in each position. In eight dogs with the balloon at the level of the renal arteries, at least one renal artery became partially occluded (flow decreased from 23% to 98%, with a mean decrease of 66%).

These researchers cited additional studies suggesting that collateral blood flow at subfiltration pressures may preserve the glomerulus for a while, but irreversible renal tubular atrophy and acute tubular necrosis are likely if total occlusion persists longer than 4 hours. In the St. Louis study, there was not a total loss of renal blood flow; therefore the affected kidneys remained viable, yet virtually nonfunctional. Renal blood flow and urine output measurements clearly demonstrated renal insufficiency while the IAB was in the renal position. Several kidneys with ischemia and little urine output began producing more urine when the IAB was repositioned proximally from the renal artery position. This suggested that the injury was reversible once the occlusion was relieved and normal renal blood flow was restored.

In an effort to minimize hemolysis and to prevent aortic wall damage, it is recommended that the IAB occlude no more than 90% of the aorta. "Balloon sizing" is further discussed in Chapter 14.

PUMP CONSOLE AND COUNTERPULSATION

To ensure proper synchronization between counterpulsation and the patient's hemodynamics, complex console logic computer systems are in operation. Phasic balloon gas volume changes are effected by computer control systems. Timing logic, which is further discussed in Chapters 17 and 18, describes methods of synchronizing balloon counterpulsation. The ECG is usually used as a "trigger signal" from which the computer references systole and diastole.

IMPACT OF COUNTERPULSATION ON THE ARTERIAL PRESSURE WAVEFORM

Elevation of intraaortic pressure during diastole is termed *diastolic augmentation*. This action is reflected on the arterial pressure wave as an increase in diastolic pres-

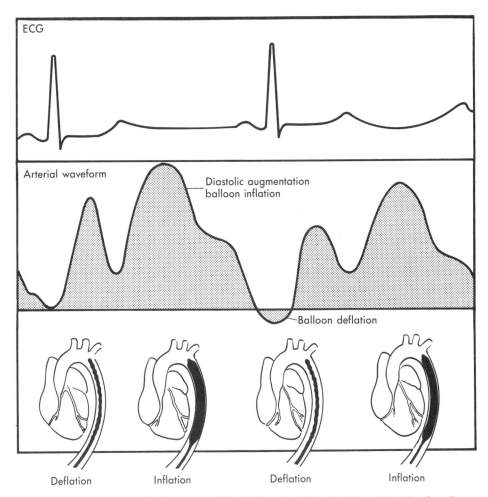

ECG

Arterial waveform

Diastolic augmentation
balloon inflation

Balloon deflation

Deflation   Inflation   Deflation   Inflation

Fig. 6-6. Two counterpulsation cycles. The balloon is inflated during diastole, thus "augmenting" diastolic pressure. Deflation occurs during isovolumetric contraction. Because balloon inflation displaced intraaortic balloon volume, aortic end-diastolic pressure is "lowered" during IAB deflation.

sure, which now becomes the highest pressure point of the arterial waveform. Two counterpulsation cycles are schematically depicted in Fig. 6-7. Console instrumentation allows the operator to adjust points of inflation-deflation manually within defined safety limits in an effort to maximize hemodynamic benefits to the patient. Although the ECG is used in triggering the pump, it is the arterial pressure waveform that must be used to "time" counterpulsation and assess its effect on the patient's hemodynamics.

REFERENCES

1. Chiles C, Vail CM, Coblerntz CL et al: Intra-aortic balloon pumps: an update on radiographic recognition, *Can Assoc Radiol J* 42:257, 1991.
2. McBride LR, Miller LW, Naunheim MD et al: Axillary artery insertion of an intraaortic balloon pump, *Ann Thorac Surg* 48:874, 1989.
3. Gueldner TL, Lawrence GH: Intra-aortic balloon assist through cannulation of the ascending aorta, *Ann Thorac Surg* 19:88, 1975.
4. Bonchek MD, Olinger G: Direct ascending aortic insertion of the "percutaneous" intra-aortic balloon catheter in the open chest: advantages and precautions, *Ann Thorac Surg* 32:512, 1981.
5. Kantrowitz A: Technique of femoral artery cannulation for phase-shift balloon pumping, *J Cardiovasc Surg* 86:219, 1968.
6. Bregman D: Percutaneous intra-aortic balloon pumping: a time for reflection, *Chest* 82:397, 1981.
7. Moulopoulos S, Topaz S, Kolff W: Diastolic balloon pumping (with carbon dioxide) in the aorta-A mechanical assistance to the failing circulation, *Am Heart J* 63:669, 1962.
8. Holinger WA: The intra-aortic balloon pump and other mechanical cardiac assist devices, *CVP* 9:19, 1981.
9. Rushmer RF: *Cardiovascular dynamics*, ed 4, Philadelphia, 1976, WB Saunders.
10. Tyson GS, Davis JW, Rankin JS: Improved performance of the intra-aortic balloon pump in man, *Surg Forum* 37:214, 1986.
11. Nichols AB: Left ventricular function during intra-aortic balloon pumping assessed by mitigated cardiac blood pool imagery, *Circulation* 58 (suppl I): Entire issue, 1978.
12. Swartz MT, Sakamoto T, Arai H et al: Effects of intraaortic balloon position on renal artery blood flow, *Ann Thorac Surg* 53:604, 1992.

CHAPTER 7

Interactive hemodynamics of IABC

Susan J. Quaal

Intraaortic balloon counterpulsation (IABC) acts as an auxiliary pump to the heart and will not provide adequate circulation in the absence of a significant contribution from the patient's own left ventricle.[1] Balloon inflation increases diastolic pressure and therefore potentially contributes to coronary, cerebral, and systemic circulation. Presystolic deflation lowers the impedance to systolic ejection and the next systolic pressure. Myocardial work and oxygen requirements are therefore reduced.[1]

The increase in cardiac output observed with IABC is between 0.5 and 1.0 L per min.[2] Freedman [1] states "This small increase in cardiac output also reminds us that the balloon pump best functions as an assisting circulatory support device."

EFFECTS OF IABC ON MYOCARDIAL OXYGEN SUPPLY AND DEMAND

The primary physiological impact of IABC is on myocardial oxygen supply/demand. Oxygen supply is determined by patency of the coronary arteries, autoregulation, diastolic perfusion gradient (aortic diastolic pressure minus left ventricular end diastolic pressure), and the diastolic pressure time index. Balloon counterpulsation's effect on improving oxygen supply is best appreciated by examining the diastolic pressure time index (DPTI) and tension time index (TTI)[2] (Fig. 7-1).

Adequacy of subendocardial perfusion can be predicted by calculating myocardial supply/demand ratio, defined as the ratio of DPTI divided by the systolic pressure TTI. DPTI describes pressure-time events during diastole and accurately estimates diastolic and subendocardial blood flow.[2] Myocardial oxygen demands are directly related to the area under the left ventricular systolic pressure curve, which is termed TTI. On-line monitoring of TTI and DPTI (myocardial oxygen supply/demand) ratios is useful as an indicator of adequate left ventricular subendocardial blood flow as impacted by IABC. Bedside monitor software advances now make such monitoring feasible.

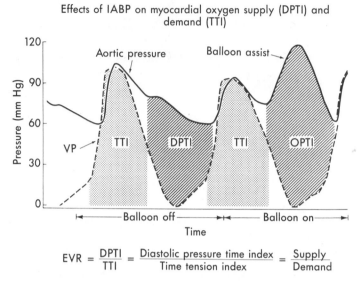

EVR $= \dfrac{\text{DPTI}}{\text{TTI}} = \dfrac{\text{Diastolic pressure time index}}{\text{Time tension index}} = \dfrac{\text{Supply}}{\text{Demand}}$

Fig. 7-1. Effects of IABC on myocardial oxygen supply (DPTI) and demand (TTI). The area beneath the systolic portion of the curve (TTI) represents myocardial oxygen consumption. The area beneath the diastolic pressure (DPTI) directly correlates with oxygen availability to the myocardium. Endocardial viability ratio (EVR) is calculated from diastolic pressure time index/tension time index. IABC lowers TTI and increases DPTI, thereby increasing EVR. (From Bolooki H: *Clinical application of intra-aortic balloon pump*, New York, 1984, Futura Publishing.)

The subendocardial layer receives most or all of its oxygen supply during diastole.[3] Intramyocardial compression during systole limits subendocardial blood flow to this area. As a response to myocardial ischemia, coronary vasodilatation occurs and subendocardial perfusion becomes pressure dependent.[3] Myocardial blood flow is regulated by forces affecting aortic diastolic pressure, left ventricular end-diastolic pressure, or diastolic duration. DPTI depends upon the pressure-time relationship of these factors and therefore can be used to estimate diastolic and subendocardial blood flow.[3]

Intraaortic balloon inflation increases DPTI and therefore myocardial oxygen delivery. In cases where balloon augmented diastolic pressure is not greater than patient's systolic pressure, DPTI may however still be increased. DPTI increases with IABC due to an increase in diastolic blood pressure and a decrease in end-diastolic pressure.

TTI decreases with balloon deflation due to a decrease in systolic blood pressure. DPTI to TTI therefore provides an accurate estimate of the adequacy of oxygen delivery to the myocardium, which is expressed as the endocardial viability ratio (EVR):

$$EVR = \frac{DPTI \text{ (oxygen supply)}}{TTI \text{ (oxygen demand)}}$$

An EVR of 1.0 signifies a normal supply/demand balance. It may demonstrate a positive response to IABC therapy on a beat-by-beat basis by indicating improvement in subendocardial perfusion. Phillips and associates introduced EVR in conjunction with IABC and cautioned "although EVR will reflect the increased blood flow occurring during augmentation, only a period of EVR observation without balloon support may assist in determining prognosis."[2]

Bolooki[4] states "With utilization of IABC, the DPTI/TTI ratio is increased mainly due to an increase in numerator and decrease in denominator. Although IABC in patients with an EVR of <0.7 postcardiac surgery has been demonstrated to improve survival, use of this index carries more of a theoretical advantage than a realistic one. This is especially true for patients in cardiogenic shock, where an improvement in this ratio does not guarantee patient survival. In certain situations, however, such as intraoperative failure, the EVR ratio can be used with greater confidence as a criterion for early utilization of IABC."

It must be understood that EVR does not reflect the beneficial effects of a reduction in ventricular volume achieved by IABC. Myocardial oxygen consumption is a function of force that is proportional to both pressure and volume. TTI only accounts for pressure. In accordance with this, if IABC produces a decrease in volume as well as pressure, then EVR will only reflect the decrease in pressure. As a consequence, the decrease in myocardial oxygen consumption will be underestimated.

IMPACT OF BALLOON INFLATION IN DIASTOLE ON CORONARY ARTERY PERFUSION

Coronary perfusion is potentially increased as the balloon inflates in diastole. Effective augmentation of coronary perfusion is, however, dependent on the degree of vasodilation within the coronary bed. Myocardial ischemia is a potent stimulus for increasing blood flow and oxygen delivery to the myocardium through vasodilation; coronary flow through vasodilated coronary arteries then becomes pressure dependent.[5] Autoregulatory vasodilation of coronary vessels is however impaired by atherosclerosis.

Balloon inflation displaces blood proximally, potentially increasing coronary perfusion. IABC thus can potentially improve coronary perfusion by increasing diastolic pressure and the diastolic perfusion gradient.[6] Coronary artery flow will increase in proportion to pressure increase.

Effect of IABC on coronary perfusion as studied in the animal model

Kern[7] summarized reports of experimental animal studies that assessed the impact of IABC on myocardial perfusion. Results were highly variable. In animals with normal systemic arterial pressure, intraaortic balloon counterpulsation reduced myocardial oxygen consumption without significantly changing total coronary flow. In ischemic animal preparations with low systemic arterial pressure, myocardial oxygen consumption became dependent on coronary flow. IABC had little effect on perfusion to myocardial regions supplied by occluded coronary vessels. In some experiments in which IABC increased perfusion, this small response was of limited functional significance.

Effect of IABC on coronary perfusion as studied in patients

In patients with severe coronary artery disease in which autoregulation is perceived to be absent, coronary flow is directly related to diastolic perfusion pressure. IABC should therefore theoretically improve coronary flow.[8] Gewirtz and associates at the University of Rhode Island[9] undertook a study to determine if IABC increased flow distal to a severe coronary stenosis. Heart rates were held constant with atrial pacing. In response to IABC, endomyocardial blood flow distal to the stenosis remained unchanged vs. control. Distal vessel mean diastolic pressure (beyond the stenosis) failed to increase with IABC.

McDonald and associates[10] found that IABC increased prestenotic but not poststenotic flow. They attributed clinical improvement associated with IABC to ventricular unloading and not to enhanced coronary perfusion. Folland,[11] however, contradicted this report. He employed IABC in patients with coronary artery disease and severe aortic valvular stenosis. IABC relieved angina in this population. These researchers concluded that because aortic stenosis was a fixed defect, negating any ventricular unloading produced by IABC, improvement in coronary flow must occur with IABC.

Collateral flow and IABC

From its position in the descending thoracic aorta, the intraaortic balloon (IAB) cannot be expected to increase blood flow through tightly stenosed or completely occluded vessels.[12] However, diastolic IAB inflation does increase blood flow through other more patent collateral vessels. Freedman[13] supported this premise by stating "Collateral circulation is a most important factor in patient outcome following myocardial infarction. Although the occluded artery is no longer able to supply oxygen and nutrients to a portion of the myocardium, resulting in cell death, the use of appropriate myoconservation techniques—and most notably the initiation of IABC to stimulate collateral circulation in the area surrounding this core of myocardial damage—can salvage many of the remaining viable cells."

Kern[14] delineated pathophysiologic mechanisms of collateral flow and rationale for IABC enhancement of collateral perfusion. He explained that collaterals act as passive conduits in which resistance depends upon mechanical factors. Enhanced collateral perfusion is dependent on a critical opening gradient for dormant closed vessels, which is achieved by IAB inflation.

IABC impact on coronary blood flow velocity

Kern also assessed intracoronary flow velocity during catheterization in 12 patients receiving IABC. Diastolic flow velocity-time integral (DFV_i) was computed from digitized waveforms. The greatest increase in DFV_i occurred in patients with a baseline systolic pressure ≤ 90 mm Hg. The researchers concluded that IABC unequivocally and significantly augments proximal coronary blood flow velocity by doubling the coronary flow velocity integral. This mechanism may be the predominant means of ischemia relief in hypotensive patients.[14]

AFTERLOAD REDUCTION

Static and dynamic work efforts are required for the myocardial transfer of energy from its metabolic substrate to the pressure developed in contraction (Fig. 7-2).

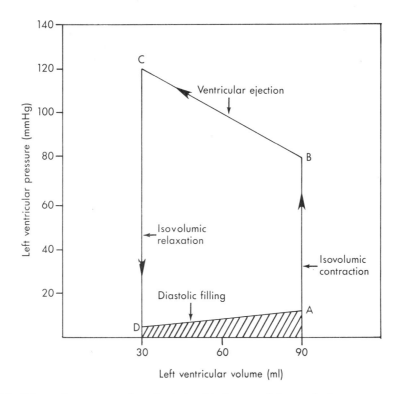

Fig. 7-2. Schematic representation of relationship between left ventricular pressure and volume during the cardiac cycle (see text for discussion).

During the isovolumic phase of ventricular contraction (**A** to **B**), pressure increases, but volume remains unchanged. Ventricular volume decreases rapidly during ventricular ejection (**B** to **C**), whereas the pressure continues to rise. Ventricular pressure falls rapidly after the aortic valve closes during isovolumic relaxation (**C** to **D**). Finally, ventricular volume rises during ventricular filling, with only a small increase in pressure (**D** to **A**).[15]

Static work refers to development and maintenance of ventricular pressure before opening of the aortic valve. *Dynamic work* occurs during ventricular ejection.[15] Little[16] described the static and dynamic work as analogous to pouring a pail of water over a fence. Static effort is constituted by lifting the pail of water to a height equal

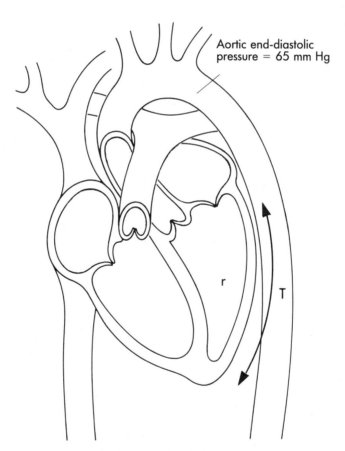

Fig. 7-3. Laplace's law: Myocardial tension (T) developed during isovolumetric contraction (static work) = ventricular radius (r) × aortic end-diastolic pressure.

to or slightly above the top of the fence. Additional energy (dynamic work) must be used to tip the pail so that water pours out of the pail and over the fence.

Laplace's law[16] further clarifies static work by delineating the relationship between ventricular tension, arterial pressure, and ventricular radius as follows (Fig. 7-3):

$$\text{ventricular tension} = \text{arterial pressure} \times \text{ventricular radius}$$

The amount of ventricular tension developed during static work is controlled by arterial pressure and ventricular radius. Ventricular hypertrophy and increased arterial pressure increase the amount of tension which must be developed during this static phase.

Intraaortic balloon deflation lowers the static component of myocardial work by reducing aortic pressure at the time of balloon deflation. Presystolic contraction produces a hypothetical void downstream from the contracting left ventricle. Thus aortic end-diastolic pressure is lowered. Applying Laplace's law (Fig. 7-4), lowering of aortic end-diastolic pressure during static work will decrease the amount of tension generated at the time the aortic valve opens. Myocardial oxygen consumption is therefore reduced.

Afterload reduction and hypotension

Akyurekli and associates[17] undertook a study to determine the systolic unloading effects of IABC, independent of diastolic augmentation. This was accomplished by counterpulsating dogs while their coronary arteries were perfused from an extracorporeal source. The perfusion pressure was lowered to produce acute cardiac failure. When IABC was instituted, systolic unloading (a reduction in left ventricular systolic pressure) was evident at normotensive states, but not in hypotensive states (coronary perfusion pressure $\leq$ 80 mm Hg).

These results suggest that balloon unloading responses may be intimately related to the functional status of the circulatory system before initiating IABC. At hypotensive states, aortic compliance increases which, as Akyurekli demonstrated, causes the aortic wall to expand with the IAB inflation, therefore blood volume displacement does not occur. If balloon inflation is not accompanied by aortic blood volume displacement, then at the time of deflation, aortic pressure will not be lowered. Static work and myocardial oxygen consumption will therefore not be lowered.[17]

IABC AND HETEROMETRIC-HOMEOMETRIC REGULATION

The terms *heterometric* and *homeometric* were coined by Sarnoff and associates.[18] *Heterometric* autoregulation refers to those adaptive mechanisms that involve changes in myocardial fiber length. *Homeometric* autoregulation refers to cardiac performance functions that are independent of changes in myocardial fiber length.

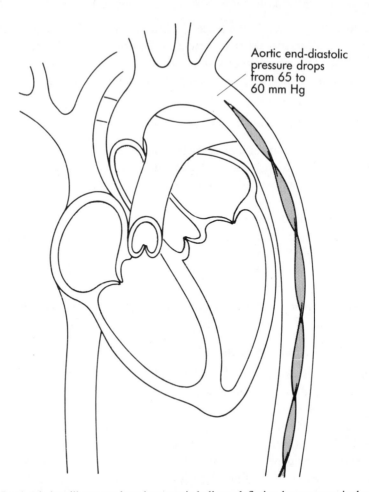

Aortic end-diastolic
pressure drops
from 65 to
60 mm Hg

Fig. 7-4. Laplace's law illustrates how intraaortic balloon deflation lowers ventricular tension. Intraaortic balloon inflation displaced stroke volume proximally and distally, which created a void in the aorta at the time of balloon deflation, thereby lowering aortic pressure. Since T = P × R, a reduction in aortic end-diastolic pressure provoked by balloon deflation lowers the amount of tension the left ventricle needs to generate to open the aortic valve.

Heterometric

Balloon deflation during isovolumetric contraction lowers aortic end-diastolic pressure. Heterometric performance is improved by decreasing the amount of static work required by the myocardium. The heart is therefore able to empty more completely and efficiently.[18]

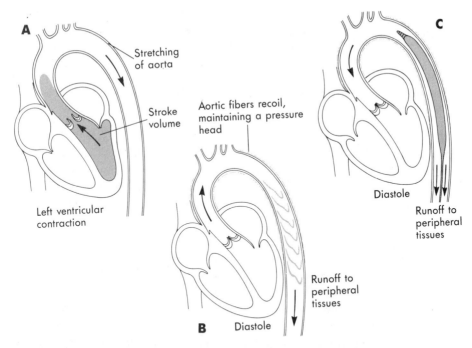

Fig. 7-5. The Windkessel effect. **A,** During systole, stroke volume is ejected and temporarily stored within the elastic aorta. This permits much of the force imparted to the blood by ventricular contraction to be stored as potential energy. **B,** During diastole, the stretched aortic fibers recoil, maintaining a pressure head, which causes a distal "run-off" of blood. **C,** Intraaortic balloon deflation during diastole enhances this intrinsic Windkessel effect.

Homeometric

An example of homeometric autoregulation occurs in response to increased afterload, termed the *Anrep effect*. As afterload increases, left ventricular diastolic pressure (LVDP) rises. Balloon deflation decreases afterload, lowering LVDP.[19]

IABC impacts another homeometric regulation by augmenting the intrinsic *Windkessel effect*, a term used to describe the temporary storage of stroke volume during the ejection period.[16] The elastic proximal aorta stretches to accommodate cardiac stroke volume in systole. This permits much of the force imparted to the blood by ventricular contraction to be stored as potential energy in the elastic arterial wall. When the heart relaxes and intravascular pressure falls, these stretched aortic fibers recoil, maintaining a pressure head. Runoff into the peripheral tissues continues in diastole under the pressure head created by energy released from the recoiling aorta. This effect serves to smooth out the flow of blood in the circulation so that flow continues during diastole. Without the Windkessel effect, blood would reach the tissues in spurts. Balloon inflation in diastole therefore augments this intrinsic Windkessel effect (Fig. 7-5).

IABC AND BARORECEPTOR RESPONSE

An inverse relationship exists between arterial blood pressure and heart rate, which was first described in 1859 by the French physician, Etienne Marey.[19] Baroreceptors are located in the aortic arch and carotid sinuses and are sensitive to stretch or distortion of vessel wall caused by increasing or decreasing systolic pressure. Baroreceptors are described as undifferentiated terminal nerve fibers, 5 μm in diameter, which branch extensively into adventitial and medial layers of the vessel wall.[16] Fibers from aortic baroreceptors articulate with the vagus nerve and end in the vasomotor area in the medulla (Fig. 7-5).

When blood pressure is gradually increased to high levels, cardiac sympathetic tone is completely suppressed after only a fraction of blood pressure elevation has been attained. Thereafter additional reduction in heart rate accompanying further increases in blood pressure is evoked entirely by an augmentation of vagal activity. The converse applies during a decrease in blood pressure. Vagal tone virtually disappears after the initial, relatively small drop in blood pressure. As pressure continues to decline, further acceleration in heart rate is ascribed solely to a progressive increase in sympathetic neural activity.[20]

As baroreceptors are stimulated by increased arterial pressure, a message is also sent to the medullary vasoconstrictor center, which inhibits peripheral vasoconstrictor activity. Total peripheral resistance is therefore reduced.[21]

Intraaortic balloon inflation elevates diastolic pressure, which stretches the baroreceptors. Heart rate is therefore lowered and systemic vascular resistance decreases with IAB inflation due to the baroreceptor response (Fig. 7-6).

PRELOAD AND HEART RATE RESPONSE

As the right atrial wall is stretched with increased preload, heart rate increases by 20% to 30%. By allowing the heart to empty more efficiently, IABC decreases right atrial preload and therefore lowers heart rate.[18]

IABC AND CHEMORECEPTOR RESPONSE

Chemoreceptors are located within the aortic arch and carotid body. They are stimulated by reduction in arterial oxygen concentration, elevation of carbon dioxide tension, and elevation in hydrogen ion concentration. Activation of the chemoreceptor invokes a reflexive sympathetic response and an increase in heart rate.[18] IABC,

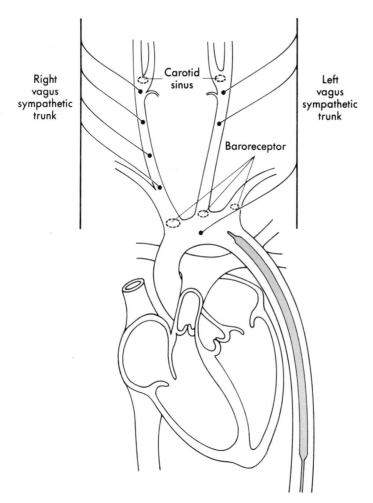

Fig. 7-6. Balloon inflation raises aortic pressure and stimulates the baroreceptors located in the aortic arch and carotid sinuses. Heart rate slows in response to baroreceptor stimulation.

by improving myocardial contractility, improves oxygen delivery proximally to the aortic arch and therefore may potentially decrease the chemoreceptor activated sympathetic response. This, however, is doubtful.

IABC AND POISEUILLE'S LAW

According to Poiseuille's law,[16]

$$Q = \frac{\pi(P_i - P_o)r^4}{8 \eta l}$$

four factors determine peripheral blood flow: pressure, resistance, length, and viscosity. A pressure difference or gradient must exist between two points for blood to flow between these two points. Blood flows from the arterial to the venous end in response to a pressure gradient.[20] The mean arterial pressure, or average driving pressure at the arterial end of the circulation, is approximately 100 mm Hg. Capillary pressure averages 25 mm Hg. Pressure at the venous end (right atrium) is 4 to 7 mm Hg. Therefore pressure progressively declines between the arterial and venous ends of the systemic circulation. The gradient is approximately 100 mm Hg.

In hypotension the gradient obviously decreases. Balloon inflation during diastole increases the arterial pressure, which increases the arterial-venous pressure gradient and thus improves flow.

Resistance is primarily determined by the radius of the blood vessel. Poiseuille's law demonstrates that resistance is inversely proportional to the fourth power of the blood vessel's radius. Reduction of the radius by one-half will increase flow resistance by sixteenfold.

Balloon inflation in diastole displaces stroke volume directly toward aortic baroreceptors, which respond by sending a message through the vagus to inhibit the medullary vasoconstrictor reflex. Peripheral resistance decreases, which, as demonstrated by Poiseuille's law, improves blood flow.

Blood viscosity and vascular length also alter resistance to flow. However, since these properties are relatively constant, their influence is normally insignificant.

LACTATE PRODUCTION

Bolooki[4] summarized the impact of IABC on lactate production as follows: "Normal myocardium utilizes glucose and breaks down lactate produced by glycolysis to pyruvate. In the normal heart at rest, there is zero lactate production in the coronary sinus blood. Once myocardial hypoxia occurs, due to either a decrease in the coronary blood supply or an unexpected increase in demand, there is a decrease in aerobic glycolysis. As a result, anaerobic metabolism will ensue causing production of lactate; this can be measured in the coronary sinus blood effluent by a positive ratio of lactate conversion to pyruvate. Decrease in lactate extraction observed in patients with myocardial ischemia or low output syndrome is usually reversed to lactate utilization when balloon assist is employed successfully. This is because of a return to aerobic myocardial metabolism due to an increase in coronary perfusion pressure and flow. IABC may not readily correct acidosis, leading to a state of irreversible failure or balloon dependence."

EFFECT OF IABC ON RENAL FUNCTION

The impact of IABC on renal blood flow has been studied in dog models.[22] Following 1 week of canine balloon counterpulsation in animals with mild to moderate failure, renal blood increased 9% to 25%. No change in serum creatinine level was observed. Postoperative improvement in human renal perfusion has also been demonstrated in humans.[23]

Effect of IAB position on renal artery flow

Recently, researchers at St. Louis University studied the effect of renal blood flow when the IAB was positioned adjacent to the renal arteries.[24] Balloon position was randomized so that it was initially placed in either control (thoracic) or experimental (at the level of the renal arteries) position. IABC was performed for 4 hours in each position. Of the 14 dogs studied, 57% had at least partial occlusion of one renal artery, with a 23% to 98% decrease in flow (mean decrease 66%) while the IAB was in the renal position.

Significance of decreased urine output

When urine output decreases after commencing IABC, the following two anatomical factors should always be considered: (1) aortic dissection and (2) juxtarenal balloon position. Persistent low cardiac output after initiating IABC is, however, the most likely cause of renal failure not attributable to iatrogenic causes.

MAGNITUDE AND DURATION OF AUGMENTATION OF DIASTOLIC PRESSURE WITH BALLOON INFLATION

Nearly 20 years ago Weber and Janicki[25] published a framework of physical and biological variables that influenced magnitude and duration of diastolic pressure augmentation during balloon inflation (see the box on p. 114). This original framework is still highly respected as a clinical reference.[26]

Physical factors

Balloon position. The closer the balloon is to the aortic valve, the greater the diastolic pressure elevation. However, positioning the balloon at the aortic root would

---

VARIABLES IMPACTING INTRAAORTIC BALLOON MAGNITUDE AND DURATION OF INFLATION

Physical (IAB)

Position
Volume
Diameter
Occlusivity
Configuration
Driving gas
Timing

Biological

Arterial pressure
Heart rate
Aortic pressure-volume relation

(From Weber KT, Janicki MS: Ann Thorac Surg 17:606, 1974.)

compromise flow to the trifurcated vessels arising from the arch at the time of balloon inflation and would pose a risk for cerebral aneurysm. Therefore the balloon is positioned distal to the aortic root, just below the bifurcation of the left subclavian artery (Fig. 7-4). If the balloon is positioned too "low," diastolic augmentation will be reduced as inflation momentum is decreased.[26]

Balloon volume. Diastolic augmentation is maximized when stroke volume is equal to balloon volume.[26] However, the volume of gas entering the balloon is usually less than the actual pump volume setting, possibly due to compressibility of gaseous material.[4] If stroke volume is <25 cc, little diastolic augmentation can be expected. On the contrary a stroke volume ≥ 100 cc is much greater than the inflated balloon's volume displacement capabilities; augmentation will therefore decrease.[26] Theoretically, if IABC is initiated in a patient with a stroke volume of 25 cc, which increases to 90 cc over a course of several days, diastolic augmentation could increase, then decrease, as stroke volume improves.

Systemic vascular resistance. As systemic vascular resistance (SVR) increases, diastolic augmentation may decrease because of the associated decrease in compliance. If the arterial system is theoretically likened to a stiff pipe with an increase in SVR, blood will be ejected out to the systemic circulation during ejection before balloon inflation. Absence of stroke volume available for displacement during balloon inflation obviously will decrease diastolic augmentation.

Balloon diameter and occlusivity. Weber, Janicki, and Walker assessed the influence of IAB diameter and occlusivity on hemodynamics.[27] Occlusivity was determined from simultaneous measurement of aortic root and abdominal aorta diastolic pressures and pressure-volume-diameter relation of a distensible IAB. For any arterial pressure or aorta size, the greatest augmentation in mean arterial diastolic pressure was observed with complete occlusion. Because of the potential aortic wall and red cell destruction at 100% occlusion, the estimated optimum occlusivity was judged to be about 90% to 95%.

Weikel et al.[28] studied aortograms from 169 patients at the Massachusetts General Hospital and found that patients' midthoracic aortic diameter, from the takeoff of the left subclavian artery to the renal artery origin, ranged from 16 to 30 mm. This factor was used in designing adult balloons.

Customizing balloon volume to appropriately occlude any given aortic state of compliance is clinically effective (refer to Chapter 14). Kantrowitz and associates[29] stated that "The significance of aortic elasticity in the patient is illustrated by the fact that aortic volume doubles between a shock mean of 30 to 40 mm Hg and a normal mean pressure of 90 to 100 mm Hg. The balloon is limited by the volume of blood contained within the aorta just before inflation. . . . further increases in pumping volume result only in distention of the aorta and not in the effective pumping of blood."

IAB configuration. Balloon shape can also affect diastolic augmentation. Studies conducted in vitro, as well as theoretical considerations, led to considerable concern about cylindrical or sausage-shaped balloons being susceptible to development of lateral wall pressure. This phenomenon was termed *bubble blowing* (see Chapter 14). In normal or high pressure, the balloon occupies most of the space within the descending thoracic aorta. At low pressure, aortic diameter decreases and a cylindrically shaped balloon develops significant lateral wall pressure, which causes the two ends of the balloon to inflate first, effectively trapping blood in the middle. This results in lower augmentation. To minimize this problem, trisegmented and dual chambered balloons were developed. Percutaneous insertion techniques requiring tightly wrapped balloons have now precluded use of these multichambered devices.

Bleifeld and associates,[30] however, questioned the occurrence of such a phenomenon in vivo, except when the IAB diameter substantially exceeds that of the aorta.

Driving gas. Carbon dioxide and helium have both been used as driving gases. Helium is currently the driving gas of choice because of its low molecular weight and therefore efficiency in balloon inflation and deflation. This is particularly advantageous during tachyarrhythmias.

Timing. Early balloon inflation prematurely terminates systole and ventricular ejection. Stroke volume available for diastolic displacement at the time of balloon inflation is therefore decreased, which limits the amount of diastolic augmentation.

Late balloon inflation allows stroke volume to run off into the periphery before inflation, again limiting stroke volume available for displacement concomitant with inflation. Diastolic augmentation is decreased. Likewise, early deflation will also decrease augmentation.

Duration of inflation is governed by heart rate. The greater the heart rate, the less the inflation duration. Elevated heart rates, by virtue of limiting duration of balloon inflation, also decrease the amount of diastolic augmentation.[26]

REFERENCES

1. Freedman RJ: The intra-aortic balloon pump system: current roles and future directions, *J Appl Cardiol* 6:313, 1991.
2. Phillips PA, Marty AT, Miyamoto AM: A clinical method for detecting subendocardial ischemia following cardiopulmonary bypass, *J Thorac Cardiovasc Surg* 69:30, 1975.
3. Alcan KE, Stertzezr SH, Wallsh E et al: Current status of intra-aortic balloon counterpulsation in critical care cardiology, *Crit Care Med* 12:489, 1984.
4. Bolooki H: *Clinical application of intra-aortic balloon pump,* 2 ed, New York, 1984, Futura Publishing.
5. Braunwald E, Sonnenblick EH, Ross J: Mechanisms of cardiac contraction and relaxation (chap 13). In Braunwald E: *Heart disease: a textbook of cardiovascular medicine,* ed 4, Philadelphia, 1992, WB Saunders.
6. Port SC, Patel S, Schmidt DH: Effects of intraaortic balloon counterpulsation on myocardial blood flow in patients with severe coronary artery disease, *J Am Coll Cardiol* 3:367, 1984.
7. Kern MJ: Intra-aortic balloon counterpulsation, *Coronary Artery Disease* 2:649, 1991.
8. Williams DO, Korr KS, Gewirtz H et al: The effect of intraaortic balloon counterpulsation on regional myocardial blood flow and oxygen consumption in the presence of coronary artery stenosis in patients with unstable angina, *Circulation* 66:593, 1982.
9. Gewirtz H, Ohley WH, Williams DO et al: Effect of intra-aortic balloon pumping on myocardial blood flow distal to a severe coronary artery stenosis, *Am J Cardiol* 49:969, 1982 (abstract).
10. MacDonald RF, Hill JA, Feldman RL: Failure of intra-aortic balloon counterpulsation to augment distal coronary perfusion pressure during percutaneous transluminal coronary angioplasty, *Am J Cardiol* 59:320, 1985.
11. Folland ED, Kemper AJ, Khuri SF et al: Intra-aortic balloon counterpulsation as a temporary support measure in decompensated critical aortic stenosis, *J Am Coll Cardiol* 5:711, 1987.
12. Fuchs R: Augmentation of regional coronary blood flow by intra-aortic balloon counterpulsation in patients with unstable angina, *Circulation* 68:117, 1983.
13. Freedman RF: Myoconservation in cardiogenic shock: use of intra-aortic balloon pumping and other treatment modalities, *Cardiac Assists* 6:1, 1992.
14. Kern MJ, Aguirre F, Penick D et al: Enhanced intracoronary flow velocity during intra-aortic balloon counterpulsation in patients with coronary artery disease, *Circulation* 84 (suppl II): II-485, 1991 (abstract).
15. Quaal SJ: The person with heart failure and cardiogenic shock (chap 11). In Guzzetta CE, Dossey BM: *Cardiovascular nursing holistic practice,* St. Louis, 1992, Mosby–Year Book.
16. Little RC: *Physiology of the heart and circulation,* ed 2, Chicago, 1989, Mosby–Year Book.
17. Akyurekli MD: Effectiveness of intra-aortic balloon counterpulsation on systolic unloading, *Can J Surg* 23:122, 1980.
18. Sarnoff SJ, Mitchell JH, Gilmroe JP et al: Homeometric autoregulation in the heart, *Circ Res* 8:1077, 1960.
19. Berne RM, Levy MN: *Cardiovascular physiology,* ed 6, (chap 8), St. Louis, 1992, Mosby–Year Book.
20. Hand HL: Direct or indirect blood pressure measurement for open heart surgery patients: an algorithm, *Crit Care Nurse* 12:52, 1992.
21. Schlant RC, Sonnenblick EH: Pathophysiology of heart failure (chap 26). In Hurst JW, Schlant RC: *The heart,* ed 7, New York, 1990, McGraw-Hill.
22. Kondratovitch MA, Ursulinko VI: The effect of intra-aortic balloon counterpulsation on regional circulation, *Kardiologiia* 19:122, 1978.
23. Hilberman M: Effect of the intra-aortic balloon pump upon postoperative renal function in man, *Crit Care Med* 9:85, 1981.
24. Swartz MT, Sakamoto T, Arai H et al: Effects of intraaortic balloon position on renal artery blood flow, *Ann Thorac Surg* 53:604, 1992.
25. Weber KT, Janicki JS: Intra-aortic balloon counterpulsation, *Ann Thorac Surg* 17:602, 1974.
26. Hanlon P: *Counterpulsation and analysis of the assisted arterial waveform,* AACN's National Teaching Institute Pre-NTI Conference Syllabus, Boston, 1991.

27. Weber KT, Janicki JS, Walker AA: The influence of balloon volume and diameter on optimal intraaortic balloon assist, *Trans Am Soc Artif Intern Organs* 2:71, 1973 (abstract).
28. Weikel AM, Jones RT, Dinsmore R et al: Size limits and pumping effectiveness of intra-aortic balloons, *Ann Thorac Surg* 12:45, 1971.
29. Kantrowitz A: *Cardiac assistance by the intra-aortic balloon pump*, 2nd Medical Physics Conference, Boston, 1969.
30. Bleifeld W, Meyer-Hartwig K, Irnich W et al: Dynamics of balloons in intraaortic counterpulsation, *Am J Roentgenol Rad Ther Nucl Med* 116:155, 1972.

CHAPTER 8

Indications

Susan J. Quaal

Percutaneous and sheathless insertion techniques as well as very user friendly instrumentation have made intraaortic balloon counterpulsation (IABC) relatively easy and quick to initiate. These advances have made balloon pumping readily accessible to the patient experiencing acute myocardial infarction, cardiogenic shock, and mechanical complications following infarction, in conjunction with percutaneous transluminal coronary angioplasty (PTCA), thrombolytic therapy, in support of the patient undergoing cardiac catheterization, as a bridge to cardiac transplantation, and to support the myocardium pre, intra, and/or postoperatively. The clinical benefits of IABC following acute myocardial infarction and its value as a circulatory assist modality in the treatment of cardiogenic shock are beyond question.[1-5] Singh and associates[6] suggested criteria for which IABC would be most successful: (1) moderately preserved left ventricular function and good opacification of the distal coronary arteries on angiography; and (2) significant mechanical lesions such as mitral insufficiency and ventricular septal defect (VSD). Patients with a large previous myocardial infarction, previous episodes of left ventricular failure, or marked cardiac enlargement are least likely to benefit; weaning and balloon dependency are higher in this patient population.

Miller[7] found that despite a series of published reports on clinical IABC experience, a survey of the literature reveals a significant lack of "hands-on" discussion of balloon insertion, reasons for patient selection, and results. Miller therefore summarized the experience at St. Louis University with a series of 50 consecutive IABC patients and follow-up ranging from 25 to 52 months. Refractory angina and/or refractory pump failure were the only selection criteria. Patients ranged in age from 25 to 76 (mean age 60.6). Of the group, 74% were male.

Indications for balloon insertion are listed in Table 8-1. Of the IABC patients reviewed, 66% underwent IABC secondary to myocardial infarction (MI). Of these MI patients, 17 experienced refractory angina; heart failure and mechanical complications were each present in 8 patients. Unstable angina with no evidence of infarction occurred in 28%; 4% had cardiomyopathy and 2% had acute mitral valve rup-

Table 8-1.   Indications for IAB insertion (St. Louis University experience)

Indication	N
Unstable angina without infarction	14 (28%)
Acute myocardial infarction	33 (66%)
Angina	17
Congestive heart failure	8
Mechanical complication	8
Cardiomyopathy	2 (4%)
Acute mitral valve failure	1 (2%)

From Miller LW: Emerging trends in the treatment of acute myocardial infarction and the role of intraaortic balloon pumping, *Cardiac Assists* 3:1, 1986.

Table 8-2.   Results of IABC (St. Louis University experience)

Outcome	N
Relief of chest pain	29/31 (93.5%)
Improved hemodynamics	46/50 (92.0%)
Patient deaths	19/50 (38.0%)
Acute myocardial infarction	13/33 (39.4%)
Unstable angina	0/4 (0%)
Cardiomyopathy	2/2 (100.0%)

From Miller LW: Emerging trends in the treatment of acute myocardial infarction and the role of intraaortic balloon pumping, *Cardiac Assists* 3:1, 1986.

ture. Table 8-2 delineates outcomes from IABC. Chest pain was totally relieved in 29 of 31 patients (94%), with improved hemodynamics in 46 of 50 patients (92%). Nineteen patients (38%) died, including 13 of 33 (40%) of those admitted for acute MI and both patients with cardiomyopathy. None of the patients who had unstable angina without evidence of MI died.[7]

All patients who survived beyond 24 hours underwent cardiac catheterization. Two-thirds of the population studied underwent coronary artery bypass surgery alone or in conjunction with valve replacement or aneurysmectomy.[7]

Fifteen patients did not undergo surgical intervention. Six patients had single vessel disease (usually occlusion of the left anterior descending coronary artery) or inoperable anatomy ($n = 4$). Seven patients who experienced myocardial pump failure and cardiogenic shock, but without mechanical complications or surgically correctable coronary artery lesions, remained on IABC for 7 to 10 days before being weaned. Two patients died waiting for surgery after IABC was initiated.[7]

Intraaortic balloon counterpulsation continued for an average of 3.3 days. Of the patients who underwent IABC, 24% required it for less than 2 days; 50% for 2 to 5 days; 18% for 5 to 10 days, and 8% for more than 10 days.[7]

Miller nicely summarized his clinical IABC experience and justification for use as follows:

The results of our clinical experience suggest that more aggressive use of IABC is likely to save the lives of coronary disease patients who develop severe complications of their disease. There have been no deaths among our patients with refractory unstable angina who had a balloon inserted and all the evidence suggests that, short of actually opening vessels to obtain relief from angina, IABC is likely to be the most effective method to treat these patients. Logistical considerations represent a significant advantage for IABC, compared with other available procedures. Both IABC and percutaneous angioplasty, for example, can be accomplished in 10-15 minutes. In emergency situations, however, where every minute is crucial, IABC is often the procedure of choice because of the time required to assemble technicians and prepare the cardiac catheterization laboratory for angioplasty. The comparative advantages of IABC are even more obvious when the hospital has no catheterization laboratory and transportation to another hospital would potentially represent a significant risk to an already unstable patient.

Continuous IABC is of great value in patients with severe coronary disease, who demonstrate rapid clinical deterioration if counterpulsation is discontinued even briefly (or develop significant arrhythmias). We have found IABC to be very effective in dealing with refractory chest pain and ischemia-related pump failure and mechanical complications (VSD, mitral insufficiency) before, during and after myocardial infarction. For these patients, we recommend initiation of IABC and cardiac catheterization, followed by a definitive surgical procedure.[7]

MYOCARDIAL INFARCTION

O'Rourke and associates[8] evaluated the effect of IABC on postmyocardial infarction (MI) pump failure. Thirty patients received IABC postinfarction. Average delay from onset of ischemic pain to initiation of IABC was 7.1 hours. Ischemic pain had subsided by the time IABC commenced. No benefit was apparent in this sample. The researchers concluded that IABC was initiated too late; myocardial damage was irreversible.

O'Rourke and associates[8] suggested that IABC was often initiated so late after an acute infarction that myocardial ischemic damage had become irreversible. These researchers tested the effects of IABC on 26 patients who experienced refractory heart failure without shock, as a complication of acute MI. One group ($n = 12$) experienced continuing myocardial ischemia, evidenced by anginal pain and S-T segment elevation. Ischemia was not persistent in the second group ($n = 14$). Though all patients demonstrated hemodynamic improvement with initiation of IABC, those with sustained ischemia (Group I) exhibited more pronounced hemodynamic improvement, reflected by pulmonary artery pressure and heart rate. Effect on ischemia was impressive; pain was abolished within minutes for 11 patients and within 12 hours for one patient. Only one hospital death attributed to low cardiac output failure occurred in Group I, 27 days after termination of IABC. Of the 14 patients in Group II, 8 died in the hospital—3 from ventricular fibrillation and 5 from heart failure.

DeWood and associates[9] compared 40 patients who were treated with IABC for cardiogenic shock following MI. Group I was treated with IABC and Group II with IABC and coronary artery bypass grafting. In-hospital mortality between Groups I and II was 71.4% vs. 47.3%. The subset of Group II that underwent reperfusion and counterpulsation within 16 hours from the onset of symptoms had a lower mortality (25.0%) than the subset that underwent surgery more than 18 hours after the onset of symptoms (71.4%).

Withdrawal of medications before removal of IABC

The St. Louis University group recommends gradually withdrawing medications (except heparin) before IAB removal. "Reinstitution of drug therapy is much easier than replacing the balloon. Withdrawal of all inotropic drugs is not always practical, of course, but it appears best to limit the dosage as much as possible before balloon removal. Since our experience suggests that patients tolerate IAB for up to 14 days without any problems, there is usually no urgency about tapering drug dosage."[7]

UNSTABLE ANGINA

Recognition and treatment of accelerating angina with threatened infarction is another proven indication for IABC.[10] By improving coronary blood flow and reducing left ventricular work, chest pain and ST-segment elevations may be ameliorated.[11] Mundth[12] reported on 24 patients who experienced accelerating chest pain and ST-T wave abnormalities. IABC abolished the pain and normalized the ECG changes in 20 patients.

In another study,[13] 25 patients with accelerating angina were treated with combined IABC and bypass grafting. Of 25 patients who were treated with the combined technique, 22 made a complete recovery. Three patients sustained definitive MI and one patient expired. Of five patients who underwent bypass grafting without supportive IABC, all suffered intraoperative infarction; three expired.

Some patients continue to experience severe angina following MI, despite aggressive medical therapy. Bardet's group in France[14] studied the effects of IABC combined with revascularization surgery in 21 patients whose chest pain reappeared after a pain-free interval of more than 24 hours, but less than 15 days following the initial episode and accentuation or reappearance of ST-T wave abnormalities. These patients underwent a period of stabilization with balloon pumping, followed by coronary angiography. Of these, 15 patients achieved a totally pain-free status following revascularization when balloon pumping was used to stabilize them at the time of recurrence of angina following MI. Such success depends upon whether the coronary lesions are amenable to surgery.

MYOCONSERVATION

Freedman[15] comprehensively summarized the concept of *myoconservation*, which he described as "a particularly useful concept, to describe the combined treatment measures designed to provide hemodynamic support within the crucial window of opportunity, ensuring that sufficient myocardium will remain viable to permit resumption of normal functioning following definitive coronary artery therapy. One of the treatment modalities that has proven most effective in accomplishing this objective is intraaortic balloon counterpulsation. The unique physiological balance of benefits of IABC include support of the coronary circulation, support of the systemic circulation, reduction in left ventricular stress, and reduction in cardiac workload." The following vignette on balloon counterpulsation and myoconservation is paraphrased (with permission) from Freedman's account.

Initiation of mechanical counterpulsation support promptly following myocardial infarction can play a major role in helping to maintain blood flow and preserving the patient's organ systems and a significant proportion of the damaged myocardium. As confirmed by many investigative groups, mechanical counterpulsation, combined with appropriate medical therapy and followed by definite corrective treatment to eliminate the cause of ischemia, can dramatically reduce mortality among these critically ill patients.

One study compared the results of survival in cardiogenic shock patients treated according to varying protocols. Investigators found that when IABC was initiated within 24 hours of the development of symptoms of cardiac failure, patient survival reached 80%. By comparison, the survival rate for those patients who were treated medically and did not receive hemodynamic support with IABC until more than 24 hours after appearance of the symptoms of heart failure (HF) was only 20%.[16]

Early intervention during a "therapeutic window of opportunity" is therefore critical to reduce myocardial oxygen demands, followed by those additional steps necessary to correct the underlying pathological condition before ischemia leads to massive cell death and permanent loss of function in large areas of myocardium.

The necessity for immediate initiation of treatment for acute myocardial ischemia is further supported by studies relating to ischemia-induced myocardial "stunning".[17] This phenomenon occurs when the myocardium has not yet suffered irreversible damage, but remains acutely unable to function. In this situation, scarring may occur in only a portion of the myocardium, while much of the heart muscle may retain the potential to return to functional status. However, this circumstance requires restoration of sufficient coronary circulation and support to the ventricular myocardium until more definitive corrective treatment can be accomplished. Again, prompt action is essential because survival of the patient requires that at least 60% of the left ventricular myocardium retain the ability to function.

Myoconservation, the use of mechanical and/or pharmacological means to preserve jeopardized myocardium from irreparable ischemic damage, is therefore most important. Restoration of arterial patency is an essential step in patient survival. However, the affected vessel must be able to provide adequate circulation to, and perfusion of, potentially viable myocardium. Intraaortic balloon counterpulsation has been most effective in accomplishing this goal.

From its position in the descending thoracic aorta (proximal tip below the left subclavian artery branch), the IAB cannot be expected to stimulate increased blood flow through vessels that are tightly stenosed or completely occluded. However, diastolic inflation of the balloon increases blood flow through other more patent coronary arteries.[18]

Collateral circulation is an important factor in patient outcome following myocardial infarction. Although the occluded artery is no longer able to supply oxygen and nutrients to a portion of the myocardium, resulting in cell death, the use of IABC as a myoconservation technique to stimulate collateral circulation in the area surrounding this core of myocardial damage can salvage many of the remaining viable cells.

VENTRICULAR IRRITABILITY

Researchers at Massachusetts General Hospital undertook a study of 22 patients with medically refractory ventricular irritability after myocardial infarction. These patients underwent IABC in an attempt to control ventricular irritability, which improved in 19 of the 22 patients and totally resolved in 12 patients.[19]

ACUTE MITRAL REGURGITATION AND VENTRICULAR SEPTAL DEFECT

Acute mitral regurgitation (MR) (Fig. 8-1) from papillary muscle rupture caused by a myocardial infarction may lead to rapid clinical deterioration with pulmonary

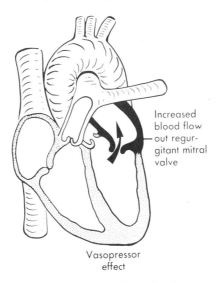

Increased blood flow out regurgitant mitral valve

Vasopressor effect

Fig. 8-1. Mitral regurgitation following myocardial infarction as a result of papillary muscle rupture. Infusion of a vasopressor agent may actually increase afterload, which causes more left ventricular stroke volume to flow out the regurgitant mitral valve lesser resistant pathway.

edema, hypotension, and death. Vasopressor agents that increase afterload and resistance to left ventricular ejection can aggravate mitral regurgitation.[20] Vasoconstriction occurs with infusion of vasopressor agents, thereby directing more of the stroke volume out the lesser resistant regurgitant mitral valve pathway, rather than through the aortic valve into the systemic circulation.

A ventricular septal defect (VSD) may arise following an anterior septal myocardial infarction if wound healing has failed to transform the infarct into a stable scar. Necrotic septal tissue may actually rupture, creating a hole between the right and left ventricles.[21] Pulmonary artery oxygen saturation is unusually high compared with the systemic arterial sample, as oxygenated blood from the left ventricle is shunted to the right ventricle through the VSD.[22] Infusion of an agent that strengthens contraction, such as an inotropic agent, may increase systemic output. However, a concomitant increase in left-to-right shunting also occurs, with a resultant increase in left ventricular work (Fig. 8-2).

Gold and associates[10] utilized IABC in patients who deteriorated into cardiogenic shock following sudden onset of MR or VSD postmyocardial infarction. Although IABC produced clinical and hemodynamic improvement in all patients, a completely satisfactory correction of the impaired circulatory dynamics could not be obtained.

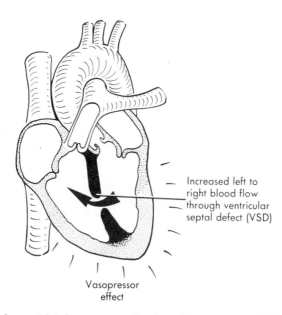

Increased left to right blood flow through ventricular septal defect (VSD)

Vasopressor effect

Fig. 8-2. Ventricular septal defect as a complication of acute myocardial infarction. Oxygenated blood is shunted from the left ventricle through the septal defect. Left ventricular stroke volume is decreased. Infusion of inotropic agents increases the force of left ventricular contraction and increases this left-to-right shunt.

The peak improvement occurred within the first 24 hours of IABC. In no patient did prolonged IABC produce further hemodynamic benefits. Intraaortic balloon counterpulsation did afford a sufficient level of hemodynamic stability to permit left ventricular cineangiography in these critically ill patients. Reduction of afterload, achieved by IABC, lowers the impedance to left ventricular ejection. Stroke volume is thereafter more easily ejected out the aorta, rather than through the regurgitant mitral valve (Fig. 8-3) or VSD (Fig. 8-4).

The effect of IABC was studied in dogs with iatrogenically induced MR and VSD.[23] Hemodynamic changes observed after creating a VSD included (1) mean arterial pressure decrease (29%); (2) left ventricular systolic pressure decrease (20%); (3) cardiac output decrease (46%); (4) right ventricular pressure increase (13%); and (5) pulmonary artery pressure increase (11%). Initiation of IABC produced a 7% increase in mean aortic pressure, a 13% increase in cardiac output, a 10% decrease in right ventricular pressure, and a 7% decrease in pulmonary artery pressure.

Hemodynamic deterioration after iatrogenic creation of MR included (1) decrease in mean arterial pressure (35%); (2) decrease in left ventricular pressure (36%); (3) decrease in cardiac output (36%); (4) increase in left atrial pressure (30%); and (5) increase in pulmonary artery wedge pressure (50%). Initiation of balloon counterpulsation produced increases of 9% in mean aortic pressure and 18% in cardiac output. Left ventricular pressure decreased by 7%, left atrial pressure decreased by 13%, and pulmonary artery pressure decreased by 9%.

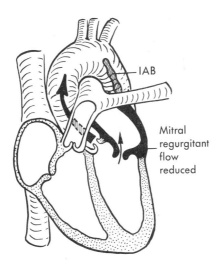

Fig. 8-3. IABC effect on acute mitral regurgitation. Balloon deflation reduces aortic end-diastolic pressure, thereby reducing afterload, which improves forward stroke volume flow.

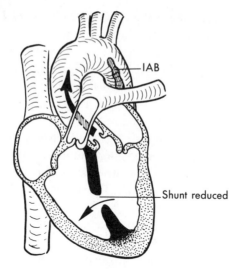

Fig. 8-4. IABC effect on an acute ventricular septal defect. Balloon deflation reduces aortic end-diastolic pressure, which lowers the amount of left-to-right shunting. A greater amount of stroke volume is directed forward, out the aortic valve.

This study suggested that IABC was effective in improving hemodynamics for both VSD and MR following acute myocardial infarction, unless the mean left atrial pressure was greater than 30 mm Hg.[23]

THROMBOLYSIS AND IABC

Use of IABC in conjunction with thrombolytic therapy has demonstrated its effectiveness and safety. Potential benefits are listed in the box below. Nearly 15% of

---

POTENTIAL BENEFITS OF IABC IN REPERFUSION THERAPY

1. Increased flow
   (Diastolic augmentation)
   Decreased thrombus formation
   Mechanical effect on intimal dissection
2. Improved collateral perfusion
3. Reduced afterload
4. Support of the "stunned myocardium"

Modified from Califf RM, Ohman EM: Reocclusion after thrombolytic therapy and percutaneous transluminal coronary angioplasty, *Cardiac Assists* 5:1, 1990.

Table 8-3.   Bleeding complications in thrombolytic therapy patients with and without concomitant IABC

Location of bleed	IABC ($n = 95$)	No IABC ($n = 612$)
Retroperitoneal	1/94 (1.1%)	8/612 (1.8%)
Intracranial	0/93 (0%)	5/612 (0.8%)
Groin	48/94 (51.1%)	292/612 (47.7%)
GI	20/94 (21.3%)	71/612 (11.6%)

Modified from George BS: Thrombolysis and intraaortic balloon counterpulsation following acute myocardial infarction. Experience in four TAMI studies, *Cardiac Assists* 4:1, 1988.

TABLE 8-4.   Blood transfusions and vascular repairs in thrombolytic therapy with and without concomitant use of IABC

Event	IABC ($n = 95$)	No IABC ($n = 612$)
>2 units PRBCs transfused	40/91 (44.0%)	99/610 (16.2%)
In-hospital vascular repair	4/93 (4.3%)	13/610 (2.1%)

Modified from George BS: Thrombolysis and intraaortic balloon counterpulsation following acute myocardial infarction. Experience in four TAMI studies, *Cardiac Assists* 4:1, 1988.

the Thrombolysis and Angioplasty in Myocardial Infarction (TAMI) study patients who required IABC experienced only minor bleeding problems.[24] In the approximately one in six patients from the first four TAMI studies who required IABC, no serious bleeding problems attributed to thrombolytic therapy occurred. Table 8-3 contrasts bleeding complications between IABC and no IABC groups from the TAMI studies. Blood transfusions were, however, greater in the IABC group (Table 8-4). The majority of these patients did require bypass surgery.

Dr. George, who summarized IABC in TAMI trials, further stated: "Far from regarding thrombolytic therapy as a contraindication to intraaortic balloon pumping, patients who fail to respond to thrombolytics may, in fact, be in the greatest need of IABC assistance. In the most seriously ill patients, the most urgent need is the restoration of hemodynamic stability, which can be most expeditiously accomplished by IABC. The balloon pump has proven effective before the initiation of more definitive measures—such as opening the artery by either pharmacological or mechanical means (with balloon angioplasty), or even in some cases with emergency bypass surgery."[24] Balloon counterpulsation was also deemed essential in management of those patients who failed to adequately respond to thrombolytic agents.

Dr. George also emphasized the importance of IAB technique when using IABC in conjunction with thrombolytic therapy. "Clinicians at this institution use a 'single-walled needle' technique, which involves puncturing only the anterior arterial wall of the common femoral artery, followed by careful insertion of the guide wire and sheaths. This differs from the practice of initiating IAB after inserting the needle through both the proximal and distal walls of the femoral artery, after which the trocar is retracted into the channel of the blood vessel (Seldinger technique)."[24]

No problems occurred with discontinuation of IABC. Heparin administration was discontinued 2 to 3 hours before IAB removal, and resumption occurred 3 to 4 hours after IAB removal. Pressure is applied above the insertion site at the time of balloon removal. When this is done, pressure is exerted on the patient's thigh to "milk" the superficial femoral artery and thereby extract any clots that may be downstream from the puncture site. After that, pressure is applied distally to cause the blood vessel to flush for 3 to 5 seconds.[24]

Firm pressure is then applied both above and below the wound for at least 30 minutes. It is recommended that this be done manually rather than using clamps, to ensure continuous monitoring of the site. If the patient suddenly moves his leg, rapid and significant blood loss can occur.[24]

Finally, the experience of the TAMI trials using IABC in conjunction with thrombolytic therapy suggests that barring severe peripheral vascular disease, there should be no hesitation about initiating IABC in the presence of any signs of hemodynamic deterioration that cannot readily be corrected by fluids or low dose vasopressors.[24]

A more recent study[25] retrospectively reviewed records of patients suffering anterior myocardial infarction who underwent (1) intravenous streptokinase without IABC ($n = 145$); (2) IABC without thrombolytic therapy ($n = 97$); and (3) intravenous streptokinase with IABC ($n = 48$). Analysis of variances suggested that there were no statistically significant differences between these groups in either transfusion requirement or need for postballoon removal surgical repair of the artery, thrombectomy, or embolectomy.

PERCUTANEOUS TRANSLUMINAL CORONARY ANGIOPLASTY AND IABC

The effectiveness of IABC in providing hemodynamic and clinical stability in conjunction with percutaneous transluminal coronary angioplasty (PTCA) for high-risk patients has been well documented.[26-29] Black and King[30] suggested using a "standby" IABC approach during PTCA in high-risk patients. A small-caliber sheath is placed in the contralateral femoral artery and the IABC equipment and personnel are immediately accessible. IABC therapy is instituted early during high-risk PTCA if hemodynamic instability becomes evident. Prophylactic IABC therapy is recommended in PTCA patients with limited cardiac reserve, poor left ventricular function, hemodynamic instability, and an unstable ischemic syndrome. These authors also have found that IABC therapy is an effective "bridge" to emergency coronary artery bypass graft surgery following irreversible complications during PTCA.

Dr. Lembo from Emory University in Atlanta states: "Clinical experience has shown that the initiation of IABC may well be the most effective use of the first few minutes after it has become evident that an angioplastic procedure will not be successful—the period during which active preparations for surgery are underway. This will help ensure that the patient's blood pressure is stabilized when arriving at the operating room."[31]

Further advice is given regarding assessment of peripheral perfusion before initiating PTCA in high-risk patients who may require concomitant IABC.[31] Foot and groin pulses should be examined in both legs. Patients must be questioned regarding possible symptoms of claudication. This information is extremely important if, for example, PTCA were initiated through the right femoral artery and the patient had baseline weak left peripheral pulses. If the patient then becomes hypotensive, Dr. Lembo suggests that the clinician's only option would probably be to "discontinue the procedure, remove all angioplasty equipment from the right groin, and initiate IABC from the same artery. Insertion of the IAB in the left groin of such a patient would clearly be inadvisable."[31]

The Mid-America Heart Institute retrospectively reported on their experience with IABC in high-risk PTCA patients.[32] During a 30-month period, a total of 3408 PTCA procedures were performed. IABC was prophylactically employed in 28 patients who were at increased risk for hemodynamic instability. Mean age was 66. Of the 28 patients, 23 had Class III or IV left ventricular dysfunction, with a mean left ventricular ejection fraction (LVEF) of 24%.

Results of the IABC-supported PTCA were excellent. Of the 94 attempts at lesion dilation, 90 (96%) were successful. No procedure had to be discontinued or was compromised because of hemodynamic instability. Based on this experience, criteria were developed for selection of patients who should be considered for prophylactic IABC before PTCA. These criteria are listed in the box below.

A recent pilot study[33] compared outcomes in patients undergoing percutaneous cardiopulmonary bypass (CPS) supported PTCA and a control. The intervention

---

CRITERIA FOR PROPHYLACTIC IABC BEFORE PTCA

1. LVEF $\leq$ 30%
2. Angioplasty of the only functional coronary artery
3. Multivessel angioplasty in patients with hypotension
4. Left main coronary artery angioplasty, when the left main artery is unprotected by a patent bypass

---

From Kahn JK: IABP in the high-risk coronary angioplasty patient, *Cardiac Assists* 6:1, 1991.

group had IABC initiated after PTCA and after removal from CPS compared with a control group that received no IABC. The IABC group had an average ejection fraction of 19% compared with the non-IABC group whose average ejection fraction was 34%. Although the IABC group was judged to be much sicker, they showed significantly shorter time of hospitalization postprocedure (6.7 vs. 14.3 days). The study and control groups were similar in their extent of preoperative coronary artery disease and postprocedure revascularization.

IABC FOR PROBLEMS OF REOCCLUSION FOLLOWING THROMBOLYTIC THERAPY AND PTCA

Reocclusion has been observed in 10% to 40% of patients who have successfully undergone thrombolytic therapy with streptokinase, tissue type plasminogen activator, and urokinase.[34] Reocclusion also occurs in about 30% of patients who undergo rescue angioplasty after failed thrombolytic therapy. Maintaining artery patency and prevention of reocclusion is critically important. Patency of the affected artery involving a myocardial infarction may exert an important effect on survival. Califf and Ohman[35] state "The risk of sudden death appears to be much lower in patients with a patent infarct-related artery after an acute infarction." IABC may play a vital role in preventing vessel reocclusion in patients who have undergone thrombolytic therapy and PTCA, as observed from a post hoc analysis of data compiled during the TAMI I study.

Mechanisms responsible for the beneficial effect of IABC in preventing reocclusion after thrombolytic therapy and PTCA have been suggested by Carliff and Ohman.[35] "Improved diastolic flow may be the most important factor. Enhanced flow reduces the propensity for new clot formation and increases exposure of the disrupted plaque to antiplatelet and anticoagulant drugs. Also, higher diastolic pressure resulting from IABC could help to prevent the closure of an intimal flap against the opposite wall of the blood vessel in patients who have undergone acute angioplasty, through a direct mechanical effect.

Another potentially important use of IABC involves patients with multivessel disease and significant dysfunction of noninfarcted myocardium. The normal response of the myocardium not involved in the acute event is to become hypercontractile (a phenomenon which has been called compensatory hyperkinesis). When significant stenoses limit the ability of the noninfarct area, compensatory hyperkinesis does not occur. These patients are especially prone to sudden hemodynamic collapse, even in the absence of previous evidence of low output state. Either reocclusion or sudden arrhythmia (which can be compensated for in patients with intact noninfarct zone myocardium) may produce a clinical event from which the patient cannot recover. IABC may thus provide enhanced coronary flow through the noninfarct-related arteries in these patients, thereby improving their tolerance to clinical events.

In patients with marginal hemodynamics, another advantage of IAB may occur through support of the "stunned" myocardium. Animal and human data have demonstrated that severely ischemic myocardium does not resume maximal function for an extended period following reperfusion. Data from both the GISSI[36] and ISIS-2[37] trials have now convincingly documented that the risk of death during the first 24 hours after thrombolytic therapy is higher than with conservative treatment, perhaps due to even greater dysfunction induced by reperfusion injury.

Generalization from this limited retrospective sample should be avoided. Future experience is likely to demonstrate that some patients who undergo IABC following PTCA and thrombolytic therapy still develop reocclusion. Further studies are needed.

RESUSCITATION

IABC has been employed during a sudden cardiac arrest. Approximately 10% of IABC patients reported from the St. Louis University series fell into this category.[7] The recommendation from this group is to reserve use of IABC in resuscitation for relatively young, viable adults (e.g., a man in his 50s brought into the emergency room with a documented acute infarction who suddenly experiences cardiac arrest). If standard resuscitative measures do not yield results, IABC-assisted resuscitation is suggested.

The St. Louis group also reports that improvement in cerebral perfusion as a result of employing IABC during resuscitation has been remarkable. "This is readily explicable in view of studies showing that standard closed-chest compression results in about 50% of normal cardiac output, which may be equal to about 60 mm Hg systolic blood pressure. Although comparative data are lacking, it seems clear that IABC leads to greater cerebral and coronary perfusion. Clinically, balloon inflation certainly brings about dramatic enhancement of cerebral blood flow. Several patients in this series, who had remained flaccid during closed-chest massage, had to be restrained when compression was timed to coincide with balloon deflation."[7]

Balloon counterpulsation should be "triggered" from the patient's arterial line during resuscitation so that counterpulsation is synchronized with chest compressions.

Wesley and Morgon[38] examined hemodynamics during cardiopulmonary resuscitation in open-chest animal studies. They found that during balloon inflation, aortic systolic pressure increased 50% to 70%, aortic diastolic pressure increased 40% to 58%, epicardial blood flow improved 44% to 57%, mesocardial blood flow increased from 40% to 56%, endocardial blood flow increased from 36% to 50%, and carotid blood flow increased 32% to 51%, with cerebral blood flow increasing 67% to 88% during balloon inflation of more than 150 seconds. There were no effects on right atrial pressure. Therefore IABC appeared to be hemodynamically beneficial during cardiopulmonary resuscitation.

BRIDGE TO CARDIAC TRANSPLANTATION*

"The rationale for the use of IABC in end-stage cardiomyopathy is based upon providing afterload reduction. Since the contractile reserve of the failing heart is limited, any increase in peripheral vascular resistance represents an increase in the impedance to ejection. The failing heart, consequently, is not very efficient at providing systemic circulation. As the disease progresses, cardiac output begins to fall, resulting in a deleterious effect on end-organ function, deteriorating renal and cerebral perfusion with associated accumulation of blood in the left atrium, increase in left atrial pressure (pulmonary capillary wedge pressure), and pulmonary edema. One method to counteract this is to reduce the afterload, to allow the heart with limited contractile reserve to pump more blood into the circulation.

Intraaortic balloon counterpulsation represents the ultimate in afterload reduction without resorting to more invasive ventricular assist devices. Vasodilators certainly reduce impedance to flow, but these drugs unfortunately also tend to reduce mean arterial pressure, which is important for maintaining peripheral perfusion. This limits the usefulness of these drugs. The use of the IAB is not associated with these drawbacks, as it reduces afterload while maintaining (perhaps even increasing) the patient's mean arterial pressure. It also increases cardiac output to the cerebral and systemic circulation, improving mentation and renal blood flow and ultimately renal function. In addition, by inflating during diastole, the IAB augments diastolic flow and blood pressure with a consequent increase in coronary blood flow that may in turn aid contractility in the failing heart. These theoretical aspects of IABC make its use a logical expedient, for a limited period, to counteract the physiological consequences of the failing heart. But the balloon cannot be left in place indefinitely; the longer it is in place, the greater the risk of potential complications that could lead to postponement of cardiac transplantation. The major complication is septicemia from infection at the balloon insertion site or from indwelling lines used to monitor the patient during support.

The timing of insertion then becomes critical as one does not want to proceed in a cavalier fashion with a procedure that could have consequences that preclude transplantation. However, one does not want to delay inserting the IAB until irreversible end-organ dysfunction has set in. One of the factors to bear in mind is the importance of preserving the patient's renal function because of the nephrotoxicity of drugs used for immunosuppression after transplantation, particularly cyclosporine. There can only be rough guidelines as to the timing of insertion as there is a tremendous amount of individual variability. In general the decision can be based upon the daily fall in blood pressure, weight gain despite diuretics, progressive oli-

---

*Material on bridge to cardiac transplantation is reproduced from Kormos RL: The role of the intraaortic balloon as a bridge to cardiac transplantation, *Cardiac Assists* 3:1, 1987.

guria, and confusion. A mean blood pressure consistently below 60 Torr, cool extremities, creatinine greater then 2.0 mg/dl, and urine output less than 300 ml in 8 hours are all warning signs. These signs or measurements together with an increasing demand for dobutamine and dopamine should indicate the necessity for IAB insertion. In a few cases, IABC has been used as an adjunct to transplantation as a way to control pain, rather than as a method to achieve hemodynamic stability. This is generally done in patients with angina pectoris who have coronary artery anatomy, which is not amenable to repeat revascularization procedures.

Patients with end-stage heart failure who are waiting for cardiac transplantation have a very short life expectancy. Any delay can have fatal consequences. Under the most sterile conditions, IABC initiation introduces a potential portal of entry for infection, and once the balloon is in place it represents one more piece of hardware that can harbor organisms that may have entered the patient through another portal. Therefore strict attention is paid to dressing the balloon site carefully, pulmonary toilet is emphasized through chest physiotherapy, and invasive lines and transducers are fastidiously capped when not in use. The sheath is left in place since this gives a better seal around the puncture with improved hemostasis and reduced danger of infection. In theory the sheath can interfere with arterial flow, but this is a less important consideration in patients with a low incidence of atheromatous disease.

All dressings and all tubing that lead to the transducer and then to the balloon are changed on a daily basis to reduce the danger of infection. Antibiotics are not given routinely or prophylactically to avoid the development of resistant strains of microorganisms and the problems associated with an adverse drug reaction. The patients all undergo systemic heparinization. They first receive a bolus of 5000 units and then a maintenance infusion of 600 to 1000 units/hour to maintain a partial thromboplastin time of 1.5 to 2.0 times normal. As a result of this routine the incidence of bleeding and thrombolytic complications has been minimal.

In summary, cardiac transplantation has become the treatment of choice for a specific subset of patients with end-stage cardiomyopathy. The use of inotropic drugs and finally IABC forms a logical therapeutic progression that has helped to preserve end-organ function in a large number of patients who develop refractory cardiac failure while awaiting transplantation. At the same time one must be judicious in the use if IABC in this population because the tolerance of the patient is much lower and the opportunities for correction of complications more limited. Cardiac transplantation is not planned as is other elective cardiac surgery, since the actual moment of the procedure is timed to the availability of a donor organ. Therefore one must avoid sepsis at all costs since it is unlikely that a patient will survive having the balloon removed. By the same token, a heart, if available, will not be offered to a patient with sepsis and it is unlikely that the patient will survive until another heart is available.

Clinical results from the University of Pittsburgh[39]

Between January 1982 and December 1986, 274 heart transplants were performed at the Presbyterian University Hospital. Thirty-seven, or 28%, required IABC as a bridge-to-transplant. Another 13 (10%) required more invasive support in the form of the Jarvik-7 total artificial heart or a ventricular assist device. These balloon insertions in transplant candidates represent less than 20% of all IABs inserted during that interim at Presbyterian University Hospital. There were no major vascular complications but two patients did develop line-related bacteremia due to staphylococcus and other skin organisms.

IABC SUPPORT BEFORE CARDIAC SURGERY

Intraaortic balloon counterpulsation provides preoperative hemodynamic stability for the high-risk cardiac surgical patient.[40,41] Suggested criteria for use of IABC before cardiac surgery are listed in the box below. Accelerating angina, poor left ventricular function, severe aortic and coronary obstruction, left main coronary lesion with concomitant right coronary disease, or presence of acute infarction and its complications all have been suggested as potential indications for preoperative IABC.[42,43]

A study at Charing Cross Hospital in London[44] compared two groups of patients who underwent coronary artery bypass grafting for impending myocardial infarction, defined by (1) anginal pain continuing despite bed rest, sedation, coronary vasodilators, and beta blockade; (2) ST-T wave changes on an electrocardiogram (ECG) during pain; (3) no ECG evidence of infarction; (4) no elevation in the serum level of cardiac muscle enzyme; and (5) clear evidence of coronary disease on an angiogram.

CRITERIA FOR ELECTIVE USE OF IABC BEFORE CARDIAC SURGERY

1. Severe left ventricular dysfunction (CI* < 1.8, EF† < 30%, EDP‡ 22)
2. Presence of moderate left ventricular dysfunction (CI < 2.2, EF 40%, EDP > 18) in patients with the following:
   a. Severe aortic stenosis (gradient > 80 mm Hg)
   b. Acute myocardial infarction or its complications
   c. Intermediate coronary syndrome (especially caused by LMC§)
   d. Valvular heart disease and coronary obstruction

Modified from Sturm JT et al: *Am J Cardiol*, 45:1333, 1980.
*CI, Cardiac index in liters per minute per square meter
†EF, Ejection fraction.
‡EDP, End-diastolic pressure of left ventricle in millimeters of mercury.
§LMC, Left main coronary stenosis.

One group of patients was treated with a combination of coronary artery bypass grafting and IABC. The positive value of cardiac support by IABC before revascularization for impending myocardial infarction was suggested by this study. Those patients in the group (88%) who were treated with combined balloon support and revascularization successfully recovered from surgery and were discharged without evidence of infarction. In the second group of patients managed by coronary artery grafting alone because IABC was not possible, 62% suffered a myocardial infarction.

Therefore the combined regimen of IABC and coronary grafting seems to offer certain advantages.

1. It protects against ischemic damage as soon as counterpulsation is instigated and reduces the need for extreme urgency in further management.
2. Counterpulsation affords protection during the critical period of anesthetic induction before the patient is placed on cardiopulmonary bypass.

LEFT MAIN CORONARY DISEASE AND IABC

Left main coronary disease carries a significant risk factor for operative mortality and perioperative myocardial infarction in coronary bypass surgery. Operative mortality has been reported to be two to five times greater and perioperative myocardial infarction over 50% more common in patients with left main lesion.[45,46] Tahan and associates[46] have documented a reduction in perioperative infarction in patients with left main coronary disease who underwent bypass surgery. These researchers did a retrospective analysis of 91 patients who underwent revascularization for an angiographically defined left main coronary lesion of 50% or greater luminal narrowing. Preoperative IABC yielded a significantly lower incidence of perioperative myocardial infarction (3%) compared with patients who underwent correction of a left main coronary lesion without pumping (23% incidence of perioperative myocardial infarction).

In contrast, Kaplan and associates[47] from Emory University proclaimed that elective preoperative insertion before cardiopulmonary bypass is most controversial. Kaplan did not concur that the routine use of IABC in the period before bypass for all patients with left main coronary disease, angina (before infarction or unstable), or moderately depressed left ventricular function was necessary. Conservative use of IABC was proposed by Kaplan, who argued that most patients with the above surgically treatable disorders can be safely anesthetized with careful use of modern monitoring and anesthetic techniques without the complications associated with balloon pumping.

Windle and Farha[48] supported Kaplan's position of selective use of counterpulsation in the period before bypass, taking the stance that it was unnecessary to initiate elective prophylactic IABC routinely in all patients with left main disease, unstable angina, or decreased left ventricular function. They supported conservative use of IABC with careful anesthetic management, adequate monitoring, and appropriate pharmacological intervention.

POSTOPERATIVE IABC SUPPORT

Buckley and colleagues[49] reported on the success of IABC as an interim organ support for patients who were unable to be weaned from cardiopulmonary bypass. Postoperative low-output syndrome was successfully corrected with balloon assist. The Texas Heart Institute[50] reported 419 cases of low-output syndrome following cardiac surgery treated with IABC. Overall, 226 patients (54%) were weaned from the balloon, and 188 (45%) were subsequently discharged from the hospital. Patients who underwent aortocoronary bypass surgery had significantly better survivial rates than patients who underwent combined aortocoronary bypass and valve procedures. Hemodynamic classification of these patients is presented in Table 8-5.

Class A hemodynamic status patients (cardiac index [CI] greater than 2.1 L/min and systemic vascular resistance [SVR] less than 21,000 dynes $\cdot$ sec $\cdot$ cm^{-5}) were all successfully weaned from the pump. The mortality of Class B hemodynamic status patients (CI greater than 1.2 but less than 2.1 L/min and SVR less than 2100 dynes $\cdot$ sec $\cdot$ cm^{-5}) was 46.3%. Class C hemodynamic status patients failed to progress beyond a CI less than 1.2 L/min or SVR greater than 2100 dynes $\cdot$ sec $\cdot$ cm^{-5}. The mortality of this class of patients was 96.6% during balloon pumping. Differences in survival rates among patient classifications of A, B, and C during balloon counterpulsation were statistically significant ($p < 0.001$).

Duration of support averaged 60.2 $\pm$ 44.7 hours in survivors compared to 10.9 $\pm$ 21.1 hours in nonsurvivors, suggesting an early high attrition rate for unsuccessful postoperative support. Patients receiving assist with balloons of 30 and 40 cc

Table 8-5. Successful treatment of postoperative low cardiac-output syndrome with balloon pumping in 263 patients at the Texas Heart Institute

Class	N	Highest hemodynamic level achieved with balloon pumping	Outcome
A	134	CI* > 2.1 SVR† < 2,100	All successfully weaned from balloon pump
B	41	CI 1.2-2.1 SVR < 2,100	Mortality 46.3%
C	88	CI < 1.2 SVR > 2,100	Mortality 46.3%

From Sturm JT et al: *Am J Cardiol* 45:1033, 1980.
*CI, Cardiac index, liters per minute per meter^2.
†SVR, Systemic vascular resistance dynes per second per centimeter^{-5}.

demonstrated significantly better survival rates (52% and 67%, respectively) than patients with 20 cc balloons (47%). Thus survival in postoperative low-output syndrome treated with IABC correlates with postoperative hemodynamic classification and trajectories of improvement or deterioration.

A review of Stanford University's[51] postoperative use of IABC over 7 years revealed the following stringent indications: (1) unsuccessful discontinuation of cardiopulmonary bypass, (2) postoperative low cardiac output, or (3) intractable ventricular tachyrhythmias. These patients were compared with a control group similar in postoperative symptoms except for a mean older age and ejection fraction in the control group. Operative mortality was 45% and 62% for the group who received IABC and the control group respectively. Two years postoperatively the actuarial survival was 45 ± 3% for the IABC group and 23 ± 20% for the control group.

In the IABC group, timing of insertion appeared to significantly influence outcome. Patients in whom balloon support was instituted before discontinuation of cardiopulmonary bypass was attempted sustained a lower operative mortality than those in whom balloon support was begun after an unsuccessful attempt at weaning (34% versus 54%, $p < 0.01$). A cause-and-effect relationship could not be imputed. These researchers concluded that balloon counterpulsation was a therapeutic adjunct in the surgical management of some patients, but the long-term survival was poor and warranted continued development of more effective methods of mechanical circulatory assist and heart replacement.

The need for escalating the degree of mechanical support after cardiopulmonary bypass in certain patients was documented by the Texas Heart Institute in a 44-month study of patients undergoing IABC for failing circulation after cardiopulmonary bypass. 3% ($n = 14,168$) required more profound mechanical support (i.e., use of the left ventricular assist device) after being weaned from cardiopulmonary bypass.[52]

According to the Texas Heart Institute's criteria for a successful outcome with IABC management of postcardiotomy low-output syndrome, the best results were achieved if SVR was maintained less than 2000 dynes $\cdot$ sec $\cdot$ cm^{-5} and the CI maintained greater than 2.0 L/min/m^2.[52]

The Texas Heart Institute's research documented the efficacy of combined nitroprusside and dopamine therapy as adjuncts to balloon counterpulsation therapy for postcardiotomy low-output syndrome. The rationale for this approach is that nitroprusside provides a vasodilator and afterload reduction effect but should not be initiated until intravascular volume is sufficient. If this precaution is not taken, the cardiac index can decrease and profound hypotension may ensue. If volume loading and nitroprusside therapy do not increase cardiac index to more than 2.0 L/min/m^2, it is recommended that dopamine be added to augment the cardiac index with its inotropic effects.[41]

This classification for hemodynamic performance has been used to predict the likelihood of success of balloon counterpulsation for postcardiotomy low-output syndrome and to assess the efficacy of individual therapeutic interventions. When combined balloon counterpulsation and nitroprusside/dopamine pharmacological support failed to improve the hemodynamic status above Class C (CI < 1.2 L/min/m^2 or SVR > 2000 dynes $\cdot$ sec $\cdot$ cm^{-5}) within 12 to 24 hours postoperatively, mortality was greater than 95%. If hemodynamic performance could be improved to Class B (CI > 1.2 but < 2.1 L/min/m^2 and SVR > 2000 dynes $\cdot$ sec $\cdot$ cm^{-5}), mortality would be approximately 45%. Patients who achieved Class A status (CI > 2.1 L/min/m^2 and SVR < 2000 dynes $\cdot$ sec $\cdot$ cm^{-5}) were usually able to be weaned from both mechanical and pharmacological support.

BALLOON COUNTERPULSATION AS AN ADJUNCT TO ABDOMINAL AORTIC ANEURYSMECTOMY IN HIGH-RISK PATIENTS

Surgical indications for the use of balloon counterpulsation have expanded to include trials as an adjunct to abdominal aortic aneurysmectomy. Patients with coronary artery disease that is not amenable to bypass grafting face an operative mortality approaching 80% for elective resection of an abdominal aortic aneurysm.[53] Attempts to reduce this mortality have centered primarily on coronary artery bypass performed before the aneurysmectomy.[54] There remains a population of patients who require emergency aneurysmectomy, which does not allow for coronary grafting before the surgery; other patients simply have severe inoperable coronary disease. IABC may afford a margin of safety for these patients who otherwise would be subjected to unacceptable surgical risk associated with the aneurysm resection procedure.

Hollier and associates[55] at Mayo Clinic reported on their experience with IABC following abdominal aortic aneurysm resection. Balloon counterpulsation was activated as a supportive measure after resection of the abdominal aortic aneurysm, replacement of that segment of the aorta, and declamping of the aorta with a graft prosthesis. The balloon was inserted via a Dacron side-arm graft through the femoral artery, passed through the segment of aorta prosthesis, and positioned in the thoracic aorta just distal to the left subclavian artery (Fig. 8-5). Improvement was documented with a 1:1 balloon assist ratio until the patient could eventually be completely weaned.

BALLOON SUPPORT IN NONCARDIAC SURGERY

The spectrum of balloon counterpulsation in the surgical field has broadened beyond interim organ support after discontinuation of extracorporeal circulation. Counterpulsation has also been suggested as playing a useful role in lowering the

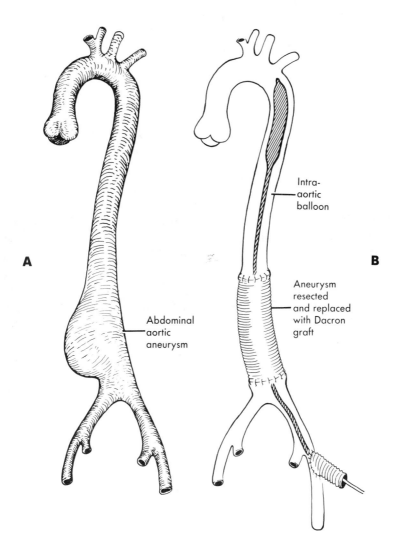

Fig. 8-5. A, Illustration of abdominal aortic aneurysm. **B,** Aneurysm resected and replaced with Dacron graft. After resection of aneurysm, intraaortic balloon is inserted through a femoral artery Dacron side-arm graft and passed retrogradely through the segment of aortic graft into the descending thoracic aorta. The balloon is positioned just below the left subclavian artery.

formidable surgical mortality observed in patients with acute myocardial injury who require emergency noncardiac operations. Such a case has been reported by the Beth Israel Hospital.[56] A major abdominal procedure was required for a patient who had suffered a myocardial infarction 5 days earlier. Anticipating that cardiac work would be substantially increased by the stress of anesthesia and surgery, the surgeon elected to use balloon counterpulsation before laparotomy. With the initiation of IABC, a marked improvement occurred in all factors that represented a shock state preoperatively. The application of balloon counterpulsation for patients with myocardial ischemia who require any major surgery seems logical and an impressive approach to lower the mortality in these high-risk surgical candidates.

INTRAAORTIC BALLOON COUNTERPULSATION: PATTERNS OF USAGE AND OUTCOME IN CARDIAC SURGERY PATIENTS

St. Louis University[57] summarized their experience with IABC in cardiac surgical patients between 1986 and 1991. There were 7884 total adult cardiac surgical procedures performed. In this series, balloon counterpulsation was initiated preoperatively ($n = 240$), intraoperatively ($n = 353$), or postoperatively ($n = 79$). Recipient mean age was 65.3 years (range, 16 to 89 years). Intraaortic balloon usage increased during the study period from 6.4% of patients in 1986 to 12.7% of patient in 1990. Relative distribution between preoperative (35.7%), intraoperative (52.5%), and postoperative (11.8%) insertion remained nearly constant during the study period. When examined by percentages, preoperative insertions accounted for 35.7%, intraoperative for 52.5%, and postoperative 11.8%. This distribution is consistent with some,[58] but not all previous reports. Relative frequency of preoperative balloon insertion in other series ranges from 4% to 44% and frequency of intraoperative insertion ranges from 16% to 82%.[59-63] These differences may reflect differing philosophies regarding indications for preoperative initiation of IABC.

Mean duration of IABC support for the entire study group was 53 hours (range, 1 to 553 hours). Median duration of IABC support for preoperative IABC patients was 63 hours (range 1 to 533 hours), 48 hours for intraoperative patients (48 hours, range 1 to 433 hours), and 62 hours for postoperative (range, 1 to 283 hours).

Overall operative (30-day) mortality for patients with preoperative, intraoperative, or postoperative IABC was 19.6%, 32.3%, and 40.5% respectively. The authors suggested that preoperative IAB insertion was associated with a better survival rate because in a large percentage of patients (32.1%) IABC was initiated to stabilize angina. These patients were quickly weaned from balloon support after revascularization because their myocardial ischemia was corrected. The authors also observed that operative mortality in those patients undergoing cardiac transplantation was least for those with preoperative balloon insertion (4.25) and considerably greater for those with intraoperative (40.0%) or postoperative (25.0%) insertion. They also suggested that the higher mortality rate associated with intraoperative IABC insertion in the setting of cardiac transplantation may represent poor donor or recipient selection or inadequate donor heart preservation.[57]

A multivariate logistic regression analysis was performed to assess the influence of the following variables on operative mortality (30-day): age, sex, preoperative NYHA classification, history of recent MI (within 14 days of operation), history of peripheral vascular disease, history of diabetes mellitus (DM) indication for balloon insertion. Age and history of DM were predictive of operative mortality in the preoperative IABC insertion subgroup. No significant predictors were detected for either the intraoperative or postoperative IABC subgroups.

The rate of IABC weaning was highest in the preoperative IABC insertion group (85.8%) and perhaps reflected the reversible nature of the hemodynamic compromise associated with unstable angina. Rates of IABC weaning for intraoperative and postoperative IABC were similar at 78.8% and 73.5%.

The authors concluded that although use of IABC in the intraoperative and postoperative settings is accompanied by a favorable outcome in most patients, the high associated mortality suggests the need for earlier intervention or other supportive measures such as the ventricular assist device.

REFERENCES

1. Kantrowitz A, Tjonneland S, Freed PS et al: Initial clinical experience with intra-aortic balloon pumping coronary flow and metabolism in man, *JAMA* 203: 135, 1968.
2. Leinbach RC, Buckley MJ, Austen WG et al: Effects of intra-aortic balloon pumping on coronary flow and metabolism in man, *Circulation* 43(suppl I):77, 1971.
3. Schneidt S, Colins M, Goldstein J et al: Mechanical circulatory assistance with the intra-aortic balloon pump and other counterpulsation devices, *Prog Cardiovasc Dis* 25:55, 1982.
4. Weintraub RM, Thurer RL: The intra-aortic balloon pump: a ten year experience, *Heart Transpl* 3:8, 1983.
5. McEnany MT, Kay HR, Buckley MJ et al: Clinical experience with intra-aortic balloon pump support in 725 patients, *Circulation* 58(suppl I):124, 1978.
6. Singh JB, Connelly P, Kocot S et al: Interhospital transport of patients with ongoing intra-aortic balloon pumping, *Am J Cardiol* 56:59, 1985.
7. Miller LW: Emerging trends in the treatment of acute myocardial infarction and the role of intra-aortic balloon pumping, *Cardiac Assists* 3:1, 1986.
8. O'Rourke MF: Randomized controlled trial of intra-aortic balloon counterpulsation in early myocardial infarction with acute heart failure, *Am J Cardiol* 47:8, 1981.
9. DeWood MA: Prevalance of total coronary occlusion during the early hours of transmural myocardial infarction, *N Engl J Med* 303:897, 1980.
10. Gold KK: Intra-aortic balloon pumping for control of recurrent myocardial ischemia, *Circulation* 47:197, 1973.
11. Weintraub RM: Treatment of pre-infarction angina with intra-aortic balloon counterpulsation and surgery, *Am J Cardiol* 34:809, 1974.
12. Mundth ED: Surgical treatment of cardiogenic shock and of mechanical complications following myocardial infarction, *Cardiovasc Clin* 8:273, 1977.
13. Harris PL: The management of impending myocardial infarction using coronary artery by-pass grafting and an intra-aortic balloon pump, *J Cardiovasc Surg* 21:405, 1980.
14. Bardet J: Treatment of post-myocardial infarction angina by intra-aortic balloon pumping and emergency revascularization, *J Thorac Cardiovasc Surg* 74:299, 1977.

15. Freedman RJ: Myoconservation in cardiogenic shock: the use of intra-aortic balloon pumping and other treatment modalities, *Cardiac Assists* 6:1, 1992.
16. Alcan KE, Stertzer SH, Wallsh E et al: Current status of intra-aortic balloon counterpulsation in critical care cardiology, *Crit Care Med* 12:489, 1984.
17. Bolli R: Mechanism of myocardial "stunning," *Circulation* 82:723, 1990.
18. Fuchs R: Augmentation of regional coronary blood flow by intra-aortic balloon counterpulsation in patients with unstable angina, *Circulation* 68:117, 1983.
19. Hanson EC: Control of post-infarction ventricular irritability with the intra-aortic balloon pump, *Circulation* 62 (suppl I):130, 1980.
20. Brundage BHJ: The role of aortic balloon pumping in post-infarction angina—a different perspective, *Circulation* 62 (suppl I):119, 1980.
21. Estrada-Quintero T, Uretsky BF, Murali S et al: Prolonged intraaortic balloon support for septal rupture after myocardial infarction, *Ann Thorac Surg* 53:335, 1992.
22. Gold HK: Wedge pressure monitoring in myocardial infarction, *N Engl J Med* 285:230, 1977, (editorial).
23. Okada M: Experimental and clinical studies on the effect of intra-aortic balloon pumping in cardiogenic shock following acute myocardial infarction, *Artif Organs* 3:271, 1979.
24. George BS: Thrombolysis and intra-aortic balloon pumping following acute myocardial infarction: experience in four TAMI studies, *Cardiac Assists* 4:1, 1988.
25. Goodwin M, Hartmann J, McKeever L et al: Safety of intraaortic balloon counterpulsation in patients with acute myocardial infarction receiving streptokinase intravenously, *Am J Cardiol* 64:937, 1989.
26. Alcan KE, Stertzer SH, Wallsh E et al: The role of intra-aortic balloon counterpulsation in patients undergoing percutaneous transluminal coronary angioplasty, *Am Heart J* 105:527, 1983.
27. Szatmary LJ, Marco J, Fajadet J et al: The combined use of diastolic counterpulsation and coronary dilation in unstable angina due to multivessel disease under unstable hemodynamic conditions, *Int J Cardiol* 19:59, 1988.
28. Kahn JK, Rutherford BD, McConahy DR et al: Supported "highrisk" coronary angioplasty using intra-aortic balloon pump counterpulsation, *J Am Coll Cardiol* 15:1151, 1990.
29. Voudris V, Marco J, Marice MC et al: High-risk percutaneous transluminal coronary angioplasty with preventive intra-aortic balloon counterpulsation, *Cathet Cardiovasc Diagn* 19:160, 1990.
30. Black AR, King SB III: Strategies for support during high-risk PTCA, *Counterpulse* 2:1, 1991.
31. Lembo NJ: Failed angioplasty and intra-aortic balloon pumping, *Cardiac Assists* 5:5, 1989.
32. Kahn JK: IABP in the high-risk coronary angioplasty patient, *Cardiac Assists* 6:1, 1991.
33. Freedman RJ: The intra-aortic balloon pump system: current roles and future directions, *J Appl Cardiol* 6:313, 1991.
34. Schaer DH, Ross Am, Wasserman AG: Reinfarction, recurrent angina, and reocclusion after thrombolytic therapy, *Circulation* 72 (suppl II):II57, 1987.
35. Califf RM, Ohman EM: Reocclusion after thrombolytic therapy and percutaneous transluminal coronary angioplasty, *Cardiac Assists* 5:1, 1990.
36. Gruppo Italiano per lo Studio della Streptochinasi nell'Infarto miocardico (GISSI): Effectiveness of intravenous thrombolytic treatment in acute myocardial infarction, *Lancet* i:397, 1986.
37. ISIS-2 (Second international study of infarct survival) Collaborative Group: Randomized trial of intravenous streptokinase, oral aspirin, both, or neither among 17,187 cases of suspected acute myocardial infarction: ISIS-2 *Lancet* ii:349, 1988.
38. Wesley RC JR, Morgan DB: Effect of continuous intra-aortic balloon inflation in canine open chest cardiopulmonary resuscitaiton, *Crit Care Med* 18:630, 1990.
39. Kormos RL: The role of the intra-aortic balloon as a bridge to cardiac transplantation, *Cardiac Assists* 3:1, 1987.
40. Cleveland JC: The role of intra-aortic balloon counterpulsation in patients undergoing cardiac operation, *Ann Thorac Surg* 110:116, 1975.
41. Golding LR: Use of intra-aortic balloon pumping in cardiac surgical patients: the Cleveland Clinic experience 1975-1976, *Cleve Clin Quarterly* 43:117, 1976.

42. Kaiser GC: Intra-aortic balloon assistance, *Ann Thorac Surg* 21:487, 1976.
43. Sturm JT: Combined use of dopamine and nitroprusside therapy in conjunction with intra-aortic balloon pumping for treatment of postcardiotomy low-output syndrome, *J Thorac Cardiovasc Surg* 82:13, 1981.
44. Goldman GS: Increasing operatility and survival with intra-aortic balloon pump assist, *Can J Surg* 19:69, 1976.
45. Kern MJ: Intra-aortic balloon counterpulsation, *Coron Arter Dis* 2:649, 1991.
46. Tahan SR: Bypass surgery for left main coronary artery disease—reduced perioperative myocardial infarction with preoperative intra-aortic balloon counterpulsation, *Br Heart J* 43:191, 1980.
47. Kaplan JA: The role of the intra-aortic balloon in cardiac anesthesia and surgery, *Am Heart J* 98:580, 1979.
48. Windle R, Farha SJ: Intra-aortic balloon pump. Limited use for maximum effectiveness in cardiac surgery, *J Kans Med Soc* 82:229, 1981.
49. Buckley MJ: Intra-aortic balloon pump assist for cardiogenic shock after cardiopulmonary bypass, *Circulation* 48 (suppl 3):90, 1973.
50. Sturm JT: Treatment of postoperative low output syndrome with intra-aortic balloon pumping: experience with 419 patients, *Am J Cardiol* 45:1033, 1980.
51. Downing TP: Therapeutic efficacy of intra-aortic balloon pump counterpulsation: analysis with concurrent "control" subjects, *Circulation* 64 (suppl 2):108, 1981.
52. Dubakey, M: Retrospective analysis of the need for mechanical circulatory support (intra-aortic balloon pump/abdominal left ventricular assist device or partial artificial heart) after cardiopulmonary bypass, *Am J Cardiol* 46:135, 1980.
53. Myhre IA: Clinical problems in the use of the intra-aortic balloon, *Int Surg* 64:57, 1979.
54. Hertzer NR: Routine coronary angiography prior to elective aortic reconstruction: results of selective myocardial revascularization in patients with peripheral vascular disease, *Arch Surg* 114:1336, 1979.
55. Hollier LH: Intra-aortic balloon counterpulsation as adjunct to aneurysmectomy in high-risk patients, *Mayo Clin Proc* 56:565, 1981.
56. Cohen SF and Weintraub R: A new application of intra-aortic balloon counterpulsation: safer laparotomy after recent myocardial infarction, *Arch Surg* 110:116, 1975.
57. Creswell LL, Rosenbloom M, Cox JL et al: Intraaortic balloon counterpulsation: patterns of usage and outcome in cardiac surgery patients, *Ann Thorac Surg* 54:11, 1992.

CHAPTER 9

Contraindications

Susan J. Quaal

THORACIC OR ABDOMINAL AORTIC ANEURYSM

Presence of a thoracic or abdominal aortic aneurysm (Fig. 9-1) precludes intraaortic balloon counterpulsation (IABC) because of the associated mechanical risk as the balloon counterpulsates against the diseased aortic wall causing aortic dissection. The majority of aortic aneurysms are actually detected at autopsy.[1]

AORTIC INSUFFICIENCY

Aortic insufficiency (AI) may be a contraindication because elevation of diastolic pressure during balloon inflation would magnify blood regurgitating into the left ventricle and worsen the patient's hemodynamic status. The severity of AI is evaluated for each individual patient before totally eliminating the possibility of IABC. With mild AI, the decision may be made to institute IABC because potential benefits outweigh the risk of increasing AI with balloon inflation and elevation of diastolic pressure.

SEVERE PREEXISTING PERIPHERAL VASCULAR DISEASE

Severe peripheral vascular disease (PVD) may be a relative contraindication because of inability to pass the balloon catheter through a tortuous and extremely atherosclerotic vessel.[2] Use of a guidewire through the balloon inner lumen and fluoroscopy have facilitated insertion in patients who previously may have been excluded because of severe PVD. Insertion through a femoral artery cut-down is also an option when percutaneous or sheathless insertion techniques are unsuccessful. Lefemine and associates noted a 12.8% failure of insertion in patients with preexisting PVD.[3] Bahn has suggested that any high-risk patient undergoing cardiac catheterization should receive one aortoiliac injection of contrast material before proceeding with coronary angiography. Information obtained regarding status of the aortoiliac system, at little additional patient risk, is extremely useful in selection of a transfem-

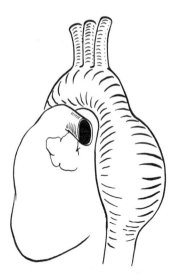

Fig. 9-1. Aortic aneurysm. Contraindications to balloon counterpulsation.

oral insertion site or totally eliminating the transfemoral approach.[4] However, routine aortoiliac arteriograms for all patients before balloon insertion are not recommended.

LACK OF DEFINITIVE THERAPY FOR UNDERLYING PATHOLOGY

IABC is one component of a master plan for definitive therapy of underlying pathology. If the underlying disease process is not amenable to definitive therapy, IABC should not be instituted.

REFERENCES

1. Benn A, Feldman T: The technique of inserting an intra-aortic balloon pump, *Clin Proc* 72:435, 1992.
2. Collier PE, Liebler GA, Park SB et al: Is percutaneous insertion of the intra-aortic balloon pump through the femoral artery the safest technique? *J Vasc Surg* 3:629, 1986.
3. Lefemine AA: Results and complications of intra-aortic balloon pumping in surgical and medical patients, *Am J Cardiol* 40:416, 1977.
4. Bahn C: Vascular evaluation for balloon pumping, *Ann Thorac Surg* 27:474, 1979.

CHAPTER 10

Complications associated with IABC

Sydney S. Lange

Since the intraaortic balloon pump's (IABP) clinical introduction by Kantrowitz in 1967, it has become the most widely used form of ventricular assist device with 65,000 to 75,000 insertions annually.[1] Technical advances have allowed percutaneous insertion on progressively smaller catheters while indications for use of intraaortic balloon counterpulsation (IABC) have broadened significantly. Although the benefits of IABC have been well documented, its use is not without risk. Complication rates reported by various clinicians range from 0%[2] to greater than 50%[3] in patients requiring counterpulsation, with most falling in the 20% to 30% range.[4-11]

As disconcerting as these statistics may be, several physicians contend that clinical studies may in fact underestimate the true frequency of IABC complications. Bregman and Cohen[12] suggest that injuries resulting from IABC may go unrecognized unless relatively catastrophic clinical consequences ensue. This position is supported by Isner[8] who found that of 20 complications in 16 patients, only 4 (20%) had been suspected before death. This data led him to believe that even studies where clinical observations were confirmed by postmortem examination could underestimate the overall frequency of IABC-related complications if they were not looked for specifically.

Other postulated reasons for underestimation of IABC complications include short survival time after actual or attempted intraaortic balloon (IAB) insertion, precluding the recognition of overt clinical symptoms and the general exclusion of patients in whom IAB insertion was unsuccessful.[8,12,13] One contention is that complication rates for unsuccessful IAB insertion attempts are likely to be equal to or greater than those patients with successful IAB placement.[14] This is supported by McCabe's[10] report of a greater incidence of complications in patients undergoing unsuccessful IAB insertion than in those patients where IAB insertion was successful.

Complications are reported to be primarily associated with the insertion process rather than pumping, removal, or postremoval monitoring.[9,10,15,16] The clinician's technical skills and experience,[16] catheter stiffness, catheter-induced arterial trauma, or thrombotic occlusion and thromboembolism[13] have been implicated in sequelae related to insertion. The advent of percutaneous insertion allows insertion that might otherwise have been unsuccessful, presumably leading to an increased incidence of limb ischemia.[15,17]

PREDISPOSING FACTORS

Now that IABC is being used for a growing variety of indications in a wider range of clinical settings, it has become increasingly important that factors placing patients at higher risk for complications be identified. This information can be used to direct the efforts of critical care personnel toward those most likely to develop sequelae from IABC, thus reducing associated morbidity and mortality.

Gender

Several research studies have reported an increased incidence of vascular IABC complications in women.[4,8,9,18-24] Some reasons suggested for this finding include the smaller femoral artery size in women,[4] and the smaller size balloon catheters frequently inserted in women.[25] The IAB catheter could be expected to occupy a greater internal vessel area in women than in men, thus increasing the chance of decreased blood flow and the risk of thrombus formation.

Funk[19] found that men who were nonsmokers, nondiabetic, and who had the IAB inserted for a reason other than cardiogenic shock had the least likelihood of developing major lower limb ischemic complications (3%). Gottlieb[20] concurred, stating that men without peripheral vascular disease had the lowest incidence of IABC-related vascular complications.

Women are 1.66 to 1.8 times more likely to experience limb ischemia/vascular complications than men simply due to their gender.[18,19,24] Gottlieb[20] found that in patients without peripheral vascular disease, females have four times more vascular complications than men. Shahian[23] reported that gender was indeed the variable having the most significant relationship to IABC morbidity. IABC patients predicted to be at greatest risk for the development of lower limb ischemia were women with peripheral vascular disease (PVD) and diabetes mellitus (83%).[19]

Age

Patient age is a variable that has been examined in several research studies; however, the findings have been inconsistent. Several clinicians have found no significant relationship between age and IABC complication rates.* Goldberger,[28]

---

*References 8, 9, 18, 20, 23, 26, 27.

Lange,[21] and Funk[19] all report a significantly increased incidence of vascular complications with increased age. This would be the more logical finding, as the atherosclerotic process progresses with age, which would presumably predispose the patient to an increased incidence of vascular complications.

Preexisting peripheral vascular disease

Although preexisting PVD would be expected to predispose a patient to vascular IABC complications, few studies have examined this possibility. Gottlieb[20] identified PVD as the most important factor for predicting major vascular IABC complications. In fact, he found that patients with a history of PVD had a threefold greater incidence in vascular IABC complications than those without PVD. Funk,[19] Iverson,[29] Kvilekval,[30] Lange,[21] and Pace[11] all found PVD positively correlated with increased risk of vascular complications. Funk,[19] Alderman,[18] and Skillman[24] have calculated that patients with PVD have 1.39 to 1.9 times the risk of developing limb ischemia when compared with those patients without PVD. Therefore it seems evident that preexisting PVD represents a significant risk factor for the development of IABC-associated morbidity.

Duration of IABC therapy

Length of IABC therapy has been a relatively well studied variable in regard to the development of IABC complications, but findings remain inconclusive. Several researchers have reported no correlation between duration of IABC therapy and the development of complications.* Prolonged duration of IABC was found to be associated with an increased incidence of fever, bacteremia, and/or local wound infection by Collier,[4] Kantrowitz,[9] and Macoviak.[36] Iverson[29] and Pelletier[37] identified an increased risk of vascular complications with longer periods of IABC. Research conducted by others[11,21,23,38-40] demonstrates an increased incidence of all types of complications with prolonged IABC.

Diabetes mellitus

Diabetes mellitus (DM) is a factor that has received incidental attention in relation to vascular IABC complications until recently. Diabetics have a more diffuse and severe atherosclerotic disease state, a higher incidence of hypertension, and a decreased resistance to bacterial contamination than nondiabetics. All of these factors would tend to increase the incidence of IABC-related morbidity.[41] Kantrowitz,[9] Wasfie,[42] and Freed[39] studied IABC complications in diabetics. They found that diabetics experienced vascular IABC complications at a significantly greater rate than nondiabetics (22% compared with 14%). An even greater complication rate was associated with insulin-dependent patients (34%). Alderman[18] and Skillman[24] have de-

---

*References 10, 13, 16, 19, 20, 26, 27, 31-35.

termined that diabetics are twice as likely as nondiabetics to develop IABC-associated limb ischemia. Funk[19] has calculated that diabetics are six times more likely to develop major lower limb ischemia than nondiabetics. The rate of local wound infection was also significantly greater in diabetic (9%) than in nondiabetic patients (4%).[42]

Methods of insertion

Although the advent of the percutaneous IAB insertion technique was expected to result in a decreased incidence of complications, that has not generally been the case. Infectious complications related to surgical IAB catheter placement were, however, reported by Collier[4] to be more frequent than with percutaneous insertion (12.3% compared with less than 1%). Even though Alcan[15] found essentially no difference in the major complication rates between the two techniques (surgical vs. percutaneous) and Iverson[29] reports a significant decrease in complications using the percutaneous technique, they are distinctly in the minority. Several studies have documented a significant increase in vascular complications with percutaneous insertion.* Goldberg[14] suggests that the difference in these rates may be due to the fact that an attempt is routinely made to retrieve thrombotic material with a Fogarty embolectomy during removal of a surgically inserted IAB catheter.

Variant placements and techniques are still being evaluated. Macoviak[36] described a decreased incidence of sequelae with IAB catheter insertion directly into the ascending thoracic aorta. These findings were supported by McGeehin in 1987.[45] Nash[46] has developed a new technique for sheathless percutaneous insertion of IAB catheters that reduces the effective catheter diameter. How this innovation will impact IABC complications has yet to be determined.

Other risk factors

Kantrowitz[9] has documented a higher incidence of vascular complications associated with IABC in hypertensive patients than in the normotensive population (27% to 20%). Patients in cardiogenic shock requiring IABC had slightly more than three times the risk (3.33) of developing major lower limb complications related to IABC than patients with other reasons for insertion.[19] Smokers were three times as likely as nonsmokers to develop major lower limb ischemia secondary to IABC.[19] Funk[19] also found obesity (20% over ideal body weight), low cardiac index, elevated systemic vascular resistance, and vasopressor use to be significantly related to the development of lower limb ischemia.

Alderman[18] and Skillman[24] have found that patients with a postinsertion ankle-brachial pressure index less than 0.8 have almost eight (7.9) times the chance of developing IABC-related ischemia than those with better circulation. Goldberg[14] deter-

---

*References 4, 5, 9, 14, 22, 28, 43, 44.

mined that most patients in the percutaneous insertion group who developed lower limb ischemic complications requiring surgical intervention also demonstrated changes on physical examination and in the ankle-arm index before catheter removal. This information may allow a more quantitative weighing of the potential risks and benefits of IABC in individual patients.

VASCULAR IABC COMPLICATIONS

Vascular complications are the most common type of sequelae associated with IABC therapy. Several studies have found only vascular complications.* Possible factors associated with the development of vascular complications include: difficult catheter insertion, preexisting peripheral vascular disease, decreased cardiac output or shock states,[53] elevated systemic vascular resistance,[19] the size of the catheter or sheath (and associated hole in the artery), the use of anticoagulant and/or antiplatelet drugs before and after the procedure, the site and method of insertion, and obesity.[6,54]

Pulse loss

Loss of peripheral pulses occurs in the IAB leg or in the ipsilateral leg in approximately 15% to 25% of all IABC patients.[19,44] This asymptomatic loss of pulses appears transiently and does not progress to threatened limb loss. Clinically, lost peripheral pulses return either spontaneously or upon IAB removal without subsequent treatment. Webster and Vesy[55] report mild limb ischemia in all 18 pediatric patients requiring IABC.

Limb ischemia

Limb ischemia is the most frequently reported IABC complication, occurring in 12% to 47% of all IABC patients.† Limb-threatening ischemia may result from decreased cardiac output and decreased flow states, elevated systemic vascular resistance, arteriosclerotic vessels, intimal injury or dissection, vessel-catheter discrepancy, thrombotic catheter occlusion, or distal thromboembolism.[10,13,54]

Signs and symptoms of limb ischemia include pain in the affected limb, pallor, cyanotic color changes, mottling, loss of distal pulses, decreased sensation, paresthesia, decreased toe temperature, and motor function loss.[13,18,26,31,60] Alderman's[18] study found limb ischemia in 42% of patients undergoing successful IAB insertion with the following incidence of signs and symptoms: abnormal limb temperature (80%), abnormal limb color (62%), abnormal motor function (9%), limb pain (8%),

---

*References 12, 13, 17, 26, 31, 47-52.
†References 5, 13, 14, 18-20, 26-28, 32, 56-59.

and limb paresthesia (24%). Limb ischemia led to premature IABC discontinuation in 27% of his patients benefiting from counterpulsation.

Vascular insufficiency occurs not only during hospitalization, but after discharge as well.[7,11,19,26,61] Chenevey[26] found that long term sequelae may occur in up to 26% of all patients undergoing counterpulsation. The posthospital discharge records documented three major categories of vascular insufficiency: (1) cramping when walking (61.5%); (2) numbness and tingling in feet (9.5%); and (3) other symptoms of claudication (13.5%). Other symptoms included ankle edema, continuous leg aching, bilateral leg pain, nocturnal leg cramps, claudication after walking 75 yards, cold lower extremities, charley horses in legs, pain or cramps in legs relieved by rest, and cellulitis in the IAB-placement leg. Funk[19] also found that gangrene and ischemic ulcers had occurred 2 to 3 weeks after IABC therapy had been initiated.

Treatment of limb ischemia varies according to its severity and may consist of IAB removal, Fogarty thrombectomy, femorofemoral crossover graft or administration of papaverine.* Opie[63] reports the results of a pilot study of eight patients who had papaverine administered high in the thoracic aorta (by means of the IAB) once severe ischemia had developed. Clinical resolution of symptoms was achieved in seven of eight patients with the addition of warming lights and a topical vasodilator (nitroglycerine ointment).

If this condition is treated unsuccessfully, gangrene and subsequent digital or limb amputation may result, or the patient may sustain neurological impairment. Although the incidence of limb ischemia progressing to gangrene and/or requiring amputation is small, many physicians report at least one occurrence.† Neurological impairment may include transient paresthesia, ischemic neuropathy, footdrop, postischemic neuritis, peroneal paralysis, and/or persistent peroneal nerve numbness.‡ Treatment generally consists of braces and physiotherapy.

Thromboembolism

The insertion of the IAB, especially percutaneously, represents a peripheral vascular insult. Atherosclerotic plaque may be disturbed during a difficult insertion or dislodged during removal. Clots are routinely seen at the time of IAB removal,[9] and fibrin and platelets may be sheared from the IAB catheter itself during removal. Symptoms of thromboembolism as well as appropriate treatment depend on the area and system affected. Cerebrovascular accidents,[9,14,20,45] renal artery occlusion(s),[69] pulmonary emboli,[4,70] peripheral emboli,§ ischemic/gangrenous bowel,[9,11,38,67,73] mesenteric infarction,[4,20,21,43] renal emboli,[3,11,47,74] splenic infarction,[75] hemianop-

---

*References 4, 9, 15, 31, 36, 49, 52, 58, 62, 63.
†References 3, 6, 7, 9, 11, 19, 20, 22, 26, 33, 35, 37-39, 42, 43, 48, 50, 54, 64-67.
‡References 4, 7, 9, 11, 13, 20, 31, 39, 42, 51, 67, 68.
§References 8, 9, 11, 13, 17, 30, 31, 33, 42, 44, 47, 52, 71, 72.

sia, coronary artery embolism,[76] and spinal cord infarction[59,71,77-80] have all been attributed to IABC.

Beckman[38] described a decrease in bowel sounds, abdominal rigidity, and leukocytosis in a patient with gangrene of the cecum with perforation. Marked left upper quadrant pain, tachycardia, hypotension, and a falling hemoglobin may indicate a splenic infarction.[75] A renal embolism may cause a sudden onset of flank pain on the affected side, hematuria, moderate renal dysfunction, and a positive renal scan.[3] Paraplegia due to a spinal cord infarction may manifest itself as severe lower back pain, decreased or absent sensation, and limb weakness progressing to complete paraplegia[71,77-79,81,82] while the patient's pulses remain palpable with brisk capillary refill.

Therapeutic anticoagulation with heparin to maintain the prothrombin time 1.5 to 2 times normal may prevent thrombotic or embolic phenomena. During the postoperative period, some clinicians prefer to use low molecular weight dextran instead to decrease the risk of hemorrhage. The "open" or surgical removal of the IAB includes routine thrombectomy and allows direct visualization and repair (if necessary) of the femoral artery at the same time. Routine surgical removal has been suggested for percutaneously placed balloons by Cutler[27] and Shahian[23] to decrease the possibility of thromboembolism.

Compartment syndrome

Compartment syndrome is a type of peripheral vascular ischemia that has been linked to IABC. The thighs, buttocks, and lower legs are made up of compartments containing bone, muscle, nerve tissue, and blood vessels that are surrounded by a fibrous membrane (fascia). Compartment syndrome is defined as a condition in which increased pressure within the closed, nondistensible fascial space reduces capillary blood41thus compromising the enclosed tissues.[83] IA patients are at increased risk for compartment syndrome because of prolonged immobilization, loss of capillary blood flow, preexisting peripheral vascular disease, vasopressor drug use, thrombus formation, and difficulty with insertion.[57,84]

In the conscious patient, the diagnosis of compartment syndrome can generally be made from the signs and symptoms of calf pain (especially on dorsiflexion of the foot), and loss of lower leg sensation or function in the presence of a tense, painful calf.[57] The deep, throbbing feeling of pressure is greater than would be expected from the primary problem. Paresthesia may progress to hypoesthesia and ultimately, anesthesia, if treatment is delayed.[83] Compartment pressure is often high enough to cause nerve and muscle damage, but not arterial occlusion or loss of peripheral pulses. This distinction can help differentiate compartment syndrome from other causes of limb ischemia.

Because many IABC patients are ventilated and sedated, the diagnosis of compartment syndrome is frequently missed. Glenville[57] describes the use of a slit catheter as "invaluable" in the early detection and possible treatment of compartment syndrome. A needle or catheter is inserted into the suspect compartment, allowing direct pressure measurement, with normal tissue pressures measuring 0-12 mm Hg.[83] The tolerance of tissue for increased pressure may be reduced by such factors as shock, arterial occlusion, and limb elevation, so compartment syndrome may occur at significantly lower tissue pressures when these problems are present.[85] Because of this variability of tissue tolerance, no "critical pressure" has been recognized as definitive in the treatment of compartment syndrome.[84]

The level of creatine phosphokinase (CPK) is often used as an index of muscle ischemia; in acute compartment syndrome, CPK levels from 1000 to 5000 IU have been reported.[83] Muscle ischemia of 4 hours duration gives rise to significant myoglobinuria, reaching a maximum level approximately 3 hours after circulation is restored.[84] Myoglobinuria is caused by the filtration and excretion of myoglobin from the damaged muscle cells, and may persist for up to 12 hours.

Once compartment syndrome is diagnosed, a fasciotomy is frequently performed to relieve the pressure.* Complications of compartment syndrome itself include persistent hyperesthesia, motor weakness, infection of the bone and soft tissue, renal failure, contractures, and amputations. Prevention is the best treatment for compartment syndrome. So many IABC patients are sedated and/or intubated that their input is negligible. Glenville advocates the use of a slit catheter in unconscious patients for early detection of compartment syndrome. The role of the critical care nurse is to assess for changes in lower limb sensation or pressures, especially when there are no changes in the patient's pulse status.

Aortic dissection

Aortic dissection is a serious complication that often goes unrecognized until IABC is discontinued.† When IABC is ultimately discontinued, hemodynamic instability ensues and may lead to death.[8,15,38,67,88]

Bolooki[88] noted an increased incidence of aortic dissection in patients undergoing percutaneous IAB insertion, possibly due to the stiffness of the introducer sheath. Aortic dissection may, in fact, occur without the clinician's knowledge, and successful balloon augmentation may be achieved. Isner[8] found evidence of aortic dissection in 36% of IABC patients on autopsy, although it was not suspected in any patient before their death. Grayzel[47] states that a common problem is the operator's failure to recognize the initiation of the intimal tear and progressive dissection as the false lumen is enlarged and extended by the advancing catheter. He cautions the physician inserting the balloon to view even minor resistance with suspicion.

Symptoms of aortic dissection include back and/or abdominal pain, falling hema-

---

*References 14, 18, 19, 31, 36, 43, 57, 65-67, 80.
†References 8, 12, 32, 38, 47, 86, 87.

tocrit, or mediastinal enlargement.[38] The critical care nurse and the physician inserting and/or removing the IAB must be prepared for this potential complication. If not acted upon quickly and aggressively, aortic dissection may prove to be a lethal sequela to IABC.

Local injury

Local vascular injury such as false aneurysm formation,* hematoma formation,† chronic serous drainage,[23,35,36,67] lymphedema,[10,67] lymph fistula,[10] wound hemorrhage,‡ and laceration of the femoral artery,[30,43] iliac artery,§ or aorta,‖ may also occur as complications of IABC.

Arteriotomy repair,[15] femorofemoral bypass, hematoma evacuation,[64] endarterectomy,[31] graft angioplasty,[31] or other surgical repairs may be necessary to treat various IABC sequelae described above. The presence of a bruit and pulsatile mass over the femoral artery almost always identifies a false aneurysm without angiography.[24] If an infected arteriovenous fistula is suspected, Archie[93] recommends that a culture and Gram stain of material obtained by needle aspiration be done before reconstructive vascular surgery.

Infective complications

Local wound infection necessitating drainage, debridement and irrigation, systemic antibiotics, and/or removal of the surgical patch graft required for IAB insertion has been reported in several studies.¶ If untreated or if treatment proves unsuccessful, wound infection may cause arterial rupture,[4] false aneurysm formation, an infected surgical patch, or bacteremia.#

Bolooki[88] suggests that improper preparation and contamination of the groin area, especially in obese patients, may lead to a higher incidence of infection in surgical IAB insertions. Rutala[98] has described two instances where the water reservoir on the SMEC IABP was presumably the source of *Pseudomonas cepacia* bacteremia. Wasfie[42] and Kantrowitz[9] have implicated the setting of IAB insertion as influencing the risk of infectious complications; the greatest incidence of infection occurred in IAB insertions in the CCU or SICU (approximately 25%) and the least in the operating room or the cardiac catheterization laboratory (12% and 17% respectively). This discrepancy may be partially due to the sterility of the setting and also to the deteriorating status of the patient.

---

*References 3, 7, 11, 21, 23, 24, 32, 37, 43, 47, 51, 67, 72, 89.
†References 3, 7, 14, 15, 18, 21, 32, 33, 44, 48, 62, 64-66, 90.
‡References 3, 6, 9, 15, 21, 30, 32, 42, 44, 47, 51, 52, 67, 71, 91, 92.
§References 7, 8, 10, 21, 23, 30, 37, 43, 64, 67.
‖References 3, 6, 12, 13, 21, 36, 50.
¶References 4, 6-11, 13-15, 20-23, 32, 35, 36, 38, 42, 44, 45, 65-67, 71, 76, 90-92, 94-96.
#References 3, 6, 9, 10, 14, 15, 21, 30, 32, 33, 38, 39, 42, 43, 67, 97.

IAB rupture and/or entrapment

Use of IABC for 327 days as a bridge-to-transplant without catheter rupture helps support the contention that IAB rupture is not a frequent occurrence. However, when it does occur, immediate recognition with subsequent IAB removal and/or catheter replacement is required.[99] Stahl[100] notes that women are three times more likely to sustain IAB rupture than men. The most commonly proposed cause is perforation caused by prolonged contact of the IAB membrane against calcific atheromatous plaque,[99,101-107] although fracture of the catheter due to chemical exposure to acetone and/or ether at the time of removal has also been implicated.[108] Finegan[109] describes an IAB rupture secondary to needle puncture while administering intraaortic protamine sulfate, recognized as such by gas bubbles in the aortic perfusion tubing accompanied by extreme hypotension. A case of intraaortic balloon rupture and impaction necessitating thoracotomy and removal through the thoracic aorta has also been described. Impaction was due to central stylet dislocation, producing a fish-hook effect (Fig. 10-1) and was diagnosed from plain abdominal radiographs.[110]

The most common sign of IAB rupture is blood in the tubing,* although Stahl[100] found that decreased IABC augmentation preceded the appearance of blood in the tubing in five of nine patients. Several clinicians report that no alarm signals or increased balloon filling were noted before the appearance of blood in the tubing to alert the clinician to this condition.[100,102,103,105,112]

IAB rupture can lead to two serious complications: (1) gas embolus and (2) entrapment of the IAB catheter. Although the IAB was changed without problems in most instances,[9,45,100,105] Pennington[65] recounts an instance where a patient received a helium embolus and subsequently suffered a cardiac arrest.

---

*References 9, 45, 92, 100, 102, 103, 105-107, 111.

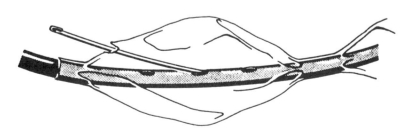

Fig. 10-1. Artist's drawing showing stylet protruding through third proximal side hole in proximal balloon chamber. (From Grotte GJ and Butchart EG: *J Thorac Cardiovasc Surg* 80:229, 1980.)

Hyperbaric oxygen therapy is the only specific treatment for gas embolism. It has been shown to reduce the volume of intravascular gas bubbles, reduce hypoxia by increasing the distance oxygen will diffuse, reduce cerebral edema by lowering the intracranial pressure, and reduce the inflammatory response caused by blood-bubble interaction.[113]

Frederiksen[113] describes a case of arterial helium embolism in which the patient suddenly became unresponsive and lost all voluntary neurological function. Blood was noted in the balloon tubing, the IAB was promptly removed, the patient was placed on 100% oxygen, and dexamethasone was administered intravenously. The patient then experienced slow, intermittent focal seizures for approximately 3 minutes, followed by total flaccidity. After several hyperbaric oxygen therapy treatments, the patient was discharged home with mild residual weakness as the only complication.

Entrapment of the IAB can occur when the rupture or perforation is small and the blood is allowed to clot within the catheter itself. Since the catheter defect is small, it may not interfere with the functioning of the device. Once entrapment occurs, immediate removal is required. Surgical removal of the IAB catheter is the treatment of choice,[102,108,110,112] despite Brodell's report of a successful percutaneous removal.[102] Millham[112] recommends a flat plate abdominal film be taken before attempting IAB removal. This is to discern the level of entrapment to prevent hemorrhage upon removal of the impacted catheter.

Hematologic changes

Increased destruction of blood cells, including a decrease in circulating platelets and red blood cells, has been noted in IABC patients.[10,62,88] The degree of decrease appears to be related to the duration of IABC therapy and subsides immediately once it is discontinued.[10,62,88] Goldberg[14] identified a difference in the percentage of IABC patients requiring blood transfusions according to method of insertion: 36% of the surgical group received blood transfusions compared to 8% of the percutaneous insertion group. IABC does not appear to preclude the safe use of intravenous streptokinase because Goodwin[114] found no increased need for transfusions or femoral surgery in these patients.

Other complications associated with IABC

Malposition of the IAB catheter occurs in 2% to 5% of the patients requiring this treatment modality.[115] If positioned too high, the IAB may compromise the origin of the carotid arteries and cause cerebral embolism,[62] occlude the left internal mammary artery,[116] (Fig. 10-2) and/or the subclavian artery, especially on the left.[33] If positioned too low, the IAB may compromise the renal arteries. The catheter may move as much as 1 to 4.5 cm as the patient sits up, even when the initial position is correct.[115]

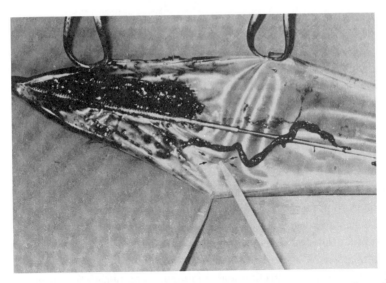

Fig. 10-2. Section of the balloon showing a 5 cm hard clot distally and a smaller soft clot in the proximity of a 5 mm longitudinal rupture. (From Rodigas PC and Bridges KG: *J Thorac Cardiovasc Surg* 91:147, 1986.)

Inability to unwrap the IAB catheter is detected by small or absent augmentation, a squared off IAB pressure curve, and/or a high pressure alarm.[3] Harvey[3] suggests correcting this by grasping the IAB catheter and sheath as a unit and turning it one-quarter turn counterclockwise (in the direction indicated by the unwrap arrow). If this is unsuccessful, manual inflation utilizing a 60 cc syringe attached to the catheter lumen may be attempted. If these efforts do not correct the problem, the IAB catheter should be removed and another one inserted.

Haykal[117] describes the physiological and clinical course of one patient sustaining an air embolism to the brain. In arterial air embolism the brain is involved more frequently than the spinal cord. Air bubbles lodging in a cerebral artery produce an immediate but transient block followed by dissipation of the air through the capillary and venous beds. Arterial spasm ensues, and is later followed by vascular dilatation and stasis of flow. Clinically, the patient experiences a sudden decrease in his level of consciousness, which may progress to coma. Generalized seizures are common and focal neurological signs may be present. Treatment consists of anticonvulsant therapy, and occasionally, hyperbaric oxygen therapy, which has shown promising results. The degree of neurological dysfunction depends on the location of the air bubbles and the degree of ischemia that ensues. Cerebral air embolism usually carries a grave prognosis, but spontaneous recovery has been reported.

Cardiac tamponade[48,76] has been mentioned as a rare result of anticoagulant therapy during IABC therapy.

A retrospective study of IABC patients conducted at Massachusetts General Hospital found delirium to be the most common complication of this therapy (34%).[118] Residual organic brain syndrome involving impairments in orientation, memory, speech, attention, or other cognitive functions was noted at discharge in 16% of the patients who experienced delirium. Patients receiving haloperidol fared better than those receiving narcotics or neuroleptic medication in regard to mortality, length of stay, and the development of organic brain syndrome and other complications.

IMPLICATIONS FOR NURSING

Despite the technical advances allowing for smaller IAB catheters and the development of various insertion techniques, the vascular complication rate associated with IABC has not decreased as expected. The importance of nursing assessment and appropriate interventions to minimize morbidity associated with IABC cannot be overemphasized. The critical care nurse, as primary care provider to IABC patients, has a key role in detecting and minimizing complications during hospitalization and after discharge.

A comprehensive vascular assessment is crucial to providing adequate care for IABC patients. This assessment should be placed on a form to be used during the remainder of the patient's hospital stay, as long-term complications are not unusual. Assessment begins by noting the skin color and temperature. Mottled, cyanotic, pale, or cool skin is an indication of poor perfusion and arterial insufficiency.[26,119] Distal limb temperature should be equal bilaterally. Loss of foot and leg hair, thickened toe nails, and pale, shiny skin are all signs of decreased perfusion. Femoral, popliteal, dorsalis pedis, and posterior tibial pulses should be palpated and marked with a felt-tip marker to facilitate later identification. The following scale is generally used to document a patient's pulse volume: 3+ (bounding, increased); 2+ (normal); 1+ (weak, thready, decreased); and 0 (absent).[26] It is important to note that 15% of the general population do not have a palpable dorsalis pedis pulse,[26] so a loss or change of pulse status is a more significant finding than the mere absence of a pulse. Chenevey,[26] Sexton-Stone,[26] and Goran[119] all recommend that after IAB insertion, lower limb circulatory assessment occur every 15 minutes for the first hour, every 30 minutes for the second hour, and hourly thereafter. From the time of IAB removal until hospital discharge, they suggest performing a circulatory assessment every 15 minutes for the first hour, every 30 minutes for the second hour, and hourly for the next 48 hours, then at least every shift.

Several clinicians advocate the inclusion of an ankle-brachial index (ABI) or ankle-arm index (AAI) as part of the vascular assessment to provide a more quantitative measure of adequate circulation. To determine the ankle-brachial ratio, the posterior tibial or dorsalis pedis pulse must be located by Doppler. A blood pressure cuff is then applied around the ankle above the malleolus and inflated in the usual manner to 20 mm Hg above the brachial pressure. As the cuff is slowly deflated, the systolic pressure is measured where the Doppler signal reappears. The normal ratio for the ABI is 0.8 to 1.2.[119]

Capillary refill time should also be included in the peripheral vascular assessment. Test capillary refill by squeezing a small area of the patient's foot or toe to cause blanching and measure the amount of time it takes for the limb to return to its usual color. It should occur almost instantaneously.

The occurrence of postural changes also indicates lower limb ischemia. Have the supine patient raise his or her legs to a 45 degree elevation and observe the color. Patients with normal circulation will continue to have pink feet, while patients with ischemia may have pale feet on elevation.[26,119]

Malposition of the IAB catheter affects 2% to 5% of the patients requiring this treatment modality and the catheter may migrate as much as 1 to 4.5 cm when the patient sits up.[115] The use of a knee immobilizer has been suggested as one means of restricting movement of the affected extremity in place of a soft restraint.[114]

Routine checks of the IAB tubing every 2 hours should be made to assess the presence of blood, indicating IAB catheter rupture. If a patient has already suffered one IAB rupture, this inspection should be increased in frequency to every 30 minutes. This first perforation should be viewed as a danger sign; the damaged balloon may indicate this patient's vasculature predisposes him to perforation or abrasion in subsequent balloons.[107]

Because IABC patients require multiple invasive lines, they are in danger of developing nosocomial infections. Many institutions do not routinely culture all invasive lines, therefore it is impossible to determine the infection source. Routine cultures of the IAB catheter when discontinued would provide important data about the actual incidence of IAB-induced septicemia.

Information about possible late vascular IABC-related complications should be communicated to the patient and his family before discharge.[7,26] A knowledgeable patient is the best informant regarding peripheral circulatory changes such as tingling, numbness, coldness, and pain. Most patients experiencing lower limb ischemia complained of claudication or pain in a muscle group brought on by ambulation. Pain at rest is a more advanced symptom, which may occur at night, especially when the legs are elevated. The patient needs to be aware that this is a serious change and requires immediate evaluation and treatment to prevent possible tissue loss.[26] The patient and/or his family should be taught to inspect his or her feet daily for redness or ulcerations, especially on the toes or around any pressure points. Additional symptoms of lower limb ischemia include numbness, coldness, pallor, or tingling. The patient must be made to understand that any of these signs, even if they seem insignificant, must be brought to the physician's attention.

SUMMARY

As health care professionals we can do a great deal to maximize the benefit the patient can receive from IABC therapy, at the same time minimizing the associated risks. Recognizing factors predisposing patients to the development of IABC complications, implementing actions specifically intended to prevent or to assess for these sequelae, and providing patient education about possible changes requiring medical intervention are integral parts of the critical care nurse's role in providing care to these complex and challenging patients.

REFERENCES

1. Cardiac assist devices: an emerging life-saving technology, *Kidder, Peabody Equity Research* 18:14, October 1988.
2. Vijayanager R, Bognolo DA, Eckstein PF et al: The role of intra-aortic balloon pump in the management of patients with main left coronary artery disease, *Cathet Cardiovasc Diagn* 7:397, 1981.
3. Harvey JC, Goldstein JE, McCabe JC et al: Complications of percutaneous intraaortic balloon pumping, *Circulation* 64(suppl II):II-114, 1981.
4. Collier PE, Liebler GA, Park SB et al: Is percutaneous insertion of the intra-aortic balloon pump through the femoral artery the safest technique? *J Vasc Surg* 3(4):629, 1986.
5. Curtis JJ, Boland M, Bliss D et al: Intra-aortic balloon cardiac assist: complication rates for the surgical and percutaneous insertion techniques, *Am Surg* 54(3):142, 1988.
6. Goldman BS, Hill TJ, Rosenthal GA et al: Complications associated with use of the intra-aortic balloon pump, *Can J Surg* 25(2):153, 1982.
7. Hedenmark J, Ahn H, Henze A et al: Complications of intra-aortic balloon counterpulsation with special reference to limb ischemia, *Scand J Thorac Cardiovasc Surg* 22(2):123, 1988.
8. Isner JM, Cohen SR, Virmani R et al: Complications of the intraaortic balloon counterpulsation device: clinical and morphologic observations in 45 necropsy patients, *Am J Cardiol* 45:260, 1980.
9. Kantrowitz A, Wasfie T, Freed PS et al: Intraaortic balloon pumping 1967 through 1982: analysis of complications in 733 patients, *Am J Cardiol* 57:976, 1986.
10. McCabe JC, Abel RM, Subramanian VA et al: Complications of intra-aortic balloon insertion and counterpulsation, *Circulation* 57(4):769, 1978.
11. Pace PD, Tilney NL, Lesch M et al: Peripheral arterial complications of intra-aortic balloon counterpulsation, *Surgery* 82(5):685, 1977.
12. Bregman D, Cohen SR: Mechanical techniques of circulation support: a percutaneous intra-aortic balloon device, *Artif Organs* 7(1):38, 1983.
13. Alpert J, Parsonnet V, Goldenkranz RJ et al: Limb ischemia during intra-aortic balloon pumping: indication for femorofemoral crossover graft, *J Thorac Cardiovasc Surg* 79:729, 1980.
14. Goldberg MJ, Rubenfire M, Kantrowitz A et al: Intraaortic balloon pump insertion: a randomized study comparing percutaneous and surgical techniques, *J Am Coll Cardiol* 9(3):515, 1987.
15. Alcan KE, Stertzer SH, Wallsh E et al: Comparison of wire-guided percutaneous insertion and conventional surgical insertion of intra-aortic balloon pumps in 151 patients, *Am J Med* 75:24, 1983.
16. Miller LW: Emerging trends in the treatment of acute myocardial infarction and the role of intra-aortic balloon pumping, *Cardiac Assists* 3(1):1, 1986.
17. Leinbach RC, Goldstein J, Gold HK et al: Percutaneous wire-guided balloon pumping, *Am J Cardiol* 49:1707, 1982.
18. Alderman JD, Gabliani GI, McCabe CH et al: Incidence and management of limb ischemia with percutaneous wire-guided intraaortic balloon catheters, *J Am Coll Cardiol* 9(3):524, 1987.
19. Funk M, Gleason J, Foell D: Lower limb ischemia related to use of the intra-aortic balloon pump, *Heart Lung* 18(6):542, 1989.
20. Gottlieb SO, Brinker JA, Borkon AM et al: Identification of patients at high risk for complications of intraaortic balloon counterpulsation: a multivariate risk factor analysis, *Am J Cardiol* 53(8):1135, 1984.

21. Lange SS: Relationship of physiologic factors to intra-aortic balloon pump complications, masters thesis (unpublished), Houston, 1988, University of Texas Health Science Center School of Nursing.
22. Sanfelippo PM, Baker NH, Ewy HG et al: Experience with intraaortic balloon counterpulsation, *Ann Thorac Surg* 41(1):36, 1986.
23. Shahian DM, Neptune WB, Ellis FH et al: Intraaortic balloon pump morbidity: a comparative analysis of risk factors between percutaneous and surgical techniques, *Ann Thorac Surg* 36(6):644, 1983.
24. Skillman JJ, Kim D, Baim DS: Vascular complications of percutaneous femoral cardiac interventions, *Arch Surg* 123(10):1207, 1988.
25. Beddermann C, McGee MG, Turner SA et al: Intraaortic balloon pumping in women: effects of balloon size on survival, *Thorac Cardiovasc Surg* 28:428, 1980.
26. Chenevey B, Sexton-Stone K: Lower limb ischemia: an iatrogenic complication of IABP, *Dimens Crit Care Nurs* 4(5):264, 1985.
27. Cutler BS, Okike ON, Van der Salm TJ: Surgical versus percutaneous removal of the intra-aortic balloon, *J Thorac Cardiovasc Surg* 86:907, 1983.
28. Goldberger M, Tabak SW, Shah PK: Clinical experience with intra-aortic balloon counterpulsation in 112 consecutive patients, *Am Heart J* 111(3):497, 1986.
29. Iverson LI, Herfindahl G, Ecker RR et al: Vascular complications of intraaortic balloon counterpulsation, *Am J Surg* 154(1):99, 1987.
30. Kvilekval KH, Mason RA, Newton GB et al: Complications of percutaneous intra-aortic balloon pump use in patients with peripheral vascular disease, *Arch Surg* 126(5):621, 1991.
31. Alpert J, Bhaktan EK, Gielchinsky I et al: Vascular complications of intra-aortic balloon pumping, *Arch Surg* 111:1190, 1976.
32. Bolooki H: Current status of circulatory support with an intra-aortic balloon pump, *Cardiol Clin* 3(1):123, 1985.
33. Kuchar DL, Campbell TJ, O'Rourke MF: Long-term survival after counterpulsation for medically refractory heart failure complicating myocardial infarction and cardiac surgery, *Eur Heart J* 8(5):490, 1987.
34. Sutorius DJ, Majeski JA, Miller SF: Vascular complications as a result of intra-aortic balloon pumping, *Am Surg* 45(8):512, 1979.
35. Vigneswaran WT, Reece IJ, Davidson KG: Intra-aortic balloon pumping: seven years' experience, *Thorax* 40:858, 1985.
36. Macoviak J, Stephenson LW, Edmunds LH et al: The intraaortic balloon pump: an analysis of five years' experience, *Ann Thorac Surg* 29(5):451, 1980.
37. Pelletier LC, Pomar JL, Bosch X et al: Complications of circulatory assistance with intra-aortic balloon pumping: a comparison of the surgical and percutaneous techniques, *J Heart Transplant* 5(2):138, 1986.
38. Beckman CB, Geha AS, Hammond GL et al: Results and complications of intraaortic balloon counterpulsation, *Ann Thorac Surg* 24(6):550, 1977.
39. Freed PS, Wasfie T, Zado B et al: Intra-aortic balloon pumping for prolonged circulatory support, *Am J Cardiol* 61(8):554, 1988.
40. Michels R, Haalebros M, Kint P-P et al: Intra-aortic balloon pumping in myocardial infarction and unstable angina, *Eur Heart J* 1:31, 1980.
41. Clement R, Rousou JA, Engelman RM et al: Perioperative morbidity in diabetics requiring coronary artery bypass surgery, *Ann Thorac Surg* 46(3):321, 1988.
42. Wasfie T, Freed PS, Rubenfire M et al: Risks associated with intraaortic balloon pumping in patients with and without diabetes mellitus, *Am J Cardiol* 61(8):558, 1988.
43. Martin RS, Moncure AC, Buckley MJ et al: Complications of percutaneous intra-aortic balloon insertion, *J Thorac Cardiovasc Surg* 85(2):186, 1983.
44. Yuen JC: Percutaneous intra-aortic balloon pump: emphasis on complications, *South Med J* 84(8):956, 1991.
45. McGeehin W, Sheikh F, Donahoo JS et al: Transthoracic intraaortic balloon pump support: experience in 39 patients, *Ann Thorac Surg* 44(1):26, 1987.

46. Nash IS, Lorell BH, Fishman RF et al: A new technique for sheathless percutaneous intraaortic balloon catheter placement, *Cathet Cardiovasc Diagn* 23(1):57, 1991.
47. Grayzel J: Clinical evaluation of the Percor percutaneous intraaortic balloon: cooperative study of 722 cases, *Circulation* 66(suppl I):I-223, 1982.
48. Lefemine AA, Kosowsky B, Madoff I et al: Results and complications of intraaortic balloon pumping in surgical and medical patients, *Am J Cardiol* 40:416, 1977.
49. Lundell DC, Hammond GL, Geha AS et al: Randomized comparison of the modified wire-guided and standard intra-aortic balloon catheters, *J Thorac Cardiovasc Surg* 81(2):297, 1981.
50. Sturm JT, McGee MG, Fuhrman TM et al: Treatment of postoperative low output syndrome with intraaortic balloon pumping: experience with 419 patients, *Am J Cardiol* 45(5):1033, 1980.
51. Todd GJ, Bregman D, Voorhees AB et al: Vascular complications associated with percutaneous intra-aortic balloon pumping, *Arch Surg* 118:963, 1983.
52. Vignola PA, Swaye PS, Gosselin AJ: Guidelines for effective and safe percutaneous intraaortic balloon pump insertion and removal, *Am J Cardiol* 48:660, 1981.
53. Scheidt S: Preservation of ischemic myocardium with intraaortic balloon pumping: modern therapeutic intervention or primum non nocere? *Circulation* 58(2):211, 1978 (editorial).
54. Mills JL, Wiedeman JE, Robison JG et al: Minimizing mortality and morbidity from iatrogenic arterial injuries: the need for early recognition and prompt repair, *J Vasc Surg* 4(1):22, 1986.
55. Webster H, Veasy LG: Intra-aortic balloon pumping in children, *Heart Lung* 14(6):548, 1985.
56. Berg GA, Reece IJ, Davidson KG et al: Recent clinical experience with percutaneous intra-aortic balloon pumping, *Life Support Sys* 4(3):249, 1986.
57. Glenville B, Crockett JR, Bennett JG: Compartment syndrome and intraaortic balloon, *Thorac Cardiovasc Surg* 34(5):292, 1986.
58. Gold JP, Cohen J, Shemin RJ et al: Femorofemoral bypass to relieve acute leg ischemia during intra-aortic balloon pump cardiac support, *J Vasc Surg* 3(2):351, 1986.
59. Harris RE, Reimer KA, Crain BJ et al: Spinal cord infarction following intraaortic balloon support, *Ann Thorac Surg* 42:206, 1986.
60. Massey JA: Diagnostic testing for peripheral vascular disease, *Nurs Clin North Am* 21:207, 1986.
61. Felix WR, Barsamian E, Silverman AB: Long-term follow-up of limbs after use of intra-aortic balloon counter-pulsation device, *Surgery* 91(2):183, 1982.
62. Limet R, Demoulin JC, Fourny J: Five years experience with intraaortic balloon pumping: the changing of indications and the emergence of prognostic indices, *Acta Cardiol* 35(2):121, 1980.
63. Opie JC, Zavitzanos J, Bell-Thompson J: A simple "solution" worth consideration to combat limb ischemia induced by intra-aortic balloon pumping, *J Thorac Cardiovasc Surg* 98(2):295, 1989.
64. Hauser AM, Gordon S, Gangadharan V et al: Percutaneous intraaortic balloon counterpulsation: clinical effectiveness and hazards, *Chest* 82(4):422, 1982.
65. Pennington DG, Swartz M, Codd JE et al: Intraaortic balloon pumping in cardiac surgical patients: a nine-year experience, *Ann Thorac Surg* 36(2):125, 1983.
66. Di Lello F, Mullen DC, Flemma RJ et al: Results of intraaortic balloon pumping after cardiac surgery: experience with the Percor balloon catheter, *Ann Thorac Surg* 46(4):442, 1988.
67. Perler BA, McCabe CJ, Abbott WM et al: Vascular complications of intra-aortic balloon counterpulsation, *Arch Surg* 118:957, 1983.
68. Golding LA, Loop FD, Peter M et al: Late survival following use of intraaortic balloon pump in revascularization operations, *Ann Thorac Surg* 30(1):48, 1980.
69. Baciewicz FA, Kaplan BM, Murphy TE et al: Bilateral renal artery thrombotic occlusion: a unique complication following removal of a transthoracic intraaortic balloon, *Ann Thorac Surg* 33(6):631, 1982.
70. Gonzalez M, Installe E, Tremouroux J: Percutaneous intraaortic balloon pumping: initial experience, *Intensive Care Med* 8:143, 1982.
71. Singh AK, Williams DO, Cooper GN et al: Percutaneous vs. surgical placement of intra-aortic balloon assist, *Cathet Cardiovasc Diagn* 8:519, 1982.
72. Kahn JK, Rutherford BD, McConahay DR et al: Supported "high risk" coronary angioplasty using intraaortic balloon pump counterpulsation, *J Am Coll Cardiol* 15(5):1151, 1990.

73. Jarmolowski CR, Poirer RL: Small bowel infarction complicating intra-aortic balloon counterpulsation via the ascending aorta, *J Thorac Cardiovasc Surg* 79:735, 1980.

74. Bardet J, Masquet C, Kahn J-C et al: Clinical and hemodynamic results of intra-aortic balloon counterpulsation and surgery for cardiogenic shock, *Am Heart J* 93(3):280, 1977.

75. Busch HM, Cogbill TH, Gundersen AE: Splenic infarction: complication of intra-aortic balloon counterpulsation, *Am Heart J* 109(2):383, 1985.

76. Meldrum-Hanna WG, Deal CW, Ross DE: Complications of ascending aortic intraaortic balloon pump cannulation, *Ann Thorac Surg* 40(3):241, 1985.

77. Rose DM, Jacobowitz IJ, Acinapura AJ et al: Paraplegia following percutaneous insertion of an intra-aortic balloon, *J Thorac Cardiovasc Surg* 87(5):788, 1984.

78. Tyras DH, Willman VL: Paraplegia following intraaortic balloon assistance, *Ann Thorac Surg* 25(2):164, 1978.

79. Riggle KP, Oddi MA: Spinal cord necrosis and paraplegia as complications of the intra-aortic balloon, *Crit Care Med* 17(5):475, 1989.

80. Orr E, McKittrick J, D'Agostino R et al: Paraplegia following intra-aortic balloon support, *J Cardiovasc Surg* 30(6):1013, 1989.

81. Scott IR, Goiti JJ: Late paraplegia as a consequence of intraaortic balloon pump support, *Ann Thorac Surg* 40(3):300, 1985.

82. Seifert PE, Silverman NA: Late paraplegia resulting from intraaortic balloon pump, *Ann Thorac Surg* 41(6):700, 1986.

83. Mubarak S, Hargens A: *Compartment syndrome and Volkman's contracture*, Philadelphia, 1981, WB Saunders.

84. Conry K, Bies C: Compartment syndrome: a complication of IABP, *Dimens Crit Care Nurs* 4(5):274, 1985.

85. Matsen F: *Compartmental syndromes*, New York, 1980, Grune & Stratton.

86. Biddle TL, Stewart S, Stuard ID: Dissection of the aorta complicating intra-aortic balloon counterpulsation, *Am Heart J* 92(6):781, 1976.

87. Myhre OA, Silverman ED, Tang D: Mechanical problems in the use of the intra-aortic balloon, *Int Surg* 64(2):57, 1979.

88. Bolooki H: Current status of circulatory support with an intra-aortic balloon pump, *Med Instrument* 20(5):266, 1986.

89. Macmanus Q, Lefrak EA: Pseudoaneurysm following balloon counterpulsation, *Virginia Med* 109:471, 1982.

90. Di Bari M, De Alfieri W, Greppi B et al: Intra-aortic balloon pumping in the elderly: percutaneous versus surgical catheter insertion, *Eur Heart J* 5:222, 1984.

91. Downing TP, Miller DC, Stinson EB et al: Therapeutic efficacy of intraaortic balloon pump counterpulsation: analysis with concurrent "control" subjects, *Circulation* 64(suppl II):II-108, 1981.

92. Lauwers E, Meese G, Adriaensen H et al: Perioperative intra-aortic balloon counterpulsation in cardiosurgery: a retrospective study, *Acta Anaesthesiol Belg* 41(1):41, 1990.

93. Archie JP, Mann JT: Infected femoral arteriovenous fistula after percutaneous insertion of an intra-aortic balloon, *South Med J* 82(6):778, 1989.

94. Grantham RN, Munnell ER, Kanaly PJ: Femoral artery infection complicating intraaortic balloon pumping, *Am J Surg* 146(6):811, 1983.

95. Hines GL, Delaney TB, Goodman M et al: Intra-aortic balloon pumping: two-year experience, *J Thorac Cardiovasc Surg* 78(1):140, 1979.

96. Youkey JR, Clagett GP, Rich NM et al: Vascular trauma secondary to diagnostic and therapeutic procedures: 1974 through 1982, *Am J Surg* 146(6):788, 1983.

97. Tamez A, Cooper DK, Novitzky D et al: Experience with cardiorespiratory support devices in patients undergoing heart and heart-lung transplantation, *J Okla State Med Assoc* 83(9):449, 1990.

98. Rutala WA, Weber DJ, Thomann CA et al: An outbreak of *Pseudomonas cepacia* bacteremia associated with a contaminated intra-aortic balloon pump, *J Thorac Cardiovasc Surg* 96(1):157, 1988.

99. Sutter FP, Joyce DH, Bailey BM et al: Events associated with rupture of intra-aortic balloon counterpulsation devices, *ASAIO Trans* 37:38, 1991.

100. Stahl KD, Tortolani AJ, Nelson RL et al: Intraaortic balloon rupture, *ASAIO Trans* 34(3):496, 1988.
101. Aru GM, King JT, Hovaguimian H et al: The entrapped balloon: report of a possibly serious complication, *J Thorac Cardiovasc Surg* 91(1):146, 1986.
102. Brodell GK, Tuzcu EM, Weiss SJ et al: Intra-aortic balloon-pump rupture and entrapment, *Cleve Clin J Med* 56(7):740, 1989.
103. Mayerhofer KE, Billhardt RA, Codini MA: Delayed abrasion perforation of two intra-aortic balloons, *Am Heart J* 108(5):1361, 1984.
104. Nishizawa J, Konishi Y, Matsumoto M et al: Intraaortic balloon entrapment: a case report and a review of the literature, *Jpn Circ J* 55(6):563, 1991.
105. Rajani R, Keon WJ, Bedard P: Rupture of an intra-aortic balloon, *J Thorac Cardiovasc Surg* 79:301, 1980.
106. Vicente JR, Moreno E, Penas L et al: Spontaneous rupture of an intra-aortic balloon pump, *Intens Care Med* 7:311, 1981.
107. How to detect if the balloon bursts? *Today's OR Nurse* 12(9):35, 1990.
108. Karayannacos PE, Shapiro IL, Kakos GS et al: Counterpulsation catheter fracture: an unexpected hazard, *Ann Thorac Surg* 23(3):276, 1977.
109. Finegan BA, Comm DG: Operative intra-aortic balloon rupture, *Can J Anaesthesiol* 35[3(pt 1)]:297, 1988.
110. Grotte GJ, Butchart EG: Impaction of intra-aortic balloon due to dislocation of central stylet, *J Thorac Cardiovasc Surg* 80(2):228, 1980.
111. Milgalter E, Mosseri M, Uretzky G et al: Intraaortic balloon entrapment: a complication of balloon perforation, *Ann Thorac Surg* 42(6):697, 1986.
112. Millham FH, Hudson HM, Woodson J et al: Intraaortic balloon pump entrapment, *Ann Vasc Surg* 5:381, 1991.
113. Frederiksen JW, Smith J, Brown P et al: Arterial helium embolism from a ruptured intraaortic balloon, *Ann Thorac Surg* 46(6):690, 1988.
114. Goodwin M, Hartmann J, McKeever L et al: Safety of intra-aortic balloon counterpulsation in patients with acute myocardial infarction receiving streptokinase intravenously, *Am J Cardiol* 64(14):937, 1989.
115. Chiles C, Vail CM, Coblentz CL et al: Intra-aortic balloon pumps: an update on radiographic recognition, *Can Assoc Radiol J* 42(4):257, 1991.
116. Rodigas PC, Bridges KG: Occlusion of the left internal mammary artery with intra-aortic balloon: clinical implications, *J Thorac Cardiovasc Surg* 91(1):142, 1986.
117. Haykal HA, Wang A-M: CT diagnosis of delayed cerebral air embolism following intraaortic balloon pump catheter insertion, *Comput Radiol* 10(6):307, 1986.
118. Delirium common in intraaortic balloon pump users, *Intern Med News* 34, December 15-31, 1991.
119. Goran SF: Vascular complications of the patient undergoing intra-aortic balloon pumping, *Crit Care Nurs Clin North Am* 1(3):459, 1989.

CHAPTER **11**

Ocular pneumoplethysmography in IABC

James F. Reed III, William Gee, and **Marie G. Witham**

Candidates for operative coronary artery bypass have the presence of asymptomatic carotid lesions of hemodynamic consequence as a risk factor. Balderman and associates described ocular pneumoplethysmography (OPG-Gee)* as a simple, rapid, economical means of screening for such lesions before cardiac operation.[1] We maintained a similar surveillance during May 1985 through October 1991, which included 158 patients who were being supported preoperatively with intraaortic balloon counterpulsation (IABC).

The principal role of the OPG has been the simultaneous bilateral measurement of ophthalmic systolic pressures (OSP) for comparison with a brachial systolic pressure (BSP) in the form of ophthalmobrachial systolic pressure (OBSP) indices, as calculated by the formula[5]

$$OBSP = OSP - 39.0 - 0.43 \, BSP$$

Of lesser importance has been the calculation of ocular blood flow (OBF) from these tests. The present report describes our observations related to OBF in these 158 patients and especially the considerable difference noted with and without IABC assistance.

METHODS AND MATERIALS

Standard OPG tests were performed in the 158 patients with the intraaortic balloon pump (IABP) turned on and then repeated with the IABP turned off. The terminal segments of the latter tests were modified by placing the decline of the intraocular pressures on hold, electronically magnifying the height of the ocular pulse waves by a factor of 3, and increasing the paper speed by a factor of 10. This re-

This work was supported by grants from the Dorothy Rider Pool Health Care Trust and the Pennsylvania Fraternal Order of Eagles—Max Baer Heart Research Grant.
*Type of OPG developed by William Gee, M.D.

sulted in an ocular pulse wave area magnification of thirtyfold. The tests were continued for a brief interval with the IABP turned on.

A Digisonics planimeter (digitized tablet) was used to measure the areas of all waves except the single waves in each eye at IABC initiation in square centimeters (cm^2). In addition, the ocular pulse waves during IABC were partitioned with a vertical line separating the areas resulting from cardiac thrust and the areas resulting from balloon thrust.

OBF is a product of the pulse rate per minute, the maximum volume-calibrated ocular pulse amplitude in millimeters and a constant derived by combining the volume calibration, the conversion factor and the surface area factor (OBF = PR × OPA × 0.00149). This geometry is described in detail elsewhere.[6] OBF during IABC was then calculated as the product of OBF off IABC times the ratio of area estimates of the ocular pulse waves on and off IABC.

At the end of each of the OPG tests in all patients, a brachial blood pressure was measured with a standard brachial cuff and stethoscope. The pulse rate and maximum ocular pulse amplitude from the initial unmagnified segments of the OPG tests without IABC were tabulated. The OSPs and the heart rates from the tests in each patient were also tabulated.

Descriptive statistics and paired t-tests were used to analyze the data. A Bonferroni-adjusted significance level of 0.005 was used to compensate for type I errors because of multiple significance tests.

RESULTS

Systemic pressure data are contained in Table 11-1. The pulse pressures equal the differences between the respective brachial systolic and diastolic pressures. The mean of the pulse pressures during IABC was 16.7% less than that without IABC.

Table 11-2 contains the ocular pulse wave areas measured with the Digisonics planimeter. The mean of the wave areas during IABC was 25% less than that with-

Table 11-1.   Systemic pressure data

	IABP-on		IABP-off	
	Mean	sem	Mean	sem
BSP	118.0	1.3	120.3	1.3
BDP	77.1	1.0	71.4*	0.9
PP	40.8	1.1	49.0†	1.1

*t = 7.49, p <0.001, IABP-on vs. IABP-off.
†t = 7.72, p <0.001, IABP-on vs. IABP-off.
sem, standard error of the mean; *BSP*, brachial systolic pressure, mm Hg; *BDP*, brachial diastolic pressure, mm Hg; *PP*, pulse pressure, mm Hg. The pulse pressure is reduced by 16.7% during IABC.

Table 11-2.   Ocular wave areas (cm^2)★

	Mean	sem
IABP-off	7.71†	0.24
IABP-on	5.78	0.24
During cardiac thrust	1.62	0.24
During balloon thrust	4.16	0.24

★Ocular pulse wave area measurements, in square centimeters (cm^2), with and without IABC. Wave areas during IABC are further partitioned into the areas attributable to the cardiac thrust vs. the areas resulting from balloon thrust.
†t = 14.09, $p < 0.001$, IABP-on vs. IABP-off.
sem, standard error of the mean.

out IABC. The partitioned areas during IABC demonstrate that only 28% was the result of cardiac thrust, whereas 72% was the result of balloon thrust.

In Table 11-3 only the OBF without IABC was calculated as previously described. The observed figure of 0.93 ml/min is 85.3% of the 1.09 ml/min noted in 531 individuals previously reported.[6] The remaining OBFs are proportional to the ocular pulse wave areas described in Table 11-2.

The mean of the OSPs, with and without IABC, were 97.2 mm Hg and 100 mm Hg, respectively. Although the difference of 2.8 mm Hg was significant ($p < 0.001$), this difference is not considered to have clinical consequence. The mean of the heart rates with and without IABC were 78.5 and 77.8, respectively. The difference of 0.7 was not significant ($p = 0.091$).

Of the 158 patients studied, 143 (110 males, 33 females) experienced an average 31.3% decline of OBF during IABC, as compared with that without IABC. Twelve patients (7 males, 5 females) had an average 13.4% increase of OBF during IABC, as compared with that without IABC. There was no change of OBF in three patients (1 male, 2 females). The example in Fig. 11-1 is from a patient in whom there was a 3% increase in OBF on IABC; Fig. 11-2 is from a patient in whom there was a 30% decrease in OBF on IABC.

Table 11-3.   OBF (ml/min/1.9 g tissue)★

	Mean	sem
IABP-off	0.93†	0.03
IABP-on	0.67	0.02
During cardiac thrust	0.19	0.01
During balloon thrust	0.48	0.01

★OBF in milliliters per minute per 1.9 g of tissue (OBF: ml/min/1.9 g tissue) without IABC was calculated as described in the text. Remaining OBFs reflect ocular pulse wave area comparisons in Table 11-2.
†t = 12.38, $p < 0.001$, IABP-on vs. IABP-off.
sem, standard error of the mean.

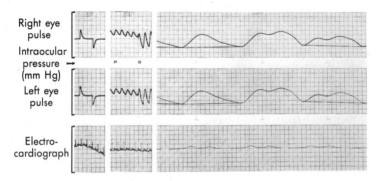

Fig. 11-1. Amplitude of ocular pulse waves typically reaches maximum about 60 mm Hg IOP. Initial segment of recording documents calibration of ocular pulse wave channels, in which first (positive) pen deflection is 10 mm, reflecting volume change of 1.0 mm^3, followed by negative wave of equal amplitude, when piston in calibrating chamber is withdrawn. Second segment of tracings focuses on IOP recording between two eye-pulse channels. IOP shown was 60 mm Hg, followed by 1 dot, with each dot interval representing 2 mm Hg. Thus IOP was maintained at 58 mm Hg during remainder of test. Thereafter *x3* symbol indicates point at which ocular pulse waves were electronically magnified by factor of 3, as shown in two ocular pulse wave channels. Thereafter paper speed was increased tenfold from 10 to 100 mm/sec. Amplitude and speed magnifications result in area magnification of ocular pulse waves by factor of 30. Third segment of test demonstrates three consecutive ocular pulse waves in both channels. First pair of waves reflect terminal waves obtained with IABC off, followed by pair of transition waves during which IABC was activated. Final pair of waves were initial waves obtained during IABC assistance. Average area for all waves during IABC exceeded average area for all waves without IABC by 3%. In 12 of 158 patients, increase of OBF during IABC was observed.

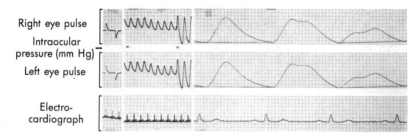

Fig. 11-2. Same sequence as in Fig. 11-1 applies here. Note that IOP of 70 mm Hg is followed by 4 dots, which indicates remainder of test was obtained at IOP of 62 mm Hg. Average area for all waves during IABC was 30% less than average area for waves noted without IABC. In 143 of 158 patients, decrease of OBF during IABC was noted.

SUMMARY

Previous observations in 56 patients not included in the present group demonstrated an overall reduction of OBF during IABC of 11.6%.[4] In the present group this overall reduction was 25%. Table 11-4 compares the previous and present groups. There is little variation in the OBF change, increased or decreased, between the two groups. However, in the present group, the percentage of patients in whom an OBF reduction was observed is considerably larger than that noted in the previous group. Conversely, the percentage of patients with unchanged or increased OBF during IABP in the previous group was over twice that observed in the present group.

The reduction of OBF during IABC does not imply a reduction of cardiac index but more probably reflects a redistribution phenomenon, which has been suggested by animal investigations in which a reduction of CBF of 10% was noted during IABC, in association with increased visceral blood flow and no change in cardiac index.[9]

In comparing the systemic and ocular hemodynamic data in the 158 patients, IABP-on/IABP-off, the two major changes noted were those of OBF and systemic pulse pressure reduction during IABC.

OBF is primarily derived from the ophthalmic arteries, the first major tributaries of the internal carotid arteries as they enter the calvarium. Unlike peripheral extremity arterial flow in which reversal of flow is noted in diastole, the low resistance to arterial flow in the ocular and cerebral circuits ensures forward flow throughout the cardiac cycle under normal circumstances. However, transcranial Doppler (TCD) spectral analysis has demonstrated reversal of intracranial arterial flow during diastole in patients with increased cerebrovascular resistance as a result of increased intracranial pressure.[7] More recently, Brass described his TCD observations in three patients supported with IABC.[3] These patients had normal TCD examinations without IABC. During IABC, two of the three patients had reversal of arterial flow in late diastole at the time of balloon deflation. Our data suggest that a larger series of patients tested with TCD would demonstrate reversal of intracranial arterial flow during IABC in more than two thirds of those studied.

Table 11-4.   OBF, IABP-on/IABP-off

	Total patients	OBF Decreased			OBF Unchanged		OBF Increased		
		Number of patients	Percent of total	OBF decreased	Number of Patients	Percent of total	Number of patients	Percent of total	OBF Increased
Previous group	56	41	73.2	24.1	2	3.6	13	23.2	26.0
Present group	158	143	90.5	31.3	3	1.9	12	7.6	13.4

Kantrowitz and associates reported on the complications associated with IABC in 733 patients.[8] Neurological complications were observed in 25 (3.4%). However, all of these complications were related to some form of peripheral nerve ischemia, and there were no central nervous system complications reported, not even in the 45 patients (6.1%) who had preexisting cerebrovascular accidents. Although gaseous and particulate emboli have been identified as causes of isolated cerebrovascular accidents in association with IABC, hypoperfusion has not been suggested as an etiological agent. In patients with well-compensated asymptomatic brachiocephalic arterial lesions of hemodynamic consequence, these lesions may remain adequately compensated even during cardiogenic shock. If symptoms of ocular or brain ischemia develop during IABC support of such patients, these symptoms may be secondary to hypoperfusion rather than emboli. The OPG test provides a rapid (45 seconds) bedside assessment of this possibility.

OBF in animals has been extensively summarized by Bill.[2] In three species of animals (rabbit, cat, and monkey), conscious and anesthetized, the average OBF was 1 ml per minute. Of this amount, only 2% is delivered to the autoregulated retinal flow, whereas 80% is routed to the choroid, which is not autoregulated. Thus the 25% reduction of ocular blood flow during IABC in the 158 patients reflects primarily the effort of IABC on a vascular bed of the internal carotid arteries, which is not autoregulated. This does not suggest that the autoregulated retinal and cerebral vascular beds are similarly affected, but a diminished autoregulatory reserve is probable.

REFERENCES

1. Balderman SC, Gutierrez IZ, Makula P, et al: Noninvasive screening for asymptomatic carotid artery disease prior to cardiac operation, *J Thorac Cardiovasc Surg* 85:427, 1983.
2. Bill A: Circulation in the eye. In Renkin EM and Michel CC, eds: *Handbook of physiology*, vol IV, American Physiological Society, 1984, Bethesda, Md.
3. Brass LM: Reversed intracranial blood flow in patients with an intra-aortic balloon pump, *Stroke* 21:484, 1990.
4. Gee W, Smith RL, Perline RK et al: Assessment of intra-aortic balloon pumping by ocular pneumoplethysmography, *Am Surg* 52:489, 1986.
5. Gee W, Lucke JF, Madden AE: Collateral compensation of severe carotid stenosis, *Eur J Vasc Surg* 3:297, 1989.
6. Gee W, Reed III Jf: Ocular pneumoplethysmographic evaluation of carotid lesions: Gee method. In Ernst CB, Stanley JC, eds: *Current therapy in vascular surgery*, ed 2, Philadelphia, 1991, BC Decker.
7. Hassler W, Steinmetz H, Gawlowski J: Transcranial doppler ultrasound in raised intracranial pressure and in intracranial circulatory arrest, *J Neurosurg* 68:745, 1988.
8. Kantrowitz A, Wasfie T, Freed PS et al: Intra-aortic balloon pumping 1967 through 1982: analysis of complications in 733 patients, *Am J Cardiol* 57:976, 1986.
9. Oster H, Stanley TH, Olsen DB et al: Regional blood flow after intra-aortic balloon pumping before and after cardiogenic shock, *Trans Am Soc Artif Intern Organs* 20:721, 1974.

CHAPTER 12

Balloon insertion techniques

Susan J. Quaal

INTRAAORTIC BALLOON REQUIREMENTS

Balloon materials, their mechanical and biological durability, threats of pyrogenicity, thrombogenicity, and hemolysis have all influenced intraaortic balloon (IAB) research, design and fabrication. Since the atherosclerotic aorta is considered a "hostile environment," the IAB must be designed with those characteristics that will allow it to perform safely and effectively in this milieu. Wolvek[1] provided a nice account of balloon requirements as follows:

The balloon does not operate in a benign environment. It is used in patients with vascular disease, whose aortas may contain considerable atheromatous plaque in various stages of calcification. On post mortem these plaques feel flat and rough to the gloved hand. Sometimes they resemble sharp spicules, not unlike broken eggshells. In a patient with a heart rate of 100 bpm the balloon may inflate 144,000 times every 24 hours. The constant abrasion of the balloon membrane against the calcific plaque lining a sick aorta may cause a pinhole penetration of the balloon membrane.

The hostile environment in which the IAB must operate, posing the threat of abrasion and of ultimate perforation, and the convolutions it must follow in that environment have created several opposing requirements for the materials employed in its fabrication. The balloon material should be thin and pliable enough to be wrapped to an extremely small diameter, yet it must not be distensible in order to insure its inflated geometry and volume. At the same time, it must be hard enough to resist abrasion, but must also possess an extremely long fatigue life. In addition, it must be highly resistant to thrombus formation. Finally, it must be biologically acceptable to the body and be capable of fabrication into the rather complex geometry of a balloon catheter.

The first decade of the IAB

By 1978 the state-of-the-art IAB was a sausage-shaped inflatable membrane approximately 24 cm long by 16 cm in diameter attached over one end of a 12-Fr catheter. The balloon was made from an extremely tough, flexible, nondistensible polyurethane membrane, which was distensible to ensure its geometry and 40 cc volume. A series of holes in the catheter lying within the balloon permitted the driving gas (initially carbon dioxide and later helium) to rapidly inflate and deflate the balloon in counterpulsation with the left ventricle, as commanded by the balloon pump consoles.[1] IAB insertion required surgical exposure of the patient's femoral artery and an arteriotomy.

SURGICAL CUTDOWN INSERTION*

After application of a local anesthesic with 2% lidocaine, the femoral pulse is felt and a longitudinal skin incision is made over the course of the vessel. The incision begins approximately 2 cm above the inguinal (Poupart's) ligament and extends for 10 to 12 cm. Dissection is directed toward the femoral pulse, and the vascular fascia (femoral sheath) is opened lateral to femoral lymph nodes and fat pad. The femoral artery is exposed above the profunda branch. At this area, the femoral artery usually has a slight dilatation. Two umbilical tapes are placed around the common femoral artery, one above the profunda branch and another just below the inguinal ligament. A few fibers of the inguinal ligament may be cut to expose the uppermost point of the common femoral artery. At this time the femoral artery is palpated to evaluate the extent of the disease within its lumen.

With a retractor on the top, pulling the inguinal ligament upward, the common femoral artery is dissected and exposed for an approximate length of 5 cm. There are usually three small arterial branches that need dissection: superficial, deep circumflex iliac arteries (dissected laterally), and external pudendal (dissected from the medial aspect of the femoral artery). These branches are preserved by a No. 2-0 black silk wrapped twice around each branch to control the retrograde bleeding. Heparin is given intravenously at this time at a dose of approximately 5 cc for a 70-kg patient and, within 4 to 5 minutes (because of slow circulation), a vascular occluding clamp is placed over the common femoral artery distally. The umbilical tape over the proximal end of the artery is passed through a rubber keeper. A longitudinal arteriotomy is done for a length of approximately 15 mm.

Before insertion of the balloon catheter, a number of precautions are taken. Always test the balloon by injecting approximately 50 cc of air into the balloon catheter and hold it for a few seconds. Second, the balloon, while inflated, is inserted in a basin of saline to check for air leaks. Third, the required length of the balloon catheter is sized. This is done by placing the tip of the balloon over the sterile drapes at the level of the sternum at the second intercostal space (the angle of Louis) and extending the balloon catheter over the umbilicus and toward the incision over the femoral artery. The point at which the balloon catheter should remain outside of the skin incision is marked with a heavy black silk tie. This tie should remain outside of

---

*Summarized with permission from Bolooki H: *Clinical application of intra-aortic balloon pump*, ed 2, Mt Kisko, NY, 1984, Futura Publishing.

the skin incision. A 10-mm woven Teflon® graft is cut at this time in a beveled fashion and is placed over the balloon catheter. Alternatively, the upper end of the saphenous vein of the same leg may be used instead of a graft. This is because the incidence of clot formation around the junction of the graft and artery is minimal, and after removal of the catheter the vein can be used as a patch over the arteriotomy.

The balloon catheter is introduced into the femoral artery after an angle is introduced over the proximal end of the catheter and while the proximal umbilical tape is released. Once the balloon catheter is within the lumen of the femoral artery, a twisting maneuver is necessary to advance it into the aorta. Depending on the extent of iliac artery disease, insertion may be smooth or impossible.

Once the balloon catheter is in the descending aorta, a few maneuvers are necessary to ensure its position. First, the balloon must be inserted until the black tie marker over the distal end of the catheter reaches the skin level. Second, at times one may feel the tip of the balloon catheter hitting the arch of the aorta. Third, once in a while, one may be able to enter the subclavian artery at which time a decrease in the pulse pressure in the left radial artery pressure line is seen on the monitor, indicating that the balloon catheter is at the junction of the aorta and the subclavian artery. In such a case, the balloon catheter should be pulled out approximately 2 cm and then tied into position. A chest x-ray examination is performed after insertion to ensure correct balloon positioning.

Once the balloon catheter is in position, balloon pumping may be initiated immediately while the graft is sewn over the femoral artery. The graft or the saphenous vein (beveled and cut longitudinally for a length of 5 to 6 mm) is sewn with a 5-0 monofilament suture taken in a standard fashion of vascular anastomosis from the base of the graft to the femoral artery, advancing proximally. To prevent bleeding, two umbilical tapes are tied around the graft (or one heavy silk tie around the vein) and the balloon catheter tightly, ensuring correct folding of the graft over the catheter. These ties are placed approximately 1 cm above the anastomosis of the graft (or vein to the artery) (Fig. 12-1). Just before tying the graft or the vein around the catheter, the distal clamp over the femoral artery should be removed to allow any clots and air to evacuate from the artery and the graft. The ties around the branches of the femoral artery are also released to allow bleeding into the graft. Once the umbilical tapes around the graft are securely tied, the proximal tape is removed. At that point the physician should attempt to palpate a distal femoral pulse from within the incision. Presence of a weak femoral pulse initially is satisfactory, because it will most likely improve in the next few hours if IABC is effective.

Before insertion of the intraaortic balloon, the area of the dorsalis pedis pulse is marked over the foot. Immediately after insertion of the balloon catheter and release of the femoral artery ties, this pulse is palpated to assess for adequacy of circulation to the foot.

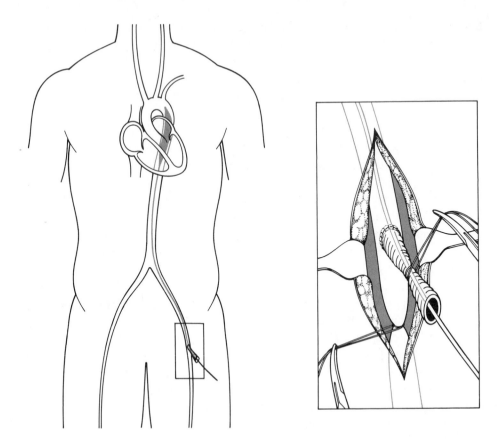

Fig. 12-1. IAB inserted through Dacron side-arm graft and passed retrogradely into descending thoracic aorta to position in situ just below bifurcation of left subclavian artery.

At this time, the groin incision is closed by standard techniques. The balloon catheter is always secured to the skin of the thigh with an additional skin suture, and one must ensure that its position will not change.

Balloon removal

Removal of an IAB inserted surgically through a femoral artery graft necessitates reopening of the surgical wound. The ligature securing the graft to balloon is cut. The balloon is disconnected from the driving console and permitted to vent to atmosphere under the impetus of central aortic blood pressure before removal. Another practice consists of evacuating the balloon by attaching a syringe to the balloon pump connector on the end of the catheter and withdrawing the plunger. After balloon removal, a Fogerty catheter is sometimes passed into the distal femoral artery to remove any suspected thrombi. After the balloon is removed, the graft is oversewn, buried in the leg incision, and the wound is surgically closed.

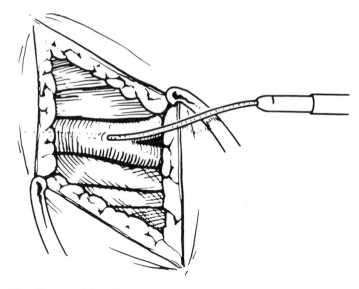

Fig. 12-2. The dilator and introducer sheath are introduced over the guidewire into the exposed common femoral artery. (From Heberle RF: *Ann Thorac Surg* 48:134, 1989.)

Simplified technique for surgical placement and removal of a percutaneous IAB

Hebeler[2] suggested that direct placement of a percutaneous sheath in the common femoral artery can be accomplished after surgical exposure of the artery, rather than placement through an end-to-side prosthetic graft. However, both the transarterial and conventional graft technique require open removal and arterioplasty. Hebeler described a simplified IAB removal technique for patients without clinically significant anterior common femoral plaques; the procedure could be done briefly in the intensive care unit. Surgical insertion and removal of a percutaneous IAB as described below and accompanying illustrations are reproduced with permission from Hebeler RF: *Ann Thorac Surg* 48:134, 1989.

The common femoral artery is exposed through an oblique groin incision and is then punctured with a Cook or Cornan needle, and the J wire is threaded up the aortic arch (Fig. 12-2). Progressive dilatation of the arteriotomy is accomplished with graded plastic cannulas, and the deflated balloon is passed up to the appropriate distance. IABC is initiated, and a mattress or purse-string 5-0 monofilament suture is carefully placed around the introducer sheath (Fig. 12-3). The sheath may be removed with a Datascope sheath stripper to allow more flow in smaller arteries. The suture is then secured with a short, 2-inch, red rubber Rummel tourniquet and is fixed in place with several metal clips placed so as not to damage the suture (Fig. 12-4). The wound is then closed over the Rummel tourniquet and suture (Fig. 12-5).

For IAB removal, the patient receives a 1% Xylocaine (lidocaine) local anesthesic. The wound is prepared, draped, and opened. Systemic heparinization is not necessary in most

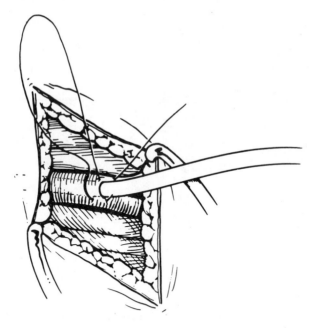

Fig. 12-3. A purse-string suture is placed around the sheath. (From Heberle RF: *Ann Thorac Surg* 48:134, 1989.)

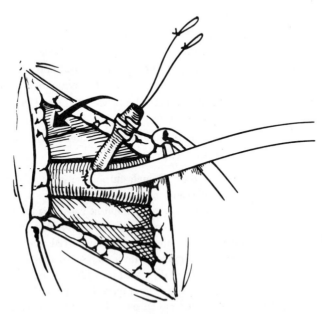

Fig. 12-4. A Rummel tourniquet securing the purse-string suture is placed into the wound. (From Heberle RF: *Ann Thorac Surg* 48:134, 1989.)

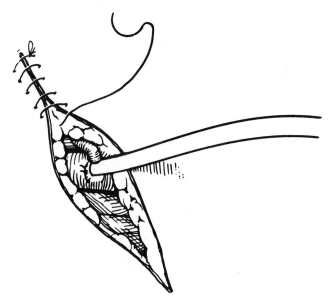

Fig. 12-5. The wound is closed over tourniquet. (From Heberle RF: *Ann Thorac Surg* 48:134, 1989.)

cases, because pumping is discontinued immediately before balloon removal. The tourniquet is released, the balloon is aspirated completely, and the balloon and sheath are then removed as a unit. The artery is flushed proximally and distally with digital pressure or vascular clamps (Fig. 12-6). The previously placed suture is then tied with minimal narrowing of the artery. If a thrombectomy is required, this can usually be performed through the arteriotomy without disruption of the suture. Additional sutures, if necessary, are easily placed.

Limitations to surgical insertion

As high as 28% of surgical cutdown insertion attempts have been unsuccessful.[3] Wolvek[1] stated:

Although the efficacy of intra-aortic balloon pumping had been established during the first decade of intra-aortic balloon pumping, the complexity, time requirements, and attendant risks of the required surgical insertion still denied balloon pumping to many patients. In addition, the limitations imposed by tortuous or atheromatous femoral/iliac arteries often prevented insertion and advancement of the relatively bulky IAB through the arteriotomy and into the thoracic aorta. It became clear that an easier method of balloon insertion was needed to make intra-aortic balloon pumping available to the large patient populations still being denied its advantages.

In the late 1970s a new catheter idea was conceived: "If one end of a balloon was allowed to rotate freely in relation to its other end, which remained fixed to its cath-

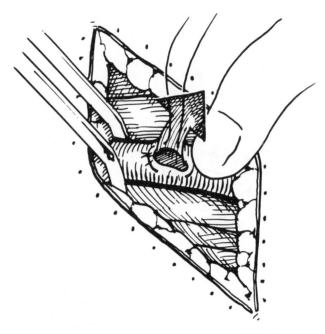

Fig. 12-6. The balloon is removed and femoral artery is flushed; suture is tied. (From Heberle RF: *Ann Thorac Surg* 48:134, 1989.)

eter, the balloon could be twisted on its own longitudinal axis to a diameter that was even smaller than that of the catheter itself."[1] This concept gave birth to the percutaneous IAB and nonsurgical insertion.

PERCUTANEOUS TECHNIQUE

Since 1979 percutaneous insertion has become the norm, offering less inherent delays in initiating IABC and extending applications to the community hospital setting,[4] where the IAB can be inserted by a cardiologist employing standard cath lab techniques. A central lumen guidewire facilitates insertion into atherosclerotic and tortuous vessels. Immediately after IAB insertion, pressure monitoring and injection of a contrast medium can be accomplished through the inner lumen of the dual catheter. Pressure monitoring permits immediate initiation of IAB pumping without having to wait for a radial artery cutdown.

Insertion

Balloon preparation and insertion should be undertaken in compliance with manufacturer's specific recommendations. The following information is provided

EQUIPMENT NEEDED FOR PERCUTANEOUS IAB INSERTION

Standard equipment	**Sterile insertion kit (items included may vary slightly among manufacturers)**
Sterile 4 × 4s	18-g angiographic needle
Ring forceps	J-tipped 120- or 145-cm guidewire
Povidone-iodine solution in sterile container	8-Fr dilator
	Introducer sheath with hemostasis valve
Sterile drapes	Introducer dilator
1% or 2% lidocaine without epinephrine	Three-way stopcock
Assorted needles and syringes	60-cc syringe
Three-way stopcock	Male leur plug
Heparinized saline in sterile bowl	Pressure tubing extension
No. 11 scalpel	Balloon pump connector
2-0 silk suture	
ECG and pressure monitoring equipment	
Defibrillator and cardiac arrest cart	
Portable fluoroscopy if insertion is at bedside	

as a tutorial guideline. Clinicians are advised to follow manufacturer's recommendations and hospital-specific procedures.

The box above suggests necessary equipment that should be assembled before insertion. The IAB is first prepared by rinsing in sterile saline solution to lubricate the IAB. The inner lumen is flushed with heparinized saline (Fig. 12-7). A 50-ml syringe is connected to the balloon port with a three-way stopcock or the one-way valve supplied in the insertion kit. The syringe plunger is gently withdrawn to cre-

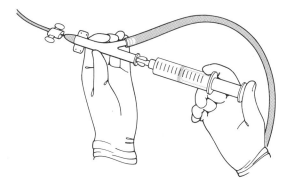

Fig. 12-7. The balloon's inner cannula is flushed with heparinized saline.

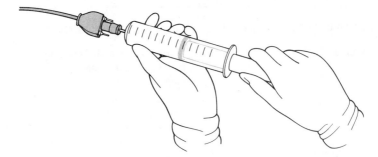

Fig. 12-8. Attach a 50 ml syringe with one-way valve (provided by manufacturer in insertion kit) or Luer-Lok syringe to balloon connector. Immediately before insertion, a vacuum is established by withdrawing plunger out of the barrel of the syringe.

ate a vacuum within the balloon, which reduces its bulk for insertion (Fig. 12-8).

Benn and Feldman[5] explicitly describe percutaneous insertion technique, which is reproduced with permission of the authors and *J Crit Illness* 7:435, 1992, and updated by Sydney Wolvek, Director of Scientific Research, Datascope Corp.

1. The ilioinguinal area is shaved, cleaned with iodine, and sterilely draped.
2. A local anesthetic is infiltrated into the area of the femoral artery just below the inguinal ligament.
3. The front wall of the artery is punctured with an angiographic needle (Fig. 12-9, *A*). The angle of the needle stick should be kept as shallow as possible. A shallow angle of entry will help prevent catheter kinking at the insertion site. Arterial penetration is immediately recognized by spurting of bright red blood from the needle hub. A J-tipped guidewire, supplied with the balloon, is then passed into the thoracic descending aorta (Fig. 12-9, *B*). The caliber of this guidewire varies from .030 to .035 inch, depending on the IAB manufacturer. The J-tip ensures that the wire will turn back on itself if it meets an obstruction or an impassable bend in the arterial vessel. Always use the guidewire supplied by the manufacturer in the insertion kit, since that guidewire has sufficient body and stiffness to ensure that the balloon will track over the wire and not take its own lead. The needle is removed over the wire while the wire position is maintained (Fig. 12-9, *C*). This guidewire is then wiped down with a wet, 4 × 4 sponge.
4. The skin at the guidewire exit point, approximately 1.5 cm below the inguinal ligament, is nicked with a No. 11 surgical blade (Fig. 12-10) to permit easier insertion of the dilator and introducer.
5. Arterial dilators of progressively increasing size are passed over the guidewire to facilitate subsequent passage of the IAB sheath. Dilators enlarge the arterial wall hole made by the needle. Wolvek[5] describes predilatation as one of the most important steps that can be taken to prevent bleeding at the insertion site,

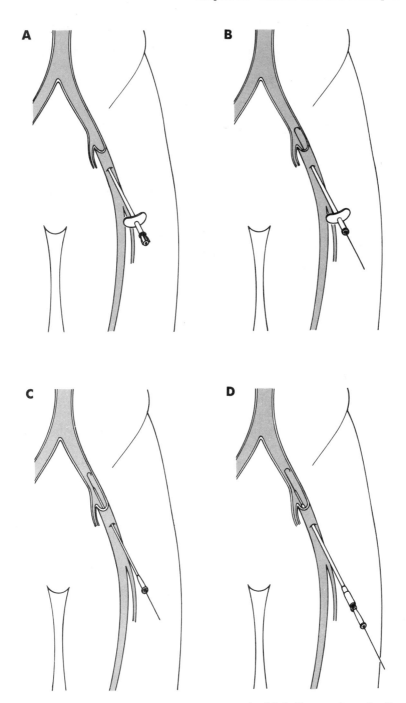

Fig. 12-9. A, Front wall of femoral artery punctured with hollow steel needle. **B,** J-tipped guidewire passed into the thoracic descending aorta. **C,** The needle is removed over the guidewire while the guidewire's position is maintained. **D,** Sheath is positioned over the guidewire.

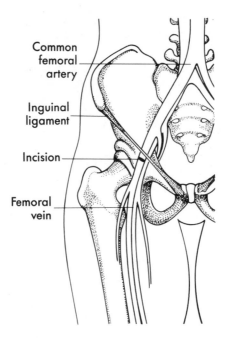

Common
femoral
artery

Inguinal
ligament

Incision

Femoral
vein

Fig. 12-10. Schematic illustration of location of skin incision approximately 1.5 cm below the inguinal ligament.

reducing the potential for hematoma and preventing the introducer sheath from crimping during entry. Careful predilatation will gently stretch the artery to permit catheter passage rather than risk its tearing. Taking time to prepare the artery to receive the catheter is most important in preventing problems. **Always wipe the guidewire with a wet lint-free gauze each time an item has been passed over it.**

6. After the guidewire has been positioned and arterial predilatation performed, the sheath through which the balloon catheter will be placed is passed over the guidewire (Fig. 12-9, *D*), through the tissue, and into the femoral artery lumen. Care must be taken at all times to control this guidewire, which must remain protruding out of the sheath. Gentle rotation of the introducer facilitates its passage through the skin and subcutaneous tissues and entry into the artery.

7. Under fluoroscopic control, advance the guidewire to a point approximately 2 cm distal to the left subclavian artery (Fig. 12-11).

8. With the introducer sheath exposed at least 1 inch above the skin line, remove the dilator from the sheath, leaving the guidewire within the sheath. After removal of the dilator, some blood leakage may be observed past the hemostasis valve, which can be controlled by pinching the sheath around the guidewire. (If the valve has been removed, pinch the sheath around the guidewire to minimize bleeding.)

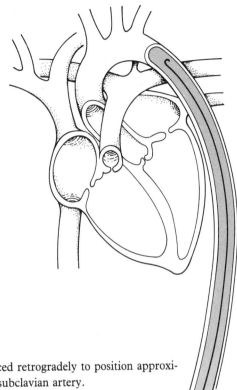

Fig. 12-11. Guidewire is advanced retrogradely to position approximately just below origin of left subclavian artery.

9. Insert the .030-inch guidewire through the central lumen opening in the tip of the IAB until it exits the female luer fitting on the IAB. Advance the IAB into the sheath while controlling the proximal end of the guidewire. Fig. 12-12 depicts the use of a guidewire preceding balloon insertion to permit retrograde navigation through a tortuous vessel with atherosclerosis.

10. The balloon is then advanced over the guidewire and passed retrogradely to a position 1 to 2 cm below the origin of the left subclavian artery (Fig. 12-13).

11. The guidewire is then removed, and a pressure monitoring set-up is connected to the inner cannula (Fig. 12-14), which either will be used to monitor arterial pressure or will be capped. This central lumen orifice may also be used to "hand inject" contrast media to verify balloon position. The sheath is sealed by sliding the "sheath seal" down the balloon catheter and onto the sheath hub. **Do not use an automatic injector. Use a manual syringe no smaller than 20 ml.**

12. The balloon is sutured to the patient's leg via two projecting tabs (see Fig. 12-14).

13. If a one-way valve had been used to create a vacuum on the balloon, this is now removed (Fig. 12-15) and the balloon connector is attached to the balloon pump

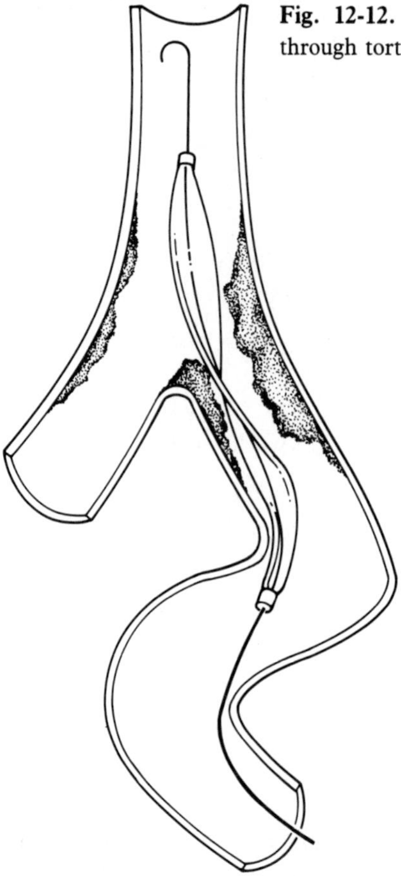

Fig. 12-12. Schematic illustration of guidewire used to navigate through tortuous, atherosclerotic vessel.

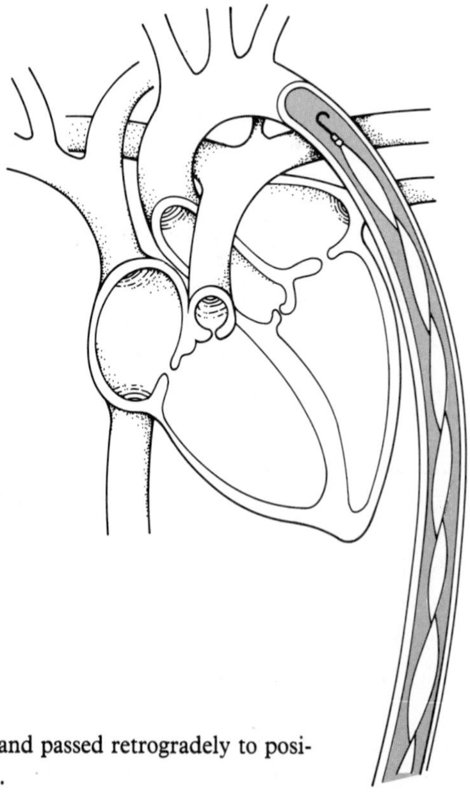

Fig. 12-13. Balloon advanced over guidewire and passed retrogradely to position just below origin of left subclavian artery.

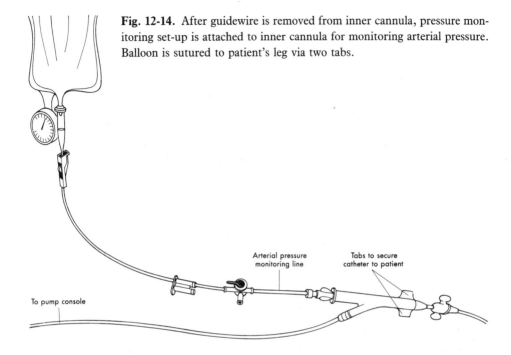

Fig. 12-14. After guidewire is removed from inner cannula, pressure monitoring set-up is attached to inner cannula for monitoring arterial pressure. Balloon is sutured to patient's leg via two tabs.

To pump console

Arterial pressure
monitoring line

Tabs to secure
catheter to patient

console. Balloon counterpulsation should then begin according to manufacturer's guidelines. Each manufacturer's guidelines should be consulted regarding procedure for a balloon that did not unwrap.

14. Balloon position should be verified by fluoroscopy. Alternatively, if fluoroscopy is not available, before beginning the procedure, lay the balloon over the draped patient. Place the tip over the sternal angle of Louis. Approximating the course of balloon within the patient, bring the catheter over the umbilicus and diagonally to the groin insertion point. Mark the balloon at the point where it will exit from the skin. At the time of IAB placement, advance the catheter until the marking is 1 inch past the sheath orifice. Following placement in this manner,

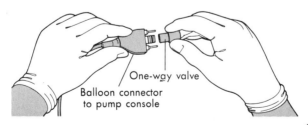

One-way valve

Balloon connector
to pump console

Fig. 12-15. If one-way valve was used to create vacuum within balloon, it is now removed and balloon connector is attached to balloon pump console.

STANDARDS OF CARE FOR PERCUTANEOUS IAB INSERTION

1. Use of fluoroscopy to confirm the position of both the guidewire and the catheter tip at all times during insertion.

2. Readiness to stop whenever the guidewire cannot be passed without great difficulty around the arch or in a reasonably straight line within the iliac vessels.

3. Use of double-lumen balloons whenever possible. It appears likely that if the J-wire does not pass easily through the vessel lumen, then neither will the dilator sheath. Under these conditions, sheath insertion may be more hazardous than balloon insertion, because the sheath is made of stiff plastic. Although its end is tapered, it could raise a flap within the blood vessel. It is then recommended to try the contralateral femoral artery.

From Miller LW: *Cardiac Assists* 3:1, 1986.

the balloon position should be determined immediately by chest x-ray film. Always observe the balloon catheter markings to make sure that the entire balloon membrane has left the insertion sheath before initiating balloon pumping.

Standards of care for percutaneous insertion

Miller[4] and associates established standards of care for percutaneous IAB insertion that supported favorable results in their series. These standards are listed in the box above. Wolvek[6] described certain technical tips also recommended to ensure successful insertion (see the box on p. 187).

Heparin administration

Miller[4] and associates also recommend the following heparin protocol. Administer a 5000-U bolus of heparin at the time of sheath insertion, followed by heparin infusion (600 to 1000 U per hour) sufficient to maintain a partial thromboplastin time of 50 to 60 seconds. No peripheral emboli or significant thrombocytopenia (platelets <100,000) has been associated with this regimen. Kantrowitz[6] recommends administering 5000 U heparin at the onset of IABC and every 4 hours until the balloon is removed, rather than a continuous infusion.

For patients with contraindications to administration of heparin, intravenous low molecular weight dextran 40 (25 ml/hour) may be substituted. Kantrowitz[7] recommends that the dose of low molecular weight dextran not exceed 10 ml/kg/24 hours. Patients in the TAMI study[8] who underwent thrombolytic therapy and IABC also received at least one aspirin tablet daily in addition to a heparin infusion to maintain the partial thromboplastin time of 1.5 to 2.0 times normal.

TECHNICAL TIPS TO FACILITATE SUCCESSFUL INSERTION

1. The angle of the needle stick should be as shallow as possible. A shallow angle of entry will help prevent catheter kinking at the insertion site, both during insertion and later in the course of therapy.

2. Always use the guidewire supplied by the manufacturer. The inner lumen of the catheter is small, and a larger wire may not be able to be successfully passed through this lumen. Also, the wire has been carefully selected to be of sufficient body and stiffness to ensure that the balloon will track over the wire and not take its own lead. Always wipe the wire with a wet lint-free gauze each time an item is passed over it.

3. Predilatation is probably one of the most important steps that can be taken to prevent bleeding at the insertion site, reduce the potential for hematoma, and prevent the sheath from crimping during entry. Because today's IABC patients are often elderly and their peripheral vascular disease is advanced, careful predilatation will gently stretch the artery to permit catheter passage, rather than risk tearing. A nick at the skin line and use of a rotary motion facilitate placement of the introducer, as well as reducing the potential for the sheath to crimp. Taking the time to prepare the artery to receive the catheter is most important in preventing problems.

4. To ensure a smooth insertion, a number of specific steps should be kept in mind. It is important to be sure that throughout the insertion procedure a vacuum is maintained on the balloon. This will ensure that it glides smoothly through the sheath. Also, the balloon should be held close to the point at which it enters the sheath and inserted with a short, rotary motion. Last, excessive force should never be used when inserting the IAB. This may result in damage to both the artery and the balloon. If resistance is met during the insertion, stop and pull the catheter and guidewire back slightly. Attempt to advance gently. If resistance is met again, stop the insertion and attempt to insert on the contralateral side.

5. Proper placement after IAB insertion is vitally important. Position the balloon in the descending thoracic aorta approximately 1 to 2 cm distal to the left subclavian artery. This position will avoid obstructing the great vessels at the proximal end of the balloon and the renal arteries at the distal end. Placement high in the aorta reduces the likelihood that the balloon will be abraded through continuing contact with calcific atherosclerotic plaque, which tends to be especially concentrated in the abdominal aorta.

6. Visualization of the location of the balloon before initiation of IABC is important. Whenever possible, fluoroscopy should be used during insertion to ensure proper placement. If fluoroscopy is not available, estimate how far to advance the balloon catheter by measuring the patient from the sternal angle of Louis to the umbilicus and then diagonally to the femoral insertion site. The catheter markings and the sheath seal on the catheter can then be used to indicate how far to advance the balloon during insertion. A chest x-ray examination must be performed. The tip of the IAB should be visualized at the level of the second to third intercostal space.

From Wolvek S: *Cardiac Assists* 6(2):9, 1992.

PERCUTANEOUS BALLOON REMOVAL

1. After counterpulsation is stopped, a syringe may be used to create a vacuum within the balloon, or the balloon can be disconnected from the console and permitted to empty by venting.

2. The balloon is then withdrawn up to the sheath. *The balloon and sheath are withdrawn as a unit. Do not attempt to withdraw the IAB through the sheath.*

3. Cover the puncture site with a sponge when removing the sheath and catheter. Firmly compress the femoral artery *distal* to the puncture site while withdrawing the balloon. Allow blood to squirt out for 1 to 2 seconds to encourage extravascular loss of clots or other debris. Then relax pressure distally to encourage back-bleeding, and while compressing the area proximal to the puncture site.[4] Good manual control of the artery, both proximal and distal to the insertion site, must be maintained.

4. Maintain firm compression directly over the site for at least 20 to 30 minutes after removal of the catheter.

5. Examine the distal limb for signs of possible emboli after balloon catheter removal.

Percutaneous balloon removal

The heparin infusion should be discontinued 2 to 4 hours before the balloon is removed.[5] Miller,[4] however, suggests that it is better to pull the balloon with some heparin effect still present than to risk clot formation and propagation with removal (see the box above).

Complications associated with percutaneous insertion

Miller[4] and associates in a 1986 publication reported an overall success rate of 50% for percutaneous insertion. Of these insertions, 74% (37/50) were accomplished on the first attempt and 16% (8/50) on the opposite side. Failed insertion has been reported as high as 4% to 10% of all attempted percutaneous placements.[7] This rate depends on both the patient's condition and the operator's experience.

Aortic dissections or perforations may occur at the time of insertion. Occlusive vascular disease becomes the primary concern once the balloon is placed. Most series show an incidence of vascular complications ranging from 20% to 30%.[9-13] Further information on complications can be found in Chapter 10.

Advances that reduce hazards. Bregman, highly experienced in percutaneous technique, offers the following guidelines to reduce morbidity associated with percutaneous technique[14,15]:

1. The percutaneous IAB *must* be inserted by a physician skilled in the Seldinger technique of cardiac catheterization.

2. Ideally the insertion procedure should be carried out under fluoroscopic control.
3. The advent of the long dilator sheath has significantly increased the success of insertion.
4. In critically ill patients who have poor ventricular function, undergoing cardiac catheterization, study of the aorta iliac system is highly desirable as a guide for subsequent balloon insertion.
5. In high-risk cardiac surgical patients undergoing open heart surgery, without IAB insertion before anesthetic induction, femoral artery access should be obtained with an arterial needle and then a guidewire, which is maintained in the sterile operative field. If IABC is subsequently required for weaning from cardiopulmonary bypass, arterial access is then already established for IABC insertion.
6. A major advance in percutaneous balloon technology has been the advent of the dual-lumen percutaneous balloon. This balloon can follow a guidewire into the aorta, virtually eliminating aortic dissection. In addition, arterial pressure monitoring can be performed through the balloon.
7. Finally, balloon removal should be carried out in the following manner: The balloon is deflated and pulled down to (but not into) the sheath. The femoral artery immediately distal to the balloon is tightly compressed, and the balloon and sheath are then removed as a unit. Blood is allowed to spurt from the artery for a few seconds, and then the compression is shifted over the puncture site for 30 minutes. Distal pulses are monitored with a Doppler, and manual compression is adjusted so that an audible pulse is registered. With this technique we have occasionally retrieved specimens of thrombus that have come out of the femoral artery and therefore have not embolized.

ANTEGRADE INSERTION TECHNIQUE

Snow and Horrigan[16] described intraaortic balloon insertion via the ascending aorta in 23 patients. Transascending aortic insertion was used, because passage via the transfemoral route had been unsuccessfully attempted or presence of severe peripheral vascular disease either preoperatively or intraoperatively prompted transaortic insertion without first opening the femoral artery. Direct insertion into the aorta within concentric purse-string sutures was utilized. Pledgeted Dacron purse-string sutures were used in each case and were tied and cut before wound closure. No partially occluding clamps were applied, and the wrapped balloons were inserted directly into the ascending aorta and advanced into the ascending thoracic aorta. The sternum was approximated with stainless steel wires in four patients, while in the remaining patients only the skin and subcutaneous tissues were closed. Repeat exploration and balloon removal were accomplished safely with the added advantage of bypass graft inspection and revision where indicated. New aortic purse-string sutures were placed at the time of removal without incident. The aorta was allowed to bleed momentarily before the sutures were tied down. One patient suffered a transient cerebrovascular deficit after balloon removal but recovered completely before discharge. After antibiotic administration and saline irrigation, conventional sternal closure was performed. No mediastinal wound infections occurred in these patients. Branchiocephalic clamping during withdrawal was not performed.

Two patients in this series required IABC in the intensive care unit after emergency resternotomy in the early postoperative period. Rapid transaortic IAB insertion was possible, with minimal equipment and operating personnel.

In the "crowded" aorta after coronary artery bypass grafting, use of aortic purse-string sutures and direct IAB insertion is the most expedient approach. Side-arm graft attachment to the aorta is time-consuming and may predispose to hemorrhagic complications at the suture line, especially in severely atherosclerotic vessels. One case has been reported where the Dacron side-arm graft became infected, and despite graft removal, the patient subsequently exsanguinated from this infected aortotomy site.[16]

Despite the lack of any anticoagulant therapy and specific measures to occlude the brachiocephalic vessels, only one embolic phenomenon was recognized.

Antegrade insertion of a percutaneous IAB

Antegrade insertion of a percutaneous IAB was described by Melvin and Goldman[17] and illustrated in Fig. 12-16.

1. With the patient on cardiopulmonary bypass, two purse-string sutures are placed in the ascending aorta proximal to the aortic cannula.
2. A small stab is made in the aorta with a No. 11 blade.
3. The smaller of the introducer dilators is inserted, then removed, and replaced with the larger introducer and the overlying plastic sheath. (It is not necessary to leave the introducer sheath in place, nor is it necessary to use the sheath at all.)[20]

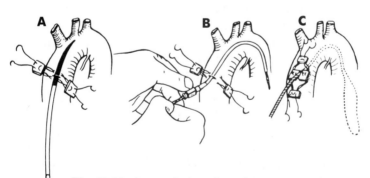

Fig. 12-16. Antegrade insertion of percutaneous IAB through ascending aorta. **A,** Insertion of introducer into ascending aorta. **B,** Introduction of IAB. **C,** IAB removal. (From Melvin KN, Goldman BS: *Ann Thorac Surg* 33:636, 1982.)

4. The introducer is removed, and free blood flow is demonstrated to rule out possible dissection.
5. The percutaneous IAB is then inserted antegradely, and the distal tip is positioned 1 to 2 cm below the left subclavian artery.
6. Removal necessitates reopening of the sternum.
7. Placement of a purse-string suture, deflation of the balloon, quick withdrawal, and tightening of the suture are all that is required.

Bonchek and Olinger[18] described another technique for IAB removal from the aortic arch. Fibrin can potentially be wiped off the IAB during removal and embolize to the brain. The innominate and left carotid arteries are occluded with tourniquets (Fig. 12-17). After removal of the IAB, the catheter insertion site is allowed to bleed momentarily before reclosing the arch vessel, releasing the tourniquets, and suturing the wound.

Kaplan, Weimar, Langen, et al.[19] described the following method of direct aor-

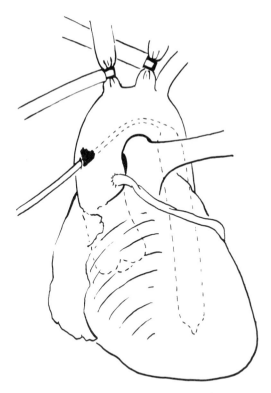

Fig. 12-17. Removal of percutaneous balloon from aortic arch. Innominate and left carotid arteries occluded with tourniquets to prevent embolization of thrombus to vessels as catheter is removed. (From Bonchek MD, Olinger G: *Ann Thorac Surg* 32:512, 1981.)

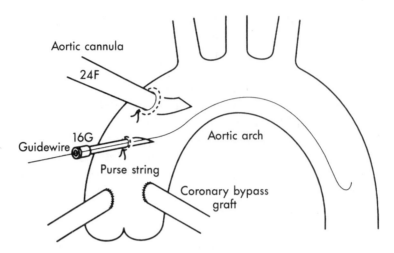

Fig. 12-18. Schematic view of ascending aorta demonstrating Seldinger technique for guidewire placement through purse-string suture. (From Kaplan LJ, Weiman DS, Langan N et al: *Ann Thorac Surg* 54:374, 1992.)

tic puncture for IAB placement using transesophageal ultrasound (TEU) as a means of avoiding intimal flap and aortic dissection:

1. With the patient on bypass, a 3-0 polyester purse-string suture is sewn on the anterior ascending aortic wall at a soft site.
2. The aorta is punctured with a 16-g needle, through which a flexible guidewire is passed (Fig. 12-18).
3. During the first two maneuvers, the aorta is visualized using TEU to ensure safe wire placement and passage. The guidewire is withdrawn and curved to match the aortic contour.
4. Reinsertion with TEU guidance offers unimpeded guidewire passage.
5. The needle is then removed and the dilator-sheath assembly passed over the wire again under TEU control.
6. The dilator is withdrawn and the IAB passed over the wire into its proper position. Accurate placement just distal to the left subclavian artery is ensured using TEU.
7. The purse-string suture is snugged down using a 12-Fr, red rubber catheter and secured with a golf tee (Fig. 12-19).
8. After the patient is successfully weaned from cardiopulmonary bypass, the IAB exists through the inferior aspect of the incision.
9. IAB removal requires repeat stenotomy.

In summary, TEU was found to facilitate accurate IAB placement and minimize insertion time, cardiopulmonary bypass time, and patient morbidity.[21]

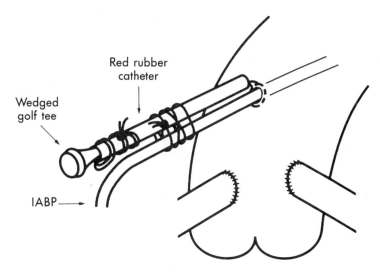

Red rubber
catheter

Wedged
golf tee

IABP——▶

Fig. 12-19. Diagram of red rubber catheter and golf tee–wedge assembly used to secure IAB in ascending aorta. Note tie securing catheter to IAB to prevent migration. (From Kaplan LJ, Weiman DS, Langan N et al: *Ann Thorac Surg* 54:374, 1992.)

SUBCLAVIAN INSERTION

Two reports describing subclavian artery insertion[20,21] have demonstrated the feasibility of using an upper extremity artery for access to the aorta. This technique may be used in an effort to avoid major surgical intervention for IAB placement when aortoiliac stenosis prevents femoral retrograde advancement or in an effort to facilitate greater patient mobility. A transverse subclavicular incision is made near the deltoid pectoralis muscle and the subclavian artery is isolated. A standard percutaneous IAB insertion kit is used. The guidewire is inserted in the subclavian artery and positioned in the descending aorta under fluoroscopic guidance. A double-lumen 9-Fr IAB is passed over the guidewire and positioned in the descending aorta so that the proximal portion of the IAB is 1 to 2 cm below the origin of the subclavian vessel. The IAB is then tunneled out to the lateral inferior aspect of the heart and secured to the skin[21] (Fig. 12-20).

TRANSAXILLARY INSERTION

McBride, Miller, Naunheim et al.[22] developed a transaxillary artery insertion technique in an attempt to improve mobility of the bridge-to-transplant patient population. This technique is described in the box on p. 196 and illustrated in Fig. 12-21.

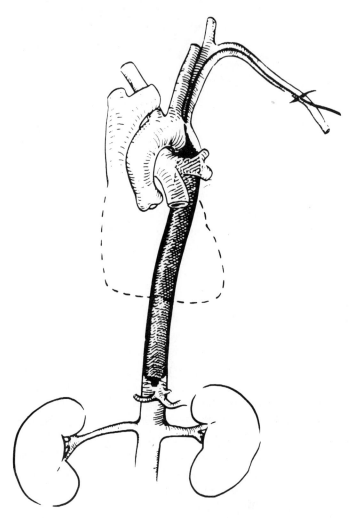

Fig. 12-20. Subclavian artery insertion of IAB. (From Reedy JE, Ruzevich SQA, Noedel NR et al: *J Heart Transplant* 9:97, 1990.)

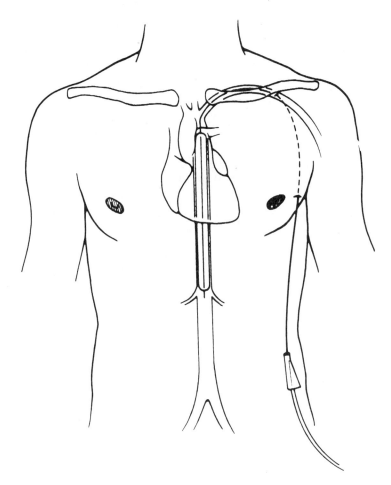

Fig. 12-21. Axillary artery IAB insertion. (From McBride LR, Miller LW, Naunheim KS et al: *Ann Thorac Surg* 48:874, 1989.)

AXILLARY ARTERY INSERTION OF IAB PUMP

1. The left or right axillary artery is exposed through a transverse infraclavicular incision extending from the deltopectoral groove to the midclavicle.

2. The pectoralis major is split in the direction of its fibers.

3. The clavipectoral fascia is divided, exposing the axillary artery and vein and the brachial plexus. The vein is gently retracted, and circumferential control of the artery is obtained by sharp dissection. Care is taken not to disrupt any of the arterial branches that may provide collateral circulation. A 4-0 polypropylene horizontal mattress stitch is placed in the vessel wall.

4. With use of the Seldinger technique, a 0.03-inch (0.76 mm) guidewire is positioned under fluoroscopic guidance into the descending aorta. If the guidewire cannot be manipulated into the descending aorta, an 8-Fr multipurpose coronary angiography catheter is used to direct the guidewire distally from the origin of the subclavian artery.

5. A 9.5-Fr double-lumen IAB (Datascope, Paramus, NJ) is inserted through a second small skin incision at the lateral pectoral margin and tunneled subcutaneously into the infraclavicular incision.

6. The balloon catheter is then passed over the guidewire and positioned in the descending aorta so that the most proximal portion of the balloon is located just beyond the origin of the left subclavian artery. In general this results in the distal end of the IAB being located at the second or third lumbar vertebral body. Fluoroscopy and arterial pressure are used to check IAB position and augmentation.

7. The management of an axillary IAB is identical to that of transfemoral IAB. Anticoagulation therapy consists of intravenous dextran sulfate or heparin.

8. With axillary insertion, the waveform is monitored using the distal port on the balloon, and counterpulsation is timed in a fashion identical to that employed with a transfemoral placement. Although arterial lines placed in the contralateral arm or either femoral artery accurately display the identical waveform, such lines are not used after IAB placement because they may impair ambulation and patient mobility. Because of the partial obstruction of the axillary artery proximal to the site of insertion, radial artery monitoring on the side of IAB placement will likely be inaccurate and should not be employed.

9. Balloon removal is usually accomplished in the operating room. The incision is reopened, and proximal and distal control are again obtained.

10. After complete balloon deflation, the IAB is withdrawn through the arteriotomy and vascular clamps are applied proximal and distal to the site.

11. Each clamp is briefly removed in turn to flush any intraarterial thrombus out through the arteriotomy.

12. The artery is then closed with a 5-0 polypropylene suture. No complications have been encountered when using this approach.

From McBride LR, Miller LW, Naunheim KS et al: *Ann Thorac Surg* 48:874, 1989.

REFERENCES

1. Wolvek S: The evolution of the intra-aortic balloon: the Datascope contribution, *J Biomater Appl* 3:527, 1989.
2. Hebeler RF: Simplified technique for open placement and removal of intraaortic balloon, *Am Thorac Surg* 48:134, 1989.
3. Lundell DC: Randomized comparison of the modified wireguided and standard intra-aortic balloon catheters, *J Thorac Cardiovasc Surg* 82:297, 1981.
4. Miller LW: Emerging trends in the treatment of acute myocardial infarction and the role of intra-aortic balloon pumping, *Cardiac Assists* 3:1, 1986.
5. Benn A, Feldman T: The technique of inserting an intra-aortic balloon pump, *J Crit Illness* 7:435, 1992.
6. Wolvek S: Technical tips, *Cardiac Assists* 6:9, 1992.
7. Kantrowitz A: Intra-aortic balloon pumping: clinical aspects and prospects. In Unger F, ed: *Assisted circulation*, ed 3, New York, 1989, Springer-Verlag.
8. George BS: Thrombolysis and intra-aortic balloon pumping following acute myocardial infarction — experience in four TAMI studies, *Cardiac Assists* 4:1, 1988.
9. Goldberg MJ, Rubenfire M, Kantrowitz A et al: Intra-aortic balloon pump insertion: a randomized study comparing percutaneous and surgical techniques, *J Am Coll Cardiol* 9:515, 1987.
10. Yuen JC, Riggs OE: Aortoiliac dissection after percutaneous insertion of an intra-aortic balloon, *South Med J* 84:1135, 1991.
11. Kvilekval KH, Mason RA, Newton GB et al: Complications of percutaneous intra-aortic balloon pump use in patients with peripheral vascular disease, *Arch Surg* 126:621, 1991.
12. Skillman JJ, Kim D, Baim DS: Vascular complications of percutaneous femoral cardiac interventions. Incidence and operative repair, *Arch Surg* 23:1207, 1988.
13. Collier PE, Liebler GA, Park SB et al: Is percutaneous insertion of the intra-aortic balloon pump through the femoral artery the safest technique? *J Vasc Surg* 3:629, 1986.
14. Bregman D: Percutaneous intra-aortic balloon pumping. A time for reflection, *Chest* 82:397, 1982.
15. Bregman D: Clinical experience with percutaneous intra-aortic balloon pumping. In Unger F, ed: *Assisted circulation*, ed 3, New York, 1989, Springer-Verlag.
16. Snow N, Horrigan TP: Intra-aortic balloon counterpulsation, *J Cardiovasc Surg* 27:337, 1986.
17. Melvin KN, Goldman BS: Intraoperative placement of the percutaneous intra-aortic balloon pump through the ascending aorta, *Ann Thorac Surg* 33:636, 1982.
18. Bonchek MD, Olinger G: Direct ascending aortic insertion of the "percutaneous" intra-aortic balloon catheter in the open chest: advantages and precautions, *Ann Thorac Surg* 32:512, 1981.
19. Kaplan LJ, Weimar DS, Langen N et al: Safe intraaortic balloon pump placement through the ascending aorta using transesophageal ultrasound, *Ann Thorac Surg* 54:374, 1992.
20. Rubenstein RB, Karhade NV: Supraclavicular subclavian technique of intraaortic balloon insertion, *J Vasc Surg* 1:577, 1984.
21. Mayer JH: Subclavian artery approach for insertion of intra-aortic balloon, *J Thorac Cardiovasc Surg* 76:61, 1978.
22. McBride LR, Miller LW, Naunheim KS et al: Axillary artery insertion of an intraaortic balloon pump, *Ann Thorac Surg* 48:874, 1989.

CHAPTER 13

Sheathless balloon insertion

Daniel J. Diver

Advances in balloon catheter design now permit percutaneous insertion of a wire-guided catheter through an introducing sheath in most patients requiring intraaortic balloon counterpulsation (IABC). These improvements in catheter design have largely eliminated the need for surgical entry of the femoral or iliac artery or operative removal of previously placed catheters. However, even the lower profile, wire-guided counterpulsation catheters commonly used today are associated with a high incidence of vascular complications.[1-3] It has been suggested that many of these vascular complications are related simply to size mismatch between the diameter of counterpulsation catheter shafts and the lumen of diseased iliac and femoral arteries.[2-4] Sheathless percutaneous insertion of intraaortic balloon catheters is a promising new technique that reduces the effective catheter diameter by elimination of the arterial sheath and may decrease the rate of vascular complications associated with balloon counterpulsation.

STANDARD PERCUTANEOUS BALLOON INSERTION

Early balloon catheter design required a surgical cutdown into the femoral or iliac artery and insertion of the balloon via a cuff of prosthetic vascular material. Intraaortic balloon insertion by surgical cutdown techniques was associated with a high rate of femoral vascular complications, reported to occur in up to 36% of patients.[5-8] Furthermore, insertion of the balloon catheter by surgical cutdown was often associated with unsuccessful insertion or with marked prolongation of insertion time and required subsequent operative removal of the surgically inserted catheters.

In the late 1970s, several groups described techniques for percutaneous insertion of balloon catheters through an arterial sheath inserted over a guidewire, with subsequent direct passage of the balloon catheter into the descending aorta through the arterial sheath.[9,10] Further improvements in technique included development of wire-guided and smaller diameter (10.5, 9.5, and, most recently, 8.5 Fr) catheters.

Percutaneous insertion of intraaortic balloons clearly represented a major advance in balloon insertion technique. The ease and speed with which balloon catheters could be inserted by this technique greatly increased the applicability of balloon counterpulsation in patients with refractory myocardial ischemia and cardiogenic shock. When performed under fluoroscopic control, percutaneous insertion was associated with a high rate of successful insertion and low rates of insertion-related complications. However, the belief that these advances in balloon insertion technique would significantly lower the rate of vascular complications proved to be unfounded. Some studies even suggested that vascular complications may be more frequent with the percutaneous technique than with surgical cutdown insertion.[1,11]

Alderman and associates at our institution reported on 103 consecutive patients who underwent placement of percutaneous wire-guided intraaortic balloon catheters between 1983 and 1986.[2] All balloon insertion attempts were successful and the average duration of counterpulsation was 3.4 ± 1.6 days. Of patients in this series, 27% developed limb ischemia severe enough to warrant premature discontinuation of counterpulsation. Development of limb ischemia was significantly correlated with diabetes, peripheral vascular disease, female gender, and the presence of a postinsertion ankle-brachial pressure index <0.8. There was no correlation between development of limb ischemia and balloon size (10.5 Fr vs. 12 Fr). Fifteen patients in this series underwent vascular surgery for treatment of balloon-related limb ischemia, with one associated operative death. Limb ischemia persisted in nine patients (7 asymptomatic, 2 symptomatic) at the time of hospital discharge. The authors concluded that although improvements in wire-guided balloon technology and balloon catheter profile increased the probability of successful balloon placement and reduced the incidence of major aortic injury, there was no evidence that these improvements had reduced the incidence of limb ischemia or severe vascular complications.

ADVANTAGE OF SHEATHLESS BALLOON INSERTION

Reduction in balloon shaft diameter should result in a decrease in the vascular complication rate associated with IABC. Little reduction in limb ischemia has occurred as catheter shaft diameter has been decreased from 12 to 9.5 (and now 8.5) Fr. However, when balloon catheters are inserted via the standard percutaneous technique, the effective occluding diameter is not that of the balloon catheter shaft but rather the outer diameter of the sheath through which the balloon catheter is inserted. Both the 10.5 and 12 Fr catheters in use at the time of the Alderman study[2] appeared to have sheath diameters (4.2 and 4.6 mm, respectively) too large to be accommodated within the femoral artery lumen of many patients. Recent progress in further reducing balloon catheter shaft diameters to as low as 8.5 Fr has not been associated with a similar reduction in sheath outer diameter, which remains at 11 Fr (3.8 mm).

Experience at our institution with balloon aortic valvuloplasty by the retrograde femoral arterial approach led to the development of techniques for sheathless percutaneous insertion of large balloon catheters inserted through the femoral artery. Our favorable experience with such techniques in the balloon valvuloplasty population led to their investigation in patients requiring percutaneous IABC. Elimination of the arterial sheath from the balloon counterpulsation insertion technique confers a significant, clinically relevant reduction in effective device diameter. For example, by eliminating the introducing sheath of a 9.5 Fr balloon catheter via sheathless insertion, the diameter of the largest device inserted in the artery decreases from 3.8 to less than 3.2 mm, reducing the effective cross-sectional area of the counterpulsation catheter from 11.5 to 7.9 mm^2.[12]

SHEATHLESS INSERTION TECHNIQUE
Preparation

Initial balloon catheter preparation should be undertaken in compliance with specific manufacturer's instructions. General preparation for most devices consists of evacuation of any residual air remaining in the balloon with a syringe/stopcock system and removal of the central obturator.

Insertion

Insertion should always be performed under fluoroscopic guidance. If arterial access has not yet been obtained, local anesthetic should be applied to the femoral insertion site and a small skin nick made with a surgical blade. Both skin and subcutaneous tissue at the femoral insertion site should be generously spread with a Kelly clamp or similar instrument. Spreading of the cutaneous and subcutaneous tissue is important to avoid subsequent snaring of the balloon catheter tip by skin or subcutaneous tissue tags. The femoral artery is then punctured percutaneously with an 18 gauge angiographic needle, and a 0.030-inch J-tip guidewire is advanced through the needle into the abdominal aorta using standard Seldinger technique. The needle is removed, leaving only the guidewire in place.

If arterial access has already been obtained (e.g., if the patient has just undergone coronary angiography) then the 0.030-inch J-tip guidewire may be advanced through the existing sheath/catheter assembly into the abdominal aorta. The catheter/sheath assembly is removed over the guidewire, leaving only the guidewire in place.

The common femoral artery and subcutaneous tissue are then predilated with a 9 Fr dilator, to establish a subcutaneous track sufficient to allow subsequent passage of the balloon catheter. With the tip of the guidewire high in the descending aorta, the balloon catheter is then advanced directly over the guidewire into the central circulation without the use of an introducing sheath. During balloon catheter insertion, the catheter shaft should always be held close to the skin insertion site, to prevent kinking of the bare wire within the femoral vasculature. Insertion may be facilitated by slight clockwise rotation of the balloon catheter shaft, although excessive rotation is likely to result in undesirable balloon wrapping. Once the catheter has been introduced into the descending aorta, the catheter tip is positioned fluoroscopically at the approximate level of the carina. The balloon is connected to a pump console in standard fashion, and counterpulsation is initiated. The catheter is secured by suturing: (1) the plastic Y connector at the proximal end of the device to the skin and (2) the exposed catheter shaft near the arterial entry site, with a skin anchor stitch and a series of locking loops around the catheter shaft. The ring designed to form a hemostatic valve when joined to the sheath during standard insertion is not used during sheathless insertion.

UNSUCCESSFUL SHEATHLESS INSERTION

Occasionally, difficulty will be encountered in attempting to pass the balloon catheter over a bare wire into the descending aorta without an arterial sheath. In most cases, this is due to trapping of the catheter tip by subcutaneous tissue/skin tags, and smooth catheter insertion is possible after further spreading of the subcutaneous tissue. However, if the balloon catheter does not advance smoothly over the guidewire, great care should be taken not to force the catheter, as this could result in guidewire kinking within the arterial system and arterial laceration. If the balloon catheter will not advance smoothly over the guidewire: (1) remove catheter from the guidewire, (2) insert sheath/dilator assembly over the guidewire, (3) remove dilator from the sheath and reinsert balloon catheter over guidewire into central circulation through the arterial sheath in standard fashion.

CONTRAINDICATIONS TO SHEATHLESS INSERTION

Sheathless intraaortic balloon insertion should not be attempted in patients with severe scarring or fibrosis at femoral access sites or with obesity severe enough to create excessive distance between the skin and femoral artery. The likelihood of successful sheathless insertion is decreased in such patients, therefore balloon catheter insertion should be attempted through a sheath by the standard percutaneous technique.

CLINICAL RESULTS OF SHEATHLESS BALLOON INSERTION

The technique of sheathless percutaneous IAB catheter insertion was first reported by Nash and colleagues at our institution in 1991.[12] This study involved prospective evaluation of 29 consecutive patients undergoing IABC catheter insertion

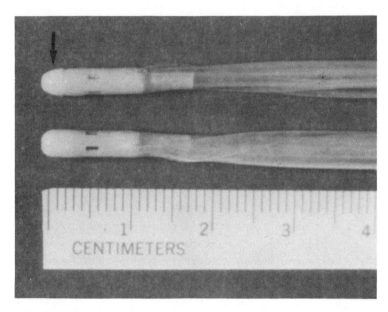

Fig. 13-1. Standard balloon catheter tip and modified "ballistic" tip of balloon catheter used in sheathless insertion study (arrow). Tack-weld, approximately 15 cm from tip, is not shown. (From Nash IS et al: *Cathet Cardiovasc Diagn* 23:57, 1991.)

between June 1, 1989 and December 1, 1989 at the Beth Israel Hospital (Boston). All patients who received counterpulsation catheters were treated with intravenous heparin to achieve a target partial thromboplastin time of 1½ to 2× control. All balloons were placed under fluoroscopic guidance in the catheterization laboratory. The intraaortic balloon catheter used for all patients was a 9.5 Fr (3.2 mm) 40 cc catheter* modified by the manufacturer in the following two ways: (1) the catheter tip was changed from the standard blunt design to a more tapered, "ballistic" profile to allow for greater ease of tissue penetration and (2) a tack-weld was added at the proximal end of the balloon to fuse the balloon more securely to the shaft and ensure enhanced pushability of the catheter without bunching up redundant balloon material (Fig. 13-1). Prewrapped catheters were inserted over a 0.030-inch guidewire,* which had a floppy end with a standard J, but a stiff core that continued along the rest of its 145 cm length to provide increased support during catheter insertion. Both the modified balloon and stiff 0.030-inch guidewire are now commercially available† for sheathless balloon insertion.

Of the 29 IABC catheters placed during the study, 22 were attempted using the

---

*Universal Medical Instrument Corporation, Ballston Spa, NY.
†Datascope Corporation, Oakland, NJ.

Table 13-1. Patient characteristics

	Sheathless	Standard
Number	20	9
Mean age	68	63
Male (%)	65	67
PVD (%)	30	33
Hypertension (%)	60	44
Diabetes mellitus (%)	30	11
Smoking (%)	65	56

From Nash IS et al: *Cathet Cardiovasc Diagn* 23:57, 1991.
PVD, Peripheral vascular disease.

new sheathless insertion technique as described. Reasons for insertion via a sheath in the remaining seven patients included the need for emergent bedside placement without fluoroscopy in one patient, temporary unavailability of the modified balloon catheter in one patient, and unspecified operator preference in the remaining 5 patients.

Balloon insertion by the sheathless technique was successful in 20 of the 22 patients in whom it was attempted. In the remaining 2 patients, initial attempts at sheathless insertion were unsuccessful because of inability to pass the balloon through subcutaneous tissue. In each case, placement of an introducing sheath over the same guidewire permitted prompt insertion of the counterpulsation catheter without complication. These two cases occurred early in our experience and suggest that there may be a learning curve associated with successful application of the sheathless technique.

Table 13-1 defines the clinical characteristics of 20 patients who underwent sheathless insertion and the 9 patients in whom standard insertion was performed (including the 2 patients in whom initial attempts at sheathless insertion were unsuccessful). The two groups appeared similar with regard to clinical characteristics, including risk factors for or actual presence of peripheral vascular disease. Indications for balloon insertion in each group are shown in Table 13-2. The most common in-

Table 13-2. Indications for IABP insertion

	Sheathless	Standard
Unstable angina	9	4
Cardiogenic shock	7	1
Failed PTCA	2	1
Instability during catheterization	1	3
Prophylaxis for surgery	1	0

From Nash IS et al: *Cathet Cardiovasc Diagn* 23:57, 1991.
IABP, Intraaortic balloon pump; *PTCA*, percutaneous transluminal coronary angioplasty.

dications for balloon insertion were severe refractory myocardial ischemia and cardiogenic shock.

Sheathless balloon catheter insertion was not associated with an increased procedure time and allowed prompt and effective counterpulsation in all patients. Catheters remained in place for a mean of 3.3 ± 2.2 days (range 1 to 9 days) in the sheathless insertion group and for a mean of 2.2 ± 1.3 days (range 1 to 4 days) in the standard insertion group. Only one balloon placed without a sheath subsequently malfunctioned because of a kink in the catheter shaft, which developed 3 days after insertion. Since in vitro testing has demonstrated that the catheter shaft is more resistant to irreversible kinking than the sheath, it is not clear whether the presence of a sheath would have prevented this complication. However, it would seem that vigorous attention to prevention of catheter kinking is appropriate following sheathless balloon insertion.

Limb ischemia, defined as a decrease in limb perfusion sufficient to warrant premature discontinuation of counterpulsation or surgical revascularization, occurred in 2 patients (10%) in the sheathless insertion group. Both patients had multiple risk factors for a vascular complication of balloon insertion, including peripheral vascular disease, hypertension, cigarette use, and diabetes. Removal of the balloon resulted in restoration of pulses in one patient; the second required vascular repair, which demonstrated that the device had been inserted through a superficial femoral artery that contained extensive thrombus. It is likely that balloon insertion in the superficial rather than the common femoral artery contributed to vascular compromise in this patient, underscoring the importance of accurate determination of anatomical landmarks during balloon insertion, regardless of insertion technique.

In summary, Nash and associates found that use of the sheathless insertion technique in conjunction with a slightly modified 9.5 Fr balloon catheter was associated with rapid and safe insertion, effective counterpulsation, and a limb ischemia rate of only 10%. Patients who did develop limb ischemia in this study had multiple risk factors for vascular complications as defined by prior studies.[2,4] Importantly, the sheathless introduction technique was *not* associated with increased bleeding at the arterial entry site.

SUMMARY

IABC catheters can be safely and effectively inserted without the use of an introducing sheath in many patients. Sheathless insertion technique is rapid and does not appear to result in bleeding around the catheter shaft at the arterial entry site. In patients in whom this method of insertion is not promptly successful, subsequent insertion via the standard technique through a sheath can be performed quickly over the same guidewire, without sacrifice of guidewire access to the central circulation. This sheathless insertion technique results in a significant reduction in the effective cross-sectional area of the counterpulsation catheter and may decrease the rate of limb ischemia and significant vascular complications. The recent introduction of 8.5 Fr balloon catheters (which require the same size introducing sheath as 9.5 Fr balloon catheters) may further increase the potential benefit of sheathless insertion. A randomized trial of standard vs. sheathless insertion is required to confirm this potential advantage.

REFERENCES

1. Goldberg MJ et al: Intraaortic balloon pump insertion: a randomized study comparing percutaneous and surgical techniques, *J Am Coll Cardiol* 9:515, 1987.
2. Alderman JD et al: Incidence and management of limb ischemia with percutaneous wire-guided intraaortic balloon catheters, *J Am Coll Cardiol* 9:524, 1987.
3. Skillman JJ, Kim DS, Baim DS: Vascular complications of percutaneous femoral cardiac interventions, *Arch Surg* 123:1207, 1988.
4. Gottlieb SO et al: Identification of patients at high risk for complications of intraaortic balloon counterpulsation: a multivariate risk factor analysis, *Am J Cardiol* 53:1135, 1984.
5. Lefemine AA et al: Results and complications of intraaortic balloon pumping in surgical and medical patients, *Am J Cardiol* 40:416, 1977.
6. McCabe JC et al: Complications of intra-aortic balloon insertion and counterpulsation, *Circulation* 57:769, 1978.
7. Isner JM et al: Complications of the intraaortic balloon counterpulsation device: clinical and morphologic observations in 45 necropsy patients, *Am J Cardiol* 45:260, 1980.
8. Kantrowitz A et al: Intraaortic balloon pumping 1967 through 1982: analysis of complications in 733 patients, *Am J Cardiol* 57:976, 1986.
9. Wolfson S et al: Modification of intraaortic balloon catheter to permit introduction by cardiac catheterization techniques, *Am J Cardiol* 41:733, 1978.
10. Bregman D et al: Percutaneous intraaortic balloon insertion, *Am J Cardiol* 46:261, 1980.
11. Goldberger M, Tabak SW, Shah PK: Clinical experience with intra-aortic balloon counterpulsation in 112 consecutive patients, *Am Heart J* 111:497, 1986.
12. Nash IS et al: A new technique for sheathless percutaneous intraaortic balloon catheter insertion, *Cathet Cardiovasc Diagn* 23:57, 1991.

CHAPTER 14

Intraaortic balloon size selection

Terrance M. Hartnett and **Theresa Gaffney**

The intraaortic balloon pump (IABP) is a circulatory assist device widely used to manage patients whose hemodynamic status may be compromised secondary to acute myocardial infarction (MI). 1991 marked the fortieth anniversary of the publication of the original experiments on diastolic augmentation by Kantrowitz and Kantrowitz.[1] Clauss et al.[2] in 1962 expanded this concept by withdrawing blood from the aorta during systole to reduce cardiac work and subsequently reinfused it during diastole to provide the augmentation. These original concepts of modern-day counterpulsation provided the impetus for extensive empirical and animal testing, which culminated in 1967 with the first human use of the IABP in the treatment of cardiogenic shock.[3]

Counterpulsation devices for increasing aortic root pressure during ventricular diastole and lowering that pressure at the onset of systole have two components: an elongated sausage-shaped balloon mounted on a long catheter and a drive console to provide synchronized inflation and deflation of the balloon. The effectiveness of a counterpulsation system depends on several factors. These include the efficiency of the drive system in sensing electrical trigger events, the system's ability to rapidly shuttle the drive gas, the hemodynamic status of the patient, the anatomical position of the balloon, and the volume of the balloon employed.

This chapter reviews IAB catheter design and sizing considerations related to adult anatomical differences.

IAB CATHETER DESIGN

IAB catheter design has evolved considerably since the first catheters were used in the 1960s. Once ideal anatomical position was established, the next consideration in balloon design was midthoracic aorta dimensions from the takeoff of the left subclavian artery to the renal artery origin.

Weikel et al[4] studied aortograms from 169 patients at the Massachusetts General

Hospital and found that "midthoracic corrected diameters varied in size from 16 to 30 mm with 90% of the patients having diameters greater than 19 mm." Paulin[5] stated "the ascending aorta has a rather constant caliber varying between 22 and 38 mm in adults. . . . Commensurate with the branching of the large arch arteries, the descending aorta has a slightly smaller caliber than the ascending aorta." Both authors infer that the size of the aorta is related to patient size, age, and weight.

Balloon design must also consider the size of the patient. The maximum elevation of aortic root pressure occurs when the balloon is as near as possible to the aortic valve.[6] However, considering the potential risks of injury or blockage to the head and neck vessels, it was determined that the optimal position of the proximal tip of the balloon is 1 to 2 cm distal to the origin of the left subclavian artery. The distal tip of the balloon should be above the origin of the renal arteries to avoid compromising renal circulation and function.

Wolvek of Datascope Corporation reported a number of findings related to patient height and sex. His data indicate that with proper proximal tip placement the distal end of the balloon will lie above the diaphragm in patients who are at least 66 inches tall. A multihospital Datascope study showed the mean height of female patients to be 62.88 inches.

In a second study, 35.7% of the female patients were under 62 inches tall (ranging from 60 to 71 inches). Wolvek also found that while the gender ratio of all IABC patients was only 31% to 35% female, the ratio of female patients who developed plaque-related leaks ranged from 57% to 62.5%. A synthesis of aortic lengths and diameters prepared from thirteen sources by the Advanced Research Group concluded that even with proper placement of a 40-cc balloon with a diameter of 15 mm, the distal portion of the balloon may lie below the celiac-renal segment where the aorta tapers from 20 mm to 13 mm in diameter in patients under 62 inches tall. Wolvek[7] states that because there is a causal relationship between height and plaque-induced leaks, as well as a generally higher incidence of calcific plaque in the abdominal than the thoracic aorta, the use of "the 34 cc Percor STAT DL 9.5 Fr balloon in the patient shorter than 62 inches will significantly reduce the balloon's contact with calcific plaque thereby reducing the possibility of balloon perforation by plaque in the smaller patient." The data of the research group are presented in Tables 14-1 and 14-2, and graphically represented in Fig. 14-1.

Another characteristics of the balloon is its shape. Studies[8,9] conducted in vitro, as well as theoretical considerations, led to considerable concern about what has come to be known as the "bubble blowing phenomena" in cylindrical balloons. At normal or high pressures, the balloon would occupy most of the space within the descending thoracic aorta. At low pressures, aortic diameter decreases and a cylindrically shaped balloon develops significant lateral wall pressure leading to selective inflation of the two ends of the balloon first, effectively trapping blood in

Table 14-1.   Aortic segment lengths related to height

Arterial segment	Length (cm)		
	Small	Medium	Large
AR-A*	2.8	3.2	3.9
AR-B	5.0	5.5	6.0
B-C	4.5	5.2	6.0
C-D	7.0	9.0	11.0
C-E	16.0	24.0	30.0
E-H	12.0	14.0	16.0
H-K	16.0	19.0	22.0
L-M	0.3	0.7	1.1
M-N	0.1	0.3	0.45
E-O	0.5	0.5	0.5
O-P	1.7	1.7	1.7
P-Q	1.3	1.3	1.3
H-I	7.0	8.0	9.0
I-J	8.0	10.0	12.0
K-L	1.0	1.0	1.0

From Datascope Corporation, Paramus, NJ.
*See Fig. 14-1 for abbreviations.

Table 14-2.   Aortic segment diameter related to height

Arterial location	Diameter (mm)		
	Small	Medium	Large
AR*	27	31	37
A	28	32	39
B	28	32	39
C	22	28	34
D	21	27	33
E	20	26	33
F	16	22	29
G	13	19	26
H	11	17	24
I	5	9	13
J	4	7	10
K	4	7	10
L	8	10	12
M	6	8	10
N	11	12.5	14
O	7	10	12
P	4	5	6
Q	2	4.5	6

From Datascope Corporation, Paramus, NJ.
*See Fig. 14-1 for abbreviations.

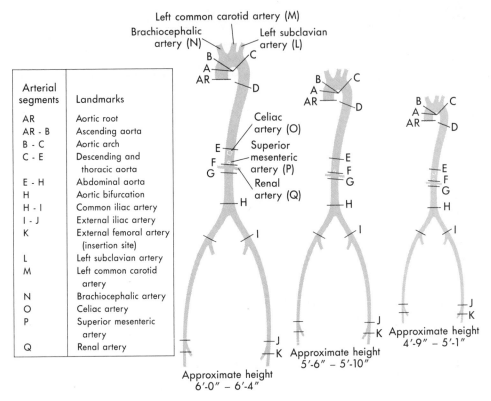

Fig. 14-1. Arterial dimensions. (Courtesy Datascope Corporation, Paramus, NJ)

the middle. This could result in lowered augmentation. To minimize this potential problem, the trisegmented AVCO balloon (Fig. 14-2) and the Datascope dual-chambered balloon (Fig. 14-3) were developed. It is important to note that the "bubble blowing" observations were made in circulation models enclosed in rigid cylinders. In future years, the development of percutaneous insertion techniques with tightly wrapped balloons precluded the use of these multichambered devices.

The diameter of the balloon is limited by aortic diameter. Weber and Janicki[10] observed that "for any arterial pressure or aorta size, the greatest augmentation of MADP was seen with complete occlusion." Concerns about red cell damage, trauma to the aortic wall, and the potential for damage to the balloon material dictated that optimal occlusivity be no more than 90% to 95%.

IAB SIZE SELECTION CONSIDERATIONS

Kantrowitz and co-workers[11] determined that the balloon is "limited by the volume of blood contained within the aorta just prior to inflation . . . further increases

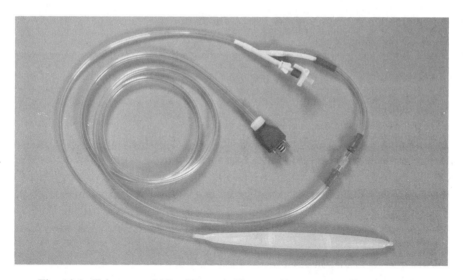

Fig. 14-2. Trisegment IAB. (Courtesy Kontron Instruments, Everett, Mass.)

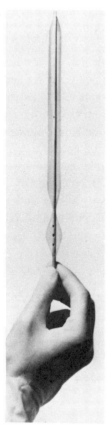

Fig. 14-3. Unidirectional IAB. (Courtesy Datascope Corporation, Paramus, NJ.)

in pumping volume result only in distention of the aorta and not in the effective pumping of blood."

From these data it can be concluded that the ideal balloon for any patient will be the following:

1. Slightly shorter than the distance from the left subclavian artery to the takeoff of the renals
2. 90% to 95% of the diameter of the aorta
3. Equal in volume to the volume of blood in the aorta at any given time

Since the use of these criteria is unrealistic in the clinical world, how is the appropriate balloon selected for any given patient? The Massachusetts General Hospital derived a formula for balloon selection based on patient weight in pounds multiplied by the patient age in years. If this product exceeds 6000, a 50-cc balloon should be used; if the product is less than 6000, a 40-cc balloon is indicated (Kontron Instruments).

Veasy and Webster, in their pediatric work, derived the following formula[12]: The balloon should have a volume of at least 50% of the stroke volume. It is assumed that cardiac output will be sufficiently low that the cardiac index (CI) will be no higher than 2.0. Accordingly, the following formula could be used:

$$\frac{2000 \ (CI) \times BSA}{heart \ rate} \times 0.5 = balloon \ size$$

Table 14-3 demonstrates the estimated balloon size calculation for adults of various heights and weights utilizing this formula with an assumed CI of 1.5 and a heart rate of 100. If one were to follow the hypothetical clinical course of a patient 6 feet tall, weighing 180 pounds (BSA, 2.04) during a period from balloon insertion through successful balloon removal, making corrections in balloon volume at intervals suggested by changes in clinical status, the results would appear in Fig. 14-4. Note that as the patient improves and CI increases while heart rate declines, the estimated balloon size necessary to maintain the same percentage of augmentation increases. These data correlate well with observations by Weber and Janicki[10] that augmentation percentage decreases as mean arterial pressure increases and by

Table 14-3.   Calculation of IAB size*

Height (in)	Weight (lb)	BSA	Calculated IAB size (cc)
60	100	1.38	23.5
64	125	1.60	27.2
68	160	1.87	31.8
72	180	2.04	34.7
74	200	2.18	37.1

*Heart rate 100 beats per minute; CI = 1.5.

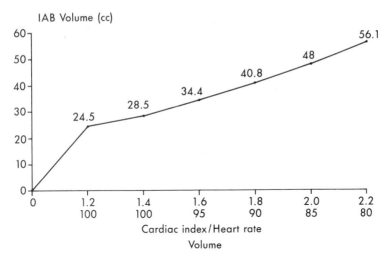

Fig. 14-4. Calculated IAB volume for a hypothetical patient 6 ft, 180 lb, BSA 2.04.

Kantrowitz et al,[11] who stated "The significance of aortic elasticity in the patient is illustrated by the fact that aortic volume doubles between a shock mean of 30 to 40 mm Hg and a normal mean pressure of 90 to 100 mm Hg." The calculations help explain one of the weaning criteria that has been observed. As the clinical status of a patient improves, augmentation decreases. When the balloon-assisted diastolic pressure is equal to or less than the patient's systolic pressure, this fact in conjunction with other clinical data may be used as an indication for balloon removal.

The standard balloon selection procedure for adults has been to opt for the largest size available and to use a smaller size balloon only if one is unable to introduce the larger. Using the data in Fig. 14-2, one could elect to introduce, for example, a 50-cc balloon in this hypothetical patient, initially pump with a volume of 24.5 cc, and increase the volume as changes in CI and heart rate indicate. This method would not only provide for optimal augmentation for the failing heart but provide ongoing optimal augmentation for the improving heart.

SUMMARY

Since the advent of percutaneous insertion, IAB catheter usage has largely been a 40-cc volume for adult patients. While in many adult clinical instances this volume is appropriate, it should be noted that IAB size can have deleterious effects when too large and reduced cardiac benefit when too small.

Currently available adult balloon sizes for each manufacturer with volumes, membrane lengths, and inflated diameters are provided in Table 14-4. We make no

Table 14-4. Balloon volumes, membrane lengths, and inflated diameters by manufacturer

Manufacturer	IAB volume (cc)	Membrane length (cm)	Inflated diameter (mm)
Aries/St. Jude Medical	30	24.1	15.6
	40	27.5	16.2
	50	27.5	18.3
Datascope Corporation	34	21.9	14.7
	40	26.3	15.0
Kontron	30	19.8	15.0
Instruments, Inc.	40	22.7	16.0
	50	22.7	18.0
Mansfield Cardiac	30	20.0	15.0
Assist	40	22.0	17.0
	40	27.0	15.0
	50	23.0	18.5

recommendation as to the selection of one balloon style or size. Contact the various manufacturers for their input and expertise in the determination of the best combination of available products to suit a specific clinical need.

REFERENCES

1. Kantrowitz A, Kantrowitz A: Experimental augmentation of coronary flow by retardation of the arterial pulse, *Surgery* 34:678, 1953.
2. Clauss RH et al: Assisted circulation. I. The arterial counterpulsation, *J Thorac Cardiovasc Surg* 41:447, 1961.
3. Kantrowitz A et al: Initial clinical experience with intra-aortic balloon pumping in cardiogenic shock, *JAMA* 203:135, 1968.
4. Weikel AM et al: Size limits and pumping effectiveness of intra-aortic balloons, *Ann Thorac Surg* 12(1):45, 1971.
5. Paulin S: Aortography. In Grossman W, Baim D, eds: *Cardiac catheterization, angiography and intervention,* Philadelphia, 1991, Lea & Febiger.
6. Gundel WD et al: Coronary collateral flow studies during variable aortic root pressure waveforms, *J Appl Physiol* 29:579, 1970.
7. Wolvek S: *Patient/balloon sizing considerations,* Paramus, NJ, 1991, Datascope Corp.
8. Laird JD et al: The dynamics of an improved intra-aortic balloon pump, 20th Annual Conference on Engineering in Medicine and Biology, Boston, Mass, 1967.
9. Laird JD et al: Theoretical and experimental analysis of the intra-aortic balloon pump, *Trans Am Soc Artif Intern Organs* XIV:338, 1968.
10. Weber KT, Janicki MS: Intra-aortic balloon counterpulsation, *Ann Thorac Surg* 17:6, 602, 1974.
11. Kantrowitz A et al: Cardiac assistance by the intra-aortic balloon pump, Second Medical Physics Conference, Boston, Mass, 1969.
12. Veasy LG, Webster H: Intra-aortic balloon pumping in infants and children, *Cardiac Assists* 2(2), 1985.

PART THREE

INTERFACING COUNTERPULSATION TO THE PATIENT'S CARDIAC CYCLE

CHAPTER 15

Supportive hemodynamic monitoring

Susan J. Quaal

Hemodynamic monitoring has been described as "repeated or continuous observations or measurements of the patient, his or her physiological status, and functions of life support equipment for the purpose of guiding management decisions, including when to make therapeutic interventions and assessment of these interventions."[1] *Hemodynamics* is a term originating from the Greek words "haima" (blood) and "dynamis" (power).[2] Hemodynamic monitoring is a most powerful adjunct in caring for the intraaortic balloon counterpulsation (IABC) patient. Direct and derived indices greatly influence clinical decision making regarding appropriateness of initiating, weaning, and withdrawing IABC therapy. Quality assurance is therefore critical to ensure that hemodynamic monitoring is a clinically accurate and supportive adjunct to IABC.

QUALITY ASSURANCE IN HEMODYNAMIC MONITORING
Static factors

A basic invasive hemodynamic monitoring system consists of a monitoring catheter inserted in a vessel from which the pressure is to be monitored, a transducer connected to this catheter, an external plumbing system with pressurized continuous flush infusion, stopcock, and fast-flush device (Fig. 15-1).

A transducer converts physiological mechanical energy in the form of pressure to an electrical signal that can be amplified and monitored on a display oscilloscope. Transducers emit their signals in response to displacements imposed by direct application of mechanical force. Pressure recording therefore involves displacement of the elastic diaphragm or transducer sensing mechanism.[3]

Zeroing. Before zeroing, the transducer should be attached to the monitor for the warm-up time recommended by the manufacturer. Gardner[4] points out that "the accuracy of blood pressure readings depends on establishing an accurate reference point from which all subsequent measurements are made." Gardner further explains

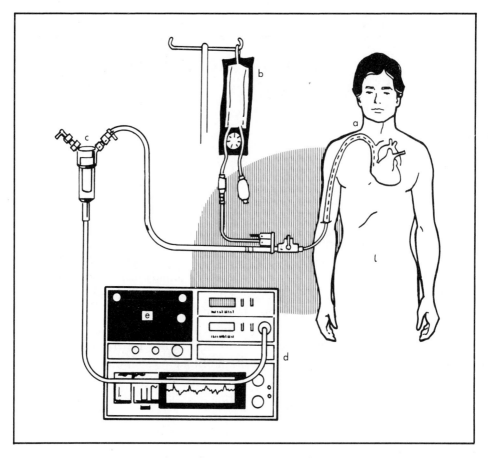

Fig. 15-1. Components of basic invasive hemodynamic monitoring system. Catheter *(a)*; pressurized continuous infusion *(b)*; transducer connects to fast-flush device *(c)*; amplifier *(d)*; oscilloscope *(e)*.

that the zeroing process is done to compensate for offset caused by hydrostatic pressure differences and offset in pressure transducer, amplifier, oscilloscope, recorder, and digital displays.[5]

Windsor and Burch[6] described the "phlebostatic axis" as an external reference point for the right atrial level. Phlebostatic axis is a point of junction between a frontal and transverse chest plane and is located by drawing an imaginary line from the fourth sternal costal space and extended around to the right side of the chest. A second imaginary line is drawn vertically from midaxillary line down to bisect with the first transverse line (Fig. 15-2).

Zeroing in a hemodynamic monitoring system is accomplished by positioning a

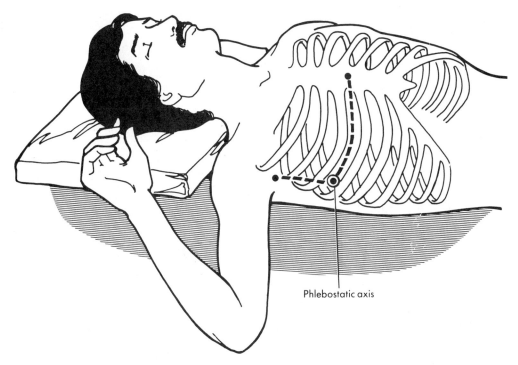

Phlebostatic axis

Fig. 15-2. Phlebostatic axis is external reference for approximating location of right atrium. One imaginary line is drawn from fourth intercostal space downward along right side of chest. Second imaginary line is drawn vertically from patient's midaxillary line down to bisect first transverse line. Junction of these two points is *phlebostatic axis.*

fluid-filled stopcock (fluid air interface) at the phlebostatic axis, turning it off to the patient or open to air, and activating the bedside monitor zero function. Zeroing the pressure system is the "single" most important step in setting up a pressure measurement system.[7]

Gardner[7] states "many pressure monitoring users erroneously assume that the location of the pressure transducer is the zero reference point. The only time such an assumption is correct occurs when the stopcock is attached to the transducer and is at the same elevation as the transducer." *It is the stopcock that is opened to air and not the transducer that is leveled to the patient's phlebostatic axis*[7-9] (Fig. 15-3). In this way, all pressure contributions from the atmosphere are negated and only pressure values that exist within the heart chamber or vessel will be measured. If the stopcock, which is opened to air, is pole mounted, a carpenter's level or improvised connecting tubing filled with water as a meniscus should be used to precisely align the stopcock opening with the patient's phlebostatic axis.

Gardner and Hollingsworth[10] suggested factors that alter the zero reference: (1)

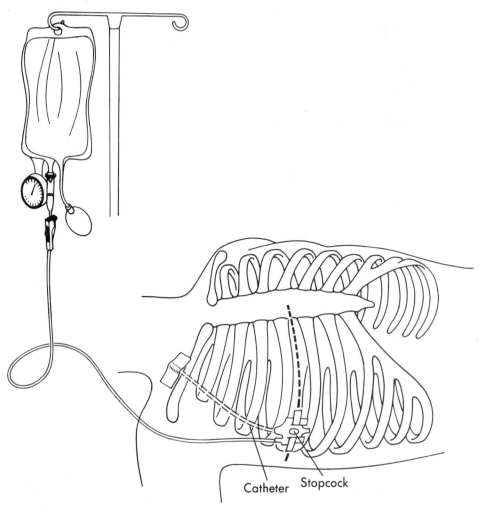

Catheter Stopcock

Fig. 15-3. Stopcock (not transducer) is opened to air and leveled to patient's hemostatic axis.

patient's vertical position in relation to the transducer (hydrostatic effect), (2) drift due to membrane dome coupling problems, (3) transducer electrical zero change, and (4) pressure amplifier drift. Pressure monitoring systems should always be zeroed before initiating treatment changes based on pressure data.

All stopcocks must be fluid filled so that no trapped air remains. Extreme care should also be taken when handling the stopcocks to ensure that contamination does not occur. After drawing blood or zeroing, stopcocks should be covered with a sterile protective cap.[11]

Table 15-1.   Steps for calibrating a transducer with mercury

1. Remove blood pressure cuff from a sphygmomanometer.
2. Attach a mercury manometer to one of the transducer dome's Luer-Lok fittings, using a short plastic tubing.
3. Attach a hand bulb to the remaining Luer-Lok fitting of the transducer dome using another short piece of plastic tubing.
4. Squeeze the hand bulb to elevate the mercury column to 200 mm Hg. Bedside monitor digital readout should also be 200 mm Hg ± 2 mm Hg.
5. Release the hand bulb and check for a return of the digital readout to zero.
6. The transducer should also be checked at a low mercury level (i.e., 10 to 20 mm Hg) to ensure linear accuracy. At low mercury levels, the bedside digital readout should not vary by more than 1 mm Hg).

Extreme care must be taken to be certain the stopcock is properly positioned so that manometer pressure is applied to the transducer. If the stopcock is positioned erroneously, a catastrophic air embolism could result.

From Daily E, Schroeder J: *Techniques in bedside hemodynamic monitoring*, St. Louis, 1989, Mosby-Year Book.

Accuracy factors

Most hemodynamic monitoring is now carried out with accurate ($\pm$1%), disposable transducers.[10] If a reusable transducer is used, it should be "calibrated." This is a process of verification that a known millimeter of mercury pressure applied to the transducer is displayed on the monitor. A sterile piece of venous tubing filled with sterile fluid can be used to microbiologically isolate the mercury manometer. However, extreme care must be taken to ensure the stopcock is properly positioned so that manometer pressure, not air, is applied to the transducer. *If the stopcock is positioned erroneously, a catastrophic air embolism to the patient could result.*[12] A procedure for transducer calibration with a mercury manometer is listed in Table 15-1 and illustrated in Fig. 15-4. At high mercury levels ($\geq$200 mm Hg), bedside monitor digital readout should not vary by more than $\pm$2 mm Hg. At low mercury levels (10 to 20 mm Hg), the bedside digital readout should not vary by more than 1 mm Hg.[8]

Dynamic factors

Quantifying hemodynamic pressure depends on the fluid-filled catheter system's ability to transmit the patient's pressure with fidelity or accuracy of reproduction. Physiological waveforms are dynamic, not static. A hemodynamic monitoring system must therefore be able to transmit pulsatile pressures through its catheter plumbing system. Transducers reliably reproduce pressure applied, no matter how distorted the signal may be. Therefore hemodynamic quality assurance must also include a dynamic factor or assessment of the instrumentation system's ability to accurately transmit a pulsatile pressure waveform to the transducer. Dynamic response

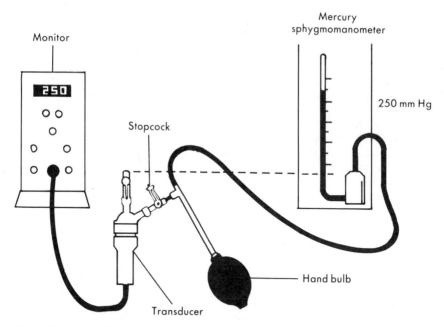

Fig. 15-4. Mercury calibration of transducer. Known value of mercury is applied to transducer, which should in turn register on oscilloscope.

characteristics are primarily determined by the system's "natural frequency" (analogous to an automobile tire bouncing on a highway) and its "damping coefficient" (how quickly the car stabilizes following each bounce).[5]

Dynamic response: natural frequency and damping coefficient. Dynamic responsiveness of a hemodynamic plumbing system depends on its "resonant or natural frequency," which refers to an oscillatory response produced by the system after it is excited. This resonant frequency response is similar to vibrations or resonate response produced by striking a bell. Another example of natural frequency is the responsiveness of a tennis ball when dropped on a hard, flat surface (Fig. 15-5). The ball bounces or oscillates and then comes to rest. With each successive bounce, the ball does not rise as high as it did on the last. Number of oscillations per second is referred to as *natural frequency*, measured in Hertz (Hz), or cycles/second. The time it takes the ball to come to rest is related to its *damping coefficient*.[3]

Long catheters with small diameters, transducer "stiffness" and entrapped air bubbles, or blood clots can distort the transmitted pressure signal and therefore distort pressure waveform fidelity. Assessment for potential technical errors within the system should be undertaken before evaluating the quantitative data measured from any transmitted pressure waveform.[13]

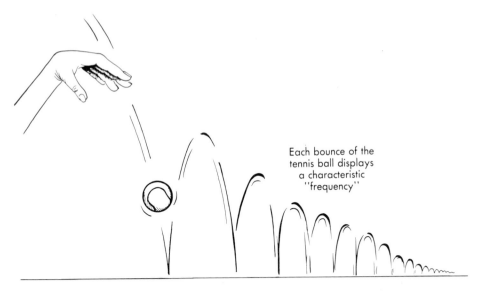

Each bounce of the
tennis ball displays
a characteristic
"frequency"

Fig. 15-5. Tennis ball dropped on hard surface bounces, or oscillates, and then comes to rest. Oscillations represent bouncing tennis ball's characteristic frequency. Time taken for ball to come to rest is referred to as damping coefficient.

Arterial pressures are less affected by technical error and are easier to measure because of their high mm Hg. Measurement of a pulmonary artery wedge pressure (PAWP) is more difficult because (1) it requires inflation of a balloon, which introduces noise, and (2) the catheter passes through two heart valves, which make contact with the catheter at the time of valve closure.

Fast-flush test

Frequency response of a catheter-plumbing hemodynamic monitoring system can be obtained by stimulating the system with high pressure and then observing the system's natural frequency and damping coefficient. The system's in-line, fast-flush device (Fig. 15-6) can be used to excite the system by opening, then quickly closing this device. A fast-flush device tests the entire system from transducer to the catheter tip.[12] This action temporarily interrupts pressure waveform transmission and applies a step change or "square wave" pressure, followed by oscillations, which revert back to the pressure waveform monitored. Measurement of these oscillating components is used to calculate both natural frequency and damping coefficient.

Natural frequency is determined by measuring the distance between two consecutive oscillatory peaks in millimeters (also called a *period*) and dividing the distance by the paper speed (usually 25 mm/sec) (Fig. 15-7). For example, if the distance between 2 consecutive oscillatory peaks is 2 small boxes, or 2 mm, and the paper

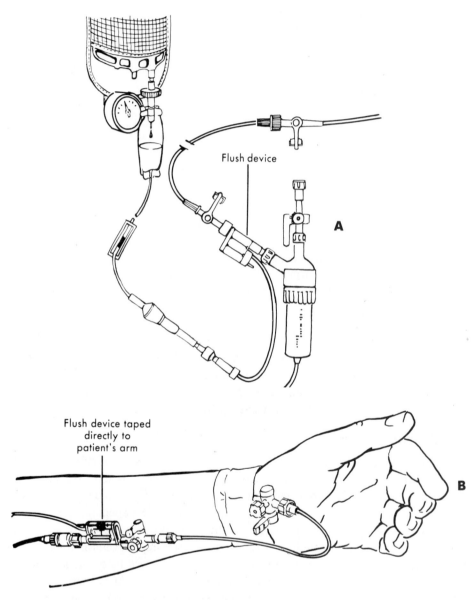

Flush device

A

Flush device taped
directly to
patient's arm

B

Fig. 15-6. A, Fast-flush device is placed in-line as part of hemodynamic monitoring system's plumbing system. **B,** Fast-flush device taped directly to patient's arm.

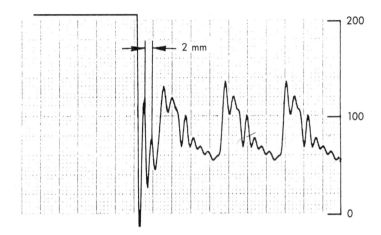

Fig. 15-7. Illustration of square wave (fast-flush) response. *Natural frequency* is estimated by dividing measured distance between two consecutive peaks (*period*) by paper speed. In this example, period is 2 mm divided by paper speed of 25 mm/sec and yields natural frequency of 12.5 Hz.

speed is 25 mm/sec, natural frequency is 12.5 Hz. Damping coefficient is calculated by measuring two consecutive peak amplitudes and dividing A2/A1 to obtain an amplitude ratio (Fig. 15-8), which is then plotted on a graph (Fig. 15-9) to obtain the damping coefficient.[12] For example, an amplitude ratio of 0.58 (right-hand side scale) corresponds to a damping coefficient (left-side scale) of 0.17.[11]

Optimal dynamic response occurs when natural frequency is high, in the range of 20 to 25 Hz and damping coefficient is between 0.5 and 0.75. The lower the natural frequency, the higher the damping coefficient required to accurately transmit physiological pulsating waveforms through the catheter-plumbing system. If natural frequency is below 7 Hz, the pressure waveform will be distorted regardless of its damping coefficient. However, if natural frequency can be increased to 24 Hz, the damping coefficient can range from 0.15 to 1.0 without waveform distortion.[14] Fig. 15-10 illustrates a fast-flush test with optimum natural frequency (25 Hz) and damping coefficient.

Fig. 15-11 illustrates an underdamped system with wide excursions above and below the baseline before oscillations come to rest. False high systolic and low diastolic readings are the consequence of a greatly underdamped system. An overdamped response is illustrated in Fig. 15-12. Overdamping reduces physiological waveform amplitude, which appears sluggish; the dicrotic notch is frequently absent. False low systolic and high diastolic readings occur with an overdamped system. However, diastolic pressures are more tolerant of dynamic response inadequacies.[14]

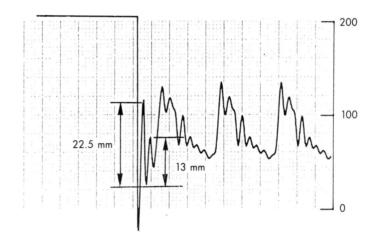

Fig. 15-8. Damping coefficient is estimated by calculating ratio of two consecutive peaks (A2/A1), which is 13/22.5 or 0.58. This ratio value is located on right-hand scale of graph pictured in Fig. 15-9.

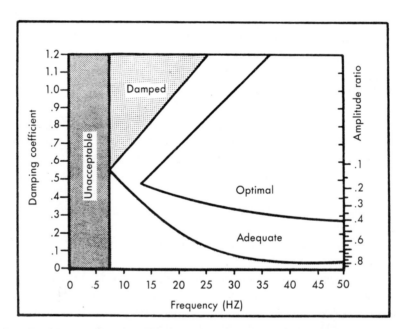

Fig. 15-9. Damping coefficient graph. Scale on right represents amplitude ratios calculated from fast flushes. Amplitude ratio is then used to locate corresponding damping coefficient on left. Amplitude ratio in Fig. 15-8 is 0.58, which corresponds to damping coefficient on left-hand scale of 0.17. (From Gardner RM, Hollingsworth KW: Optimizing the electrocardiogram and pressure monitoring, *Crit Care Med* 14:651, 1986.)

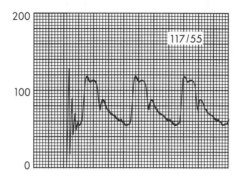

Fig. 15-10. Fast-flush test with optimum natural frequency of 24 Hz and damping coefficient of .15.

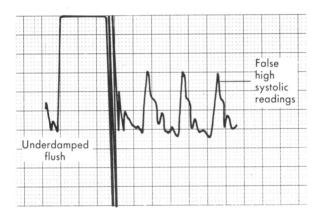

Fig. 15-11. Fast-flush illustrating underdamped system with wide excursions above and below baseline before oscillations come to rest.

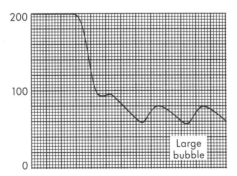

Fig. 15-12. "Overdamped" fast-flush response characterized by square wave, which does not fall below baseline on release of fast-flush device. Arterial pressure waveform appears damped with lack of any discernible dicrotic notch.

Table 15-2. Clinical recommendations for optimizing pressure monitoring dynamic response

---

1. Recommended frequency of dynamic response validation
   a. At least once each shift.
   b. After each "opening" of the system, such as for transducer zeroing, drawing blood, or changing tubing.
   c. Whenever the pressure waveform "appears" to be damped or distorted.
2. Steps to optimizing dynamic response
   a. Select monitoring "kits" that are simple, with a minimal amount of pressure tubing and relatively noncompliant tubing, flush devices, and transducer.
   b. Remove all air bubbles during setup, especially near the transducer. Air bubbles in the side ports' three-way stopcocks are invisible and can be troublesome. Eliminate them by filling all the ports of the stopcock with fluid.
   c. Minimize the potential for clot formation at the catheter tip by using a continuous flush system. Ascertain that there are no clots in the catheter by doing the fast-flushing procedure and, if necessary, aspirating blood from the catheter.
   d. Eliminate kinks in the catheter or tubing.
   e. Eliminate long lengths or compliant interconnecting tubing.
   f. Use low-volume displacement transducers and flush devices. Disposable transducers have lower volume displacement values than most of the reusable transducers.

From Gibbs NC, Gardner RM: Dynamics of invasive pressure monitoring systems: clinical and laboratory evaluation, *Heart Lung* 17:42, 1988.

Every effort should be made to maximize natural frequency by: (1) eliminating all air bubbles from the system and preventing blood clots; (2) using stiff, noncompliant tubing; (3) keeping catheter and tubing length to a minimum (no longer than 3 to 4 feet); (4) using as large a diameter possible catheters; and (5) eliminating loose fitting connections[13] (Table 15-2).

The fast-flush test also identifies free fluid flow in the catheter system.

Free flow can be impaired by blood backing up in the system, a clot at the catheter tip, catheter tip resting against a vessel wall, or a kink in the catheter or connecting tubing. Without free fluid flow in the system, pressure measurement errors will occur. To confirm free fluid flow from the fast flush test, the waveform should oscillate freely once or twice, then return directly into the pressure waveform and not "peg" or stick on the top or the bottom of the paper before going into the pressure waveform.[11]

The fast-flush test should be performed on the initial system setup, after blood withdrawal, with every recorded measurement, during troubleshooting, and at periodic intervals, such as every shift change, to document the pressure monitoring system's continued ability to accurately reflect intravascular pressure.[10-11]

PRESSURE WAVEFORMS

Placement of a pulmonary artery catheter is commonplace in conjunction with IABC (Fig. 15-13). Normal waveforms, which have been idealized for clarity, are illustrated in Fig. 15-14. It is desirable to monitor pressure waveforms from dual-channel recorders so that simultaneous electrocardiogram (ECG) and pressure waveforms can be recorded. References for normal pressures vary slightly; the most generally accepted values are presented. Common problems associated with pulmonary artery catheter monitoring, their causes, prevention, and correction are listed in Table 15-3.

Text continued on p. 233.

Table 15-3. Troubleshooting pulmonary artery catheters

Problem	Cause	Prevention	Correction
Ventricular arrhythmias	Irritation of RV endocardium by catheter on insertion or after implantation, or catheter floats back to RV after implantation	Suturing of catheter at insertion site; continuous monitoring of electrocardiogram	Ventricular irritability may require lidocaine and/or catheter repositioning
Spontaneous wedging of catheter	Migration of catheter forward, since it is flow directed and catheter material softens at body temperature	—	Spontaneous wedging leads to pulmonary infarction if not corrected; catheter must be pulled back into larger portion of PA
Right ventricular waveform appears rather than PA pressure waveform	Migration of catheter backwards into RV	Suturing of catheter at insertion site	Turning patient on his left side and having him cough may float catheter out into PA; inflating to facilitate flotation; observing for ventricular ectopy once catheter is documented to be in RV
Unable to withdraw blood from distal port	Ball clot on end of catheter	Continuous slow infusion of catheter; plumbing system with heparin drip	Clot may occasionally dissolve or dislodge, but catheter may have to be removed; no flushing with tuberculin syringe, as this blows clot off catheter and causes embolization to patient

Continued.

Table 15-3.   Troubleshooting pulmonary artery catheters—cont'd

Problem	Cause	Prevention	Correction
Unable to obtain PA wedge tracing	Insufficient air used to inflate balloon; it may be ruptured; thin latex of balloon absorbs lipoproteins from blood and gradually loses its elasticity, increasing chance of rupture	Inflating balloon gradually and not overinflating; if no resistance is felt, inflation should not be continued	Deflating and trying again; if no resistance is felt, balloon may be ruptured; discontinuing attempts to reinflate; notifying physician
Damped tracing as indicated by flush with poor ring; tracing may exhibit decreased amplitude and lower systolic readings	Most common cause is air bubbles in dome; infusion bag may have lost pressure	Flushing all bubbles out of system when assembling line; periodically checking for bubbles in tubing and stopcocks; maintaining 300 mm Hg pressure on infusion bag	Flushing bubbles in dome to outside but not to patient and reevaluating flushing and tracing
Bleeding back from catheter into connecting tubing	Patient's pressure is higher than counterpressure from pressure infusion bag; loose connections in system	Maintaining 300 mm Hg pressure on infusion bag; checking to see that all connections from patient catheter to transducer are secure	Reestablishing counterpressure in infusion bag if pressure was lost; checking all connections and stopcock positions; replacing any fractured components of software system
PAWP waveform drifts upward on scope	Balloon is overinflated	Observing monitor during inflation; not adding more air to balloon once PA waveform pattern has changed to PAWP	Deflating balloon and observing monitor on reinflation, and adding only amount of air needed to change waveform from PA tracing to PAWP
Unable to obtain pressure readings	Loose connections in system; incorrect stopcock position (transducer open to air); transducer dome is loose; malfunctioning transducer or monitor	Initiating proper system checkout according to unit/hospital biomedical protocols before activating system	Troubleshooting for loose connections; checking calibration of monitor and transducer according to unit/hospital biomedical established procedures

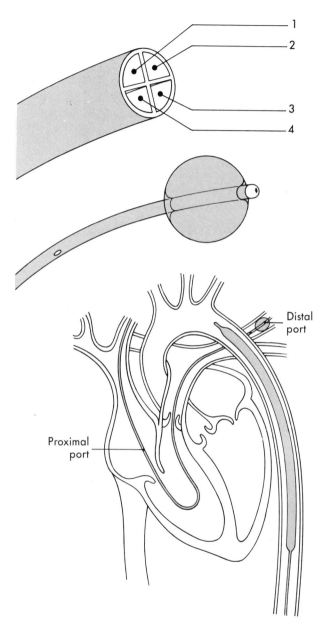

Fig. 15-13. Placement of pulmonary artery catheter in conjunction with IABC. *1*, Distal lumen; *2*, balloon inflation lumen; *3*, thermistor opening; *4*, proximal lumen.

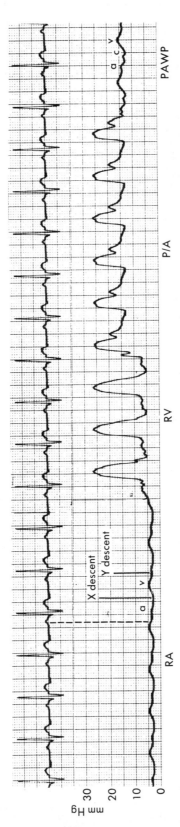

Fig. 15-14. Hemodynamic waveforms recorded during pulmonary artery catheter insertion. *RA*, Right atrium; *RV*, right ventricle; *PA*, pulmonary artery; *PAWP*, pulmonary artery wedge pressure. Right atrial "a" wave is inscribed during atrial contraction, followed by "x descent," which is atrial relaxation. Right atrial "v wave" is inscribed during filling followed by "y descent," which represents passive emptying of RA volume into RV. (Courtesy Baxter Edwards, Santa Ana, Calif.)

Right atrial pressure (normal 1-7 mm Hg)

Right atrial (RA) pressure is recorded as a mean value, since pressure in this chamber is normally low. This allows the RA to receive deoxygenated blood along a downhill pressure gradient; the vena cava serves only as a passive conduit. RA pressure should be equivalent to right ventricular (RV) systolic pressure when the tricuspid valve is open and RA and RV become common chambers. An "a wave" is produced during RA contraction, which occurs just after the atria are electrically depolarized (p wave). Following the a wave is the x descent, which occurs during atrial relaxation. The "v wave" occurs during RA filling. Following the v wave is a y descent, which represents rapid atrial emptying after the tricuspid valve opens.

Caution is extended when comparing normal RA pressure recorded from a pulmonary artery catheter in mm Hg units with a central venous pressure manometer setup, measured in centimeters of water (cm H_2O). To convert cm H_2O to mm Hg divide[8]:

$$\frac{cm \ of \ H_2O}{1.36}$$

Right ventricular pressure (normal 20-25/5-8 mm Hg)

At the time of initial insertion, the inflated balloon, which has a diameter of about 13 mm, guides the catheter through the tricuspid valve into RV and pulmonary artery. As the catheter tip enters RV, the range of pressure excursion markedly increases. Diastolic RV pressure should remain essentially the same as RA. Systolic RV pressure increases to 20 to 25 mm Hg. RV catheter location is easy to confirm because of these contrasted wide excursions in pressure. If RV presure appears when recording from the distal port, the tip of the catheter has migrated backwards from pulmonary artery (PA) to RV. If a RV waveform is recorded from the proximal catheter port, the orifice located at approximately 30 cm from the catheter tip, which should remain in the RA, has migrated through the tricuspid valve into RV.

PA pressure (normal 20-25/10-12 mm Hg)

Systolic pressure should not change between RV and PA. Diastolic pressure increases to 10 to 12 mm Hg and the PA waveform also carries a dicrotic notch landmark, representing closure of the pulmonic valve.

Pulmonary artery capillary pressure (normal <12 mm Hg)

Further progression of the catheter's distal tip inflated balloon is stopped once it migrates into a branch of a pulmonary vessel slightly smaller in diameter than the inflated balloon. Forward blood flow is terminated in that vessel. Since the pressure recording tip is just distal to the inflated balloon, only downstream pressures are recorded. Normally the pulmonary vascular bed has a low resistance. Blood flow from pulmonary capillaries to left atrium (LA) traverses a valveless course. During diastole, the normal nonstenotic mitral valve is open; pulmonary capillary bed, LA, and LV become a common chamber. The pulmonary artery capillary pressure (PACP) reflects left atrial pressure.[15]

Confirming an accurate PACP

Capillary gas. If a "wedged" pulmonary artery catheter is properly positioned in a capillary bed, blood aspirated from that pocket will reflect a high concentration of oxygen and low carbon dioxide. A wedged catheter, in essence, seals off any right ventricle and pulmonary artery venous blood from flowing into the capillary. Validation of a PACP can therefore be determined by drawing a capillary gas (with balloon inflated) and, as close as possible in time, also acquiring an arterial sample. Results are compared. PACP catheter placement is confirmed if the following is met[16]:

1. Partial pressure of capillary oxygen (P_cO_2) − partial pressure of arterial oxygen (P_aO_2) is ≥ 19 mm Hg.
2. Partial pressure of arterial carbon dioxide (P_aO_2) − partial pressure of capillary carbon dioxide (P_cO_2) is ≥ 11 mm Hg.
3. Capillary pH − arterial pH is > 0.08

Lung zone factors. PACP estimates pulmonary venous or left atrial pressure only when a continuous column of blood exists from catheter tip through the capillary bed, into left atrium.[17] If a capillary is collapsed, patency between the LA and catheter tip is interrupted, as resistance is imposed and incorrect pressures are measured.

Fig. 15-15 illustrates a pulmonary artery catheter in three different lung zones. In lung zone I, the catheter tip is positioned within a capillary located above the LA plane. Capillary inflow arterial pressure (Pa) is less than extravascular pulmonary alveolar pressure (PAl/v), which is greater than capillary outflow venous pressure (Pv). Capillaries in lung zone I are totally collapsed.[18]

Lung zone II capillaries are located horizontal to the left atrial plane (Fig. 15-15). Inflow Pa pressure is greater than PAl/v. Extravascular pulmonary alveolar pressure is however greater than Pv. Blood does enter the capillaries, but since PAl/v is greater than Pv, the capillary is partially collapsed. Therefore a pulmonary artery catheter positioned in a lung zone II capillary would be invalid, since capillaries are partially collapsed by alveolar pressure transmitted from lungs across the alveolar capillary membrane.[18]

Lung zone III capillaries are located below the left atrial plane (Fig. 15-15). Inflow Pa pressure is greater than PAl/v pressure, which is less than Pv. Therefore a continuous uninterrupted column of blood exists from left atrium back to catheter tip within a lung zone III capillary.[18]

Two factors favor spontaneous catheter positioning into lung zone III capillaries.

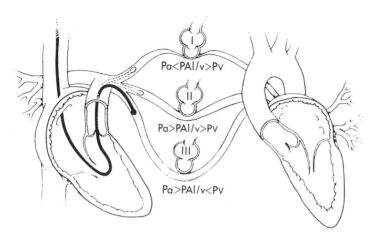

Fig. 15-15. Lung zones I, II, III. In lung zone I, capillaries are above left atrial plane. In lung zone II, capillaries are situated at level of left atrial plane. Only in lung zone III are capillaries below left atrial plane. It is only when pulmonary catheter is positioned in lung zone III that continuous column of blood exists from catheter's distal tip to left atrium, which is necessary for PACP to represent left atrial pressure. (From O'Quin R, Marini JJ: *Am Rev Respir Dis* 128:319, 1983.)

A pulmonary artery catheter is flow directed; its tendency therefore is to float to the area of greatest blood flow, which is intrinsically the dependent lung zone III capillaries. A recumbent patient position reduces lung volume situated above the left atrium. Therefore fewer capillaries will be impacted by extravascular alveolar pressure. More capillaries will fall below the left atrial alveoli, thus affording a continuous column of blood from left atrium back to catheter tip.

Interventions that increase alveolar pressure diminish lung zone III conditions. Positive end-expiratory pressure (PEEP) >10 cm H_2O induces a high alveolar pressure into lung zone III capillaries. An artificially high PACP will be recorded, reflective of alveolar pressure, rather than LA pressure.[19]

Another factor introducing a PEEP-like effect is termed *Auto PEEP*. End-expiratory alveolar pressures may rise in mechanically ventilated patients (even in the absence of PEEP) with airflow obstruction. This is caused by gas trapped behind narrow airways. Enger[20] explains that an auto PEEP-like effect may go unrecognized because the trachea, ventilator circuit, and system manometer are all downstream from the site of flow limitation and remain open to atmosphere.

Factors that lower capillary hydrostatic pressure, such as diuresis and hemorrhage, can also shift lung zone III capillaries to lung zones I or II-like conditions.

Effect of intrapleural pressure variation: where to "read" the PACP. Respiratory variation is a factor that must be taken into consideration when quantifying PACP

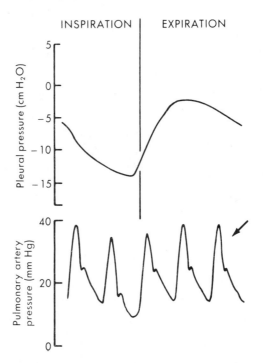

Fig. 15-16. Effect of respiration on PACP. During inspiration, intrapleural pressure decreases, which is reflected as corresponding decrease in PACP. (From Riedinger M et al: *Heart Lung* 10:675, 1981.)

waveforms. Normal inspiration-expiration changes in intrathoracic pressure cause a flux in pressure waveforms. As intrapleural pressure decreases, the pressure waveform falls (Fig. 15-16). During mechanical ventilation, pressures rise during the positive pressure inspiration and fall during exhalation (Fig. 15-17). Riedinger, Shellock, and Swan[21] suggested several techniques for reading PA and PACP waveforms with respect to respiratory variation: (1) breath-holding; (2) removing the patient from the respirator; (3) reading only mean pressure; (4) pressure averaging; and (5) reading end-expiration pressures. They concluded that the most easily obtained and accurate method was end-expiration; this is a relatively constant period of intrathoracic pressure and allows for stable pressure waveforms, which can be easily measured. They cautioned that regardless of procedure used, consistency is critical to ensure accuracy and quality assurance in pressure measurement.

Other criteria used to validate a PACP. The PACP has been reported to be an accurate reflection of LA pressure only about 75% of the time.[12] Additional criteria were proposed to validate an accurate PACP:

1. Mean PACP must be less than the mean PA pressure. The oscilloscope

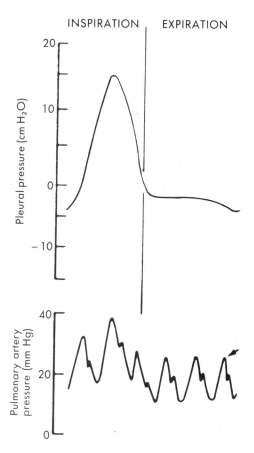

Fig. 15-17. Ventilator effect on pulmonary artery pressure. During inspiration and positive pressure generated by ventilator, pulmonary artery pressure increases and decreases during ventilator expiration. (From Riedinger M et al: *Heart Lung* 10:675, 1981.)

should be observed as the balloon is inflated to confirm a reduction in mean pressure.

2. The phasic PACP recording must be consistent with an atrial pressure waveform, which must be observed on the oscilloscope as the balloon is inflated. Care should be taken to ensure that the balloon is not overinflated, which would produce a falsely elevated PACP.

3. Free flow should be present when the catheter is in the wedge position, so that the tip is in free communication to the LA. Fast flushing the catheter in the PACP position is a reliable method of demonstrating free flow. A 1.0 second flush delivers only about 1.0 ml of fluid.

DERIVED INDICES

Hemodynamic assessment of the IABC patient should include derived indices, as well as the direct physiological pressure measurements. An indexed parameter, such as stroke volume index (SVI), is referenced to body surface area (BSA), which standardizes a normal value range that is universal for children and adults. BSA therefore becomes the denominator for any indexed parameter. The clinician is cautioned that several methods exist for calculating BSA. There have been various homograms collected from a variety of sources in different countries. The problem is that they are not representative of all patient populations. The Boyd study[22] used only white, middle-class people. Dubois[23] had only one child in his study. It has been shown that the homograms in Asian countries differ considerably from those in the United States. Fig. 15-18 illustrates the Dubois body surface chart. The DuBois formula starts to become less accurate with body surface areas less than 0.6 meter squared. It is less accurate with children (1.5% error) and is increasingly inaccurate with infants (5.77% error). The Boyd formula is more accurate across a broader range of patient sizes.[24] It is important to know which formula is utilized in bedside software. An example of possible bedside monitor software formulas is as follows[25]:

$$\text{Boyd BSA:} \quad \frac{3.207 * (\text{Weight}^{\wedge}(0.7285 - 0.0188 * \log(\text{weight}))) * \text{height}^{\wedge}0.3}{10000}$$

Dubois BSA: .007184 * ((weight/1000)$^{\wedge}$.425) * height$^{\wedge}$.725

Stroke volume[8,26,27]

Stroke volume (SV), which is the milliliters of blood ejected with each heart beat, depends on preload, afterload, and contractility. It may be affected by factors influencing total blood volume, central venous return, and resistance to forward systolic ejection. Decreased SV may be due to decreased preload or venous return, tachycardia, arrhythmias, extreme vasodilation, or cardiac tamponade. Decreased contractility, which thereby impacts SV, may be caused by hypoxemia, hypercapnia, acidosis, or changes in left ventricular diameter or wall stress. Increased SV may be the result of slower heart rates and positive inotropic pharmacological agents. SV also increases rapidly at the beginning of exercise and usually plateaus at near maximal values before less than half of maximal exercise capacity is reached.

Formula: $\dfrac{\text{Cardiac output (ml/min)}}{\text{Heart rate}}$

Normal values: 60 to 130 ml/beat

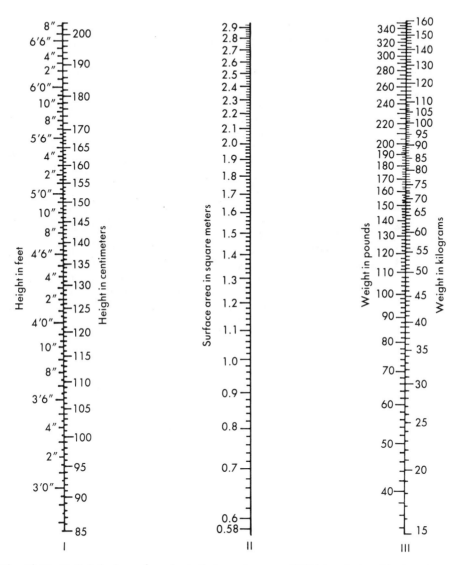

Fig. 15-18. DuBois body surface chart. Body surface area (BSA) is calculated by locating patient's height on scale I and weight on scale III. Straight edge is placed between two points, which intersect on Scale II at patient's BSA. *(From DuBois EF: Basal metabolism in health and disease*, Philadelphia, 1936, Lea & Febiger.)

Stroke volume index (SVI)[8,26,27]

Definition:	SV adjusted for BSA
Formula:	$\dfrac{SV}{BSA}$
Normal values:	41 to 51 ml/beat/m^2

Left ventricular stroke work index (LVSWI)[8,26,27]

Definition:	LVSWI measures the amount of work the left ventricle does per beat when ejecting blood. It is based on calculation of work. Work = Pressure generated × Volume of blood pumped.
Formula:*	SVI = (MAP − PACP) × SVI × 0.0136 The conversion factor of 0.0136 converts ml-mm Hg to gm-m.
Normal values:	38 to 62 g-m/beat/m^2

LVSWI is a useful calculation to assess contractility status. Stroke work index is plotted against PACP. The clinician places an "X" where these two measurements intersect. This matrix can be incorporated into the patient's balloon pump flowsheet (see Fig. 20-1B) to objectively track left ventricular performance before, during, and after IABC.

Right ventricular stroke work index (RVSWI)[8,26,27]

Definition:	RVSWI measures the amount of work the right ventricle performs per beat when ejecting blood, similar to LVSWI.
Formula:*	RVSWI = SVI × (MPAP − RAP) × 0.0136
Normal values:	7.9-9.7 gm-m/beat/^{m2}

Systemic vascular resistance (SVR)[8,26,27]

Definition:	Measurement of peripheral arteriole resistance to flow. Measures the load applied to the left ventricular muscle during systolic ejection. Vascular resistance to blood flow is calculated by an analogy to Ohm's Law: the resistance in a circuit is equal to the voltage across the circuit divided by the current.

$$\text{Resistance} = \frac{\text{voltage difference}}{\text{current flow}}$$

Vascular resistance represents the pressure difference between the proximal and distal ends of the cardiovascular system (arterial and venous) divided by the cardiac output.

---

*MAP, Mean arterial pressure; MPAP, mean pulmonary artery pressure; RAP, right atrial pressure.

Formula:

$$\frac{MAP - RA}{CO} = 12 \text{ to } 20 \text{ units}$$

or

$$\frac{MAP - RA}{CO} \times 80 = 960 \text{ to } 1500 \text{ dynes·sec·cm}^{-5}$$

Multiplied by 80, converts the units to dynes·sec·cm^{-5}.

Normal values: 15 to 20 wood units or 960 to 1500 dynes·sec·cm^{-5}

Pulmonary vascular resistance (PVR)[8,26,27]

one-sixth that of systemic vascular resistance.

Formula:

$$\frac{(PA-PACP)}{CO} = 1.87 \text{ to } 3.12 \text{ units}$$

or

$$\frac{(PA - PACP)}{CO} = 150\text{-}250 \text{ dynes·sec·cm}^{-5}$$

EJECTION FRACTION

The percentage of total ventricular volume ejected during each contraction is termed *ejection fraction*. It is computed as[15]:

$$\frac{\text{End diastolic volume (EDV)} - \text{End systolic volume (ESV)}}{\text{End diastolic volume}}$$

which is:

$$\frac{\text{Stroke volume}}{\text{End diastolic volume}}$$

Normal left ventricular ejection fraction is about 65%.[15] Opacification of the ventricular cavity with contrast medium during a heart catheterization (ventriculography) enables end-systolic and end-diastolic volumes to be determined (Fig. 15-19). Ejection fraction can also be computed from echocardiography and cardiac imaging.

The prognostic value of adding right ventricular parameters to total hemodynamic profile is well documented.[27-29] A thermal dilution technique is now available for measuring right ventricular ejection fraction by thermal dilution.[30] This method is similar to thermal dilution cardiac output, except that the catheter possesses two intracardiac electrodes to sense R-wave activity and a fast response thermistor, which potentiates sensing of changes in pulmonary artery temperature. A known quantity and temperature of injectate solution is injected into the right atrium. The injectate mixes with blood and is propelled by the right ventricle into the pulmonary artery. The thermistor, located in the pulmonary artery, senses changes in temperature resulting from this bolus of injectate. Whereas cardiac output depends on change in temperature sensed over time, right ventricular ejection fraction depends on a beat-to-beat change in temperature. The thermistor senses changes of temperature and gates them with an R-wave. By assessing the change of temperature at two

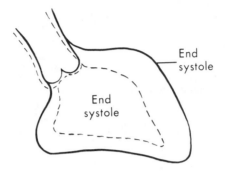

Fig. 15-19. Ejection fraction. Opacification of ventricular cavity with contrast medium during heart catheterization outlines ventricular cavity. Dimensions are obtained that permit calculation of end-systolic and end-diastolic volumes. Stroke volume is end-systolic volume subtracted from end-diastolic volume. Ejection fraction is computed by dividing stroke volume by end-diastolic volume.

different beats, as well as number of beats occurring in the interval between these two temperatures, the computer is able to calculate ejection fraction, or percent of blood ejected with each beat. Normal thermodilution right ventricular ejection fraction is between 45% to 50%.[28]

OXYGEN DELIVERY AND CONSUMPTION

The ultimate goal in hemodynamic monitoring is to evaluate components of oxygen delivery (Do_2) and oxygen consumption (Vo_2). Research has demonstrated that adequate increases in oxygen delivery improve survival.[30] Shoemaker et al[31] further supported use of hemodynamic oxygen transport parameters because:

(a) they are related to outcome, (b) they provide the essential basis for outcome predictors, and (c) they provide objective evidence that reflects the status of tissue perfusion and tissue oxygenation. In essence they may be used as "proxy" outcome measures. Moreover, changes in Do_2 and Vo_2 in response to therapy may also provide an objective measure of the realties efficacy of alternative therapies.

Do_2, Vo_2, and calculation of the mixed venous reserve are most appropriate hemodynamic indices to evaluate the impact of IABC on tissue perfusion. Formulas for each of these indices are listed in Table 15-4.

CONTINUOUS MONITORING OF VENOUS OXYGEN SATURATION

Pulmonary artery catheters contain fiberoptics, which afford continuous monitoring of mixed venous blood oxygen saturation (SVo_2) in addition to chamber pres-

Table 15-4.   Oxygen delivery and utilization parameters

Arterial oxygen delivery (Do_2)	
$*Do_2 = CO (1.34) \times Hgb \times Sao_2) 10\dagger$	Normal = 1000 ml/min
Oxygen consumption (Vo_2)	
$*Vo_2 = CO \times 1.34 \times Hgb \times (Sao_2 - Svo_2)$	Normal = 250 ml/min
Venous oxygen return	
$*CO (1.34) \times Hgb \times Svo_2) 10$	Normal = 750 ml/min

From Daily EK: Hemodynamic monitoring. In Guzzetta CG, Dossey BD, editors: *Cardiovascular nursing: holistic practice*, ed 2, St. Louis, 1992, Mosby–Year Book and White K: *The delicate balance*, 1991, Abbott Critical Care Workshop Syllabus.
*Some sources use 1.39 instead of 1.34 as oxygen carrying capacity.
†Small amount of oxygen dissolved in plasma is not included in this formula.
CO, cardiac output; *Hgb*, hemoglobin; *Sao₂*, arterial oxygen saturation; *Svo₂*, venous oxygen saturation.

sures. Optic fibers within the catheter transmit and receive reflected light from hemoglobin, according to its saturation[8]: The reflected light signal is converted to an electrical signal and transmitted to a remote data processor, which displays the signal on a screen or on a slow-speed paper recorder. A corresponding digital value is also displayed continuously and updated every 1 to 2 seconds.

Jaquith[34] further explained the benefits of continuous Svo_2 monitoring:

Continuous measurement of mixed venous oxygen saturation is important because this parameter reflects the ability of the body to satisfy tissue oxygen demands under a wide variety of clinical circumstances. The determinants of oxygen delivery are cardiac output, hemoglobin, and arterial oxygen saturation. Dysfunction of one or more of these components or an increase in oxygen consumption may cause the body to call upon its compensatory mechanisms to satisfy metabolic oxygen demand. The compensatory mechanisms immediately available to increase oxygen delivery to the tissues are increases in cardiac output and/or increases in oxygen extraction from the capillary blood. The latter results in a fall in Svo_2. The seriously compromised patient with little cardiac reserve may be unable to increase cardiac output and must then rely solely on increased oxygen extraction for improving oxygen delivery to the tissues. Therefore, desaturation of the capillary blood, reflected as a falling Svo_2, manifests the body's attempt to meet oxygen demands and prevent anaerobic metabolism and lactic acidosis. Svo_2 serves as an indicator of the relationship between oxygen delivery and oxygen demand. Changes in Svo_2 therefore alert the nurse to changes in patient status.

Svo_2 is a most useful hemodynamic index to monitor in conjunction with IABC. The normal range is between 60% to 80% or approximately 40 mm Hg.[32] Ultimately, the therapeutic goal in IABC is to increase organ survival. Its volume displacement and afterload reducing capabilities are intended to effect improved oxygen delivery to meet tissue demands. Use of Svo_2 affords a technique for continuously monitoring if oxygen supply is meeting demands in the IABC patient.

REFERENCES

1. Gravenstein JS, Paulus DA: *Monitoring practice in clinical anesthesia*, Philadelphia, 1982, JB Lippincott.
2. Thomas EL, ed: *Taber's cyclopedic medical dictionary*, ed 14, Philadelphia, 1989, FA Davis.
3. Gardner RM: Direct blood pressure measurement—dynamic response requirements, *Anesthesiology* 54:227, 1981.
4. Gardner RM: Hemodynamic monitoring. In Webster J, ed: *Encyclopedia of medical devices and instrumentation*, vol 3, 1988.
5. Gardner RM: Hemodynamic monitoring: from catheter to display, *Acute Care* 12:3, 1986.
6. Windsor T, Burch CE: Phlebostatic axis and phlebostatic reference levels for venous pressure measurements in man, *Proc Soc Exp Biol Med* 58 5:169, 1945.
7. Gardner RM, Hujcs M: Fundamentals of instrumentation principles and transducers used for physiological monitoring, *AACN's clinical issues in critical care nursing*, 1993.
8. Daily EK: Hemodynamic monitoring. In Guzzetta CG, Dossey BD, eds: *Cardiovascular nursing: holistic practice*, ed 2, St. Louis, 1992, Mosby–Year Book.
9. Quaal SJ: Quality assurance in hemodynamic monitoring, *AACN's clinical issues in critical care nursing*, 1993.
10. Gardner RM, Hollingsworth KW: Optimizing the electrocardiogram and pressure monitoring, *Crit Care Med* 14:651, 1986.
11. Gardner RM, Morris AH, Chapman RN et al: *Dynamic response and the essentials of invasive pressure monitoring*, Salt Lake City, 1986, Sorenson Publications.
12. Gardner RM: Hemodynamic monitoring: from catheter to display, *Acute Care* 12:3, 1986.
13. Gibbs NC, Gardner RM: Dynamics of invasive pressure monitoring systems: clinical and laboratory evaluation, *Heart Lung* 17:43, 1988.
14. Gardner RM: Evaluating dynamic response characteristics of pressure monitoring systems. In Armstrong PW, Baigrie Rs, Duke PC, eds: *Hemodynamic monitoring in critically ill patients*, 1984, Communications Media for Education.
15. Braunwald E: Assessment of cardiac function. In Braunwald E, ed: *Heart disease*, ed 4, Philadelphia, 1992, WB Saunders.
16. Morris AH, Chapman RH: Wedge pressure confirmation by aspiration of pulmonary capillary blood, *Crit Care Med* 13:736, 1985.
17. West JB: *Respiratory physiology: the essentials*, ed 4, Baltimore, 1989, Williams & Wilkins.
18. O'Quin R, Marini J: Occult positive end-expiratory pressure in mechanically ventilated patients with airflow obstruction, *Am Rev Respir Dis* 126:166, 1986.
19. Hotchkiss RS, Katsamouris AN, Lappas DG et al: Interpretation of pulmonary artery wedge pressure and pull-back blood flow determination after exclusion of the bronchial circulation in the dog, *Am Rev Respir Dis* 133:1019, 1986.
20. Enger R: Pulmonary artery wedge pressure: when it's valid, when it's not, *Crit Nurs Clin North Am* 3:603, 1989.
21. Reidinger MS, Shellock FG, Swan HJC: Reading pulmonary artery and pulmonary capillary wedge pressure waveforms with respiratory variation, *Heart Lung* 10:675, 1981.
22. Boyd E: *The growth of the surface area of the human body*, Minneapolis, 1935, University of Minnesota Press.
23. DuBois EF: *Basal metabolism in health and disease*, Philadelphia, 1936, Lea & Febiger.
24. Haycock GB, Schwartz GJ, Wisotsky DH: Geometric method for measuring body surface area: a height-weight formula validated in infants, children, and adults, *J Pediatrics* 93:62, 1972.
25. Weisner S: *Personal communication*, Waltham, Mass, August 10, 1992, Hewlett-Packard.
26. Pollard D, Seliger E: *An implementation of bedside physiological calculations*, Waltham, Mass, 1985, Hewlett-Packard.
27. Bustin D: *Hemodynamic monitoring for critical care*, Norwalk Conn, 1986, Appleton-Century-Crofts.
28. Headley JM, Diethorn ML: Right ventricular volumetric monitoring, *AACN's Clinical issues in critical care nursing*, 1993.

29. Pfister M, Emmenegger H, Muller-Brand J et al: Prevalence and extent of right ventricular dysfunction after myocardial infarction related to location and extent of infarction and left ventricular function, *Int J Cardiol* 28:325, 1990.
30. Ferris SE, Konno M: In vitro validation of a thermodilution right ventricular ejection fraction method, *J Clin Mon* 8:74, 1992.
31. Heard SO, Fink MP: Multiple organ failure syndrome. II. Prevention and treatment, *J Inten Care Med* 7:4, 1992.
32. Shoemaker WC, Appel PL, Kram HB: Oxygen transport measurements to evaluate tissue perfusion and titrate therapy: dobutamine and dopamine effects, *Crit Care Med* 19:672, 1991.
33. White K: *The delicate balance*, 1991, Abbott Critical Care Workshop Syllabus.
34. Jaquith SM: Continuous measurement of SV_{O_2}: clinical applications and advantages for critical care, *Crit Care Nurse* 5:40, 1985.

CHAPTER 16

Conventional timing using the arterial pressure waveform

Susan J. Quaal

TIMING DEFINED

Timing deals with beat-to-beat interaction of the balloon's inflation-deflation sequence and the patient's arterial circulatory system. Proper timing results in effective interaction between the heart's electrical activity, hemodynamic activity of the left ventricle and great vessels, and mechanical activity of intraaortic balloon counterpulsation (IABC). Kantrowitz[1] stated "The hemodynamic efficacy of balloon pumping is critically dependent on precise timing of both inflation and deflation in relation to the events of the cardiac cycle."

Timing consists of an automatic or manual regulation of inflation-deflation points in reference to systole and diastole. Balloon-pump consoles are equipped with controls that allow the operator to manually designate specific points of inflation and deflation. It is imperative that the operator learn manufacturer's specific guidelines for timing, which vary according to brand of balloon pump instrumentation used. The clinician must also understand arterial pressure waveform morphology landmarks of proper and improper timing and the hemodynamic penalties of incorrect timing.

Gould[2] stated

Interfacing mechanical events with physiological response is a skill now successfully achieved by man and machine. Terms such as "timing" and "triggering" define the response of the IABC console, as clinicians precisely regulate IABC inflation and deflation to optimize myocardial function and cardiac hemodynamics. These interactions have been carefully studied in attempts to fully realize the physiological benefit of counterpulsation.

The balloon pump console requires a "trigger signal" from which it determines systole and diastole. The most common "trigger signal" is the R wave from the patient's ECG. Most balloon pumps have a built-in default whereby inflation occurs at the T-wave midpoint (electrical index of diastole); deflation occurs before the succeeding QRS complex. The operator then manually adjusts inflation and deflation until timing is optimized.

ECG trigger signals can be obtained from a set of electrodes and lead wires that connect directly from the patient to the pump, or a phono cable can be used to output this signal from the bedside monitor and input into the balloon pump. It is imperative that the ECG signal be monophasic and artifact free to be correctly recognized by the balloon pump's logistics system. Irregular IABC may occur due to a poor quality signal. During surgery, electrocautery units may cause ECG signal interference. As an alternative, balloon triggering can also be activated from the patient's arterial pressure waveform. Some balloon pumps also offer an "internal trigger mode," which provides continuous IABC at a preselected heart rate and does not require a trigger signal. This function may be used to provide pulsatile flow during cardiopulmonary bypass.

The ECG signal is only a rough index of systole and diastole. Proper IABC must, however, be accurately related to cardiac cycle events. Therefore the arterial pressure waveform is used to fine tune IABC in relationship to systole and diastole. Balloon inflation occurs at the onset of diastole, or closure of the aortic valve, which is represented on the arterial pressure waveform as the dicrotic notch. Balloon deflation conventionally occurs during isovolumetric contraction, which is immediately before the upstroke of the next arterial systole. However, studies are ongoing to assess the therapeutic efficacy of deflating earlier or later than the conventional standard in select patient populations.

THE EFFECT OF IABC ON THE ARTERIAL PRESSURE WAVEFORM
Review of normal morphology

The normal arterial pressure waveform exhibits several points of reference that are easily understood when related to the cardiac cycle (Fig. 16-1). Aortic pressure rises at the moment of aortic valve opening when systolic ejection begins. This steeply rising component of the arterial pulse curve is termed *anacrotic limb* (Greek origin, meaning "upbeat"). Peak systolic pressure is the highest point on the arterial curve, representing left ventricular ejection. During this rapid ejection phase about 75% of that beat's stroke volume is ejected. The descending limb is termed *dicrotic limb* (Greek origin, meaning "double beat"). Aortic pressure decreases as the left ventricle relaxes. This decrease in pressure is interrupted by the *dicrotic notch*, or *incisura* (Latin origin, meaning "cutting into"). The dicrotic notch is an extremely important arterial pressure landmark for IABC timing.[3]

Left ventricular diastole begins following closure of the aortic valve. This filling phase is characterized by a continuous fall in aortic pressure as blood is perfused peripherally without further supply until the next systole. Recall from Chapter 1 that the majority of peripheral perfusion does occur during diastole because of the

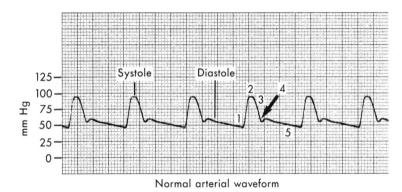

Normal arterial waveform

Fig. 16-1. Normal arterial pressure waveform. *1*, Anacrotic limb; *2*, peak systolic pressure; *3*, dicrotic limb; *4*, dicrotic notch; *5*, aortic end-diastolic pressure.

intrinsic Windkessel effect. The lowest aortic diastolic pressure point (end-diastole) represents the afterload component of cardiac work or the resistance against which the left ventricle must work during isovolumetric contraction (peripheral vascular resistance also has a significant impact on afterload).[3] Since proper IAB inflation-deflation must be related to the mechanical events of the cardiac cycle, an understanding of each of these arterial pressure landmarks as identified in Fig. 16-1 is essential.

Balloon inflation during diastole

Rapid inflation of the IAB with helium (most commonly 40 ml in an adult IAB) just after the aortic valve closes elevates the diastolic pressure, which is termed *augmented diastolic pressure* (Fig. 16-2).[4]

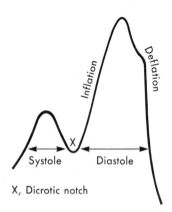

X, Dicrotic notch

Fig. 16-2. Schematic drawing of arterial pressure waveform, illustrating diastolic augmented pressure produced by IAB inflation during diastole.

Balloon inflation should occur at the beginning of diastole, or closure of the aortic valve. Thus inflation should begin right at the dicrotic notch. Ideally, an arterial pressure waveform that is used for IABC timing should be monitored from the aortic root where a dicrotic notch is inscribed in synchrony with aortic valve closure.[4] However, "central" or aortic root pressures are not monitored in the intensive care unit. Also, a delay in waveform propagation exists between the aortic root and peripheral vessels. Therefore the clinician must understand the physiology of arterial pressure waveform propagation and delay in appearance of a dicrotic notch when monitoring from a peripheral pressure line, as this must be accounted for when timing the IAB.

Adjusting for the dicrotic notch delay when timing IAB inflation. Arterial pressure is actually a "wave" of pressure that passes rapidly along the arterial system. Blood suddenly ejected into the ascending aorta during systole has insufficient energy to overcome all the inertia of the long arterial tubing system. Ejection of stroke volume during systole distends the arterial wall. Release of this distended arterial wall generates a pulse wave that travels down the arteries, analogous to the wave of a plucked violin string traveling down the string or the time it takes for a ripple in the middle of a pond to reach the shore.[5] These waves of pressure, reflected by peripheral structures, travel back toward the heart and become superimposed on the advancing pulse wave, which produces a higher peak of systolic pressure, a slurring and delay of the dicrotic notch, and a lower diastolic pressure.[5] This pulse wave velocity (4 to 5 m per second) is much faster than the velocity of blood flow (<0.5 m per second). Pulse wave velocity is determined by the compliance (elasticity) of the arterial walls.[6] The effect of the reflected wave on the impedance modulus will be minimal at a distance that is one quarter of a wavelength away from the reflection site and will be maximal at a distance one-half wavelength.[7]

As the arterial pulsation travels down the arterial system, there is an increasing lag before the beginning of the upstroke (anacrotic limb) and onset of dicrotic notch. It takes approximately 25 msec from the time of aortic valve closure for that event to be relayed to the subclavian artery. Similarly, another approximately 25 msec delay exists in retrograde transmission of the balloon pressure pulse to the aortic root. Thus the cumulative delay is about 50 msec. This delay is roughly the same when "timing" from a long subclavian arterial pressure monitoring catheter, short radial line, or the inner cannula of the percutaneous balloon catheter (Fig. 16-3). The delay is, however, about 120 msec when timing from a femoral artery catheter (Fig. 16-4). It is therefore recommended that the femoral artery not be used for pressure monitoring for the purpose of IABC timing.[7-10]

It is important to understand that the inner pressure monitoring catheter from an intraaortic balloon is *not* positioned in the aortic root. The proximal tip of the IAB resides in situ within the aorta, 1 to 2 cm below the orifice of the left subclavian artery. Therefore it is *not* a central pressure monitoring line.

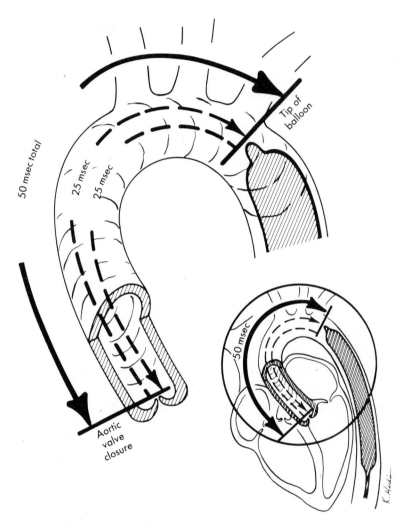

Fig. 16-3. Delay of approximately 25 msec occurs from time of aortic valve closure until effect is realized at subclavian artery. An equal delay also exists from balloon inflation at bifurcation of subclavian artery (elevation of aortic pressure at that point) until that pressure is appreciated at aortic root.

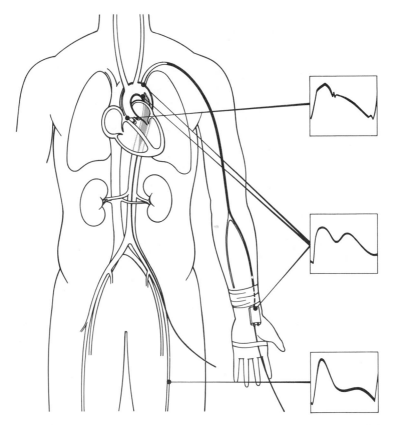

Fig. 16-4. Schematic waveforms illustrating arterial pressure waveform recorded at aortic root (*Central*), from inner cannula of percutaneous IAB (which is same as monitoring from long subclavian catheter or radial line) and from femoral line, where dicrotic notch is delayed approximately 120 msec, compared with central pressure recording.

How does this delay affect IAB timing? Inflation needs to be "timed" to occur 40-50 msec before the midpoint of the U-shaped dicrotic notch, when monitoring from the inner IAB cannula, a long subclavian or radial arterial line. At standard ECG paper speed of 25 mm/sec, 40 msec is one little box. Therefore IAB inflation should occur about 1 little box before the midpoint of the dicrotic notch, which is illustrated in Fig. 16-5.[8-10]

Adjusting inflation to occur about 40 msec earlier than the midpoint of the normal dicrotic notch changes the morphology of the dicrotic notch from a U shape to a V shape. Fig. 16-6 illustrates IABC on a 1:2 ratio of assist. Every other beat is assisted. Note the dicrotic notches of the three balloon inflation beats. The first di-

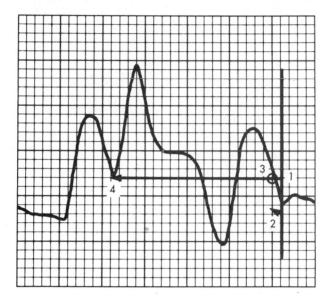

Fig. 16-5. Inflation time delay compensation. *1,* Locate midpoint of U-shaped dicrotic notch. *2,* Move to left 1 little box (40 msec). *3,* Move upward on vertical graph line until it bisects descending limb of arterial pressure waveform. *4,* Draw horizontal line from point *3* leftward to dicrotic notch of balloon-assisted beat. Point of balloon inflation *(4)* should be same as reference point *3.*

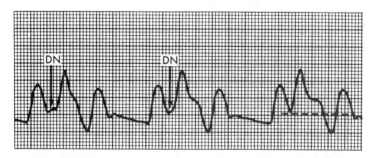

Fig. 16-6. IABC on 1:2 ratio of assistance. Inflation is adjusted with each balloon inflation until third cycle, where inflation is approximately 40 msec earlier than midpoint of normal dicrotic notch. Dicrotic notch at point of IAB inflation now assumes V shape.

crotic notch not only still depicts the U shape but also the beginning of diastole. Therefore IAB inflation is late. The second dicrotic notch is improved but still has a round, U shape. The third dicrotic notch has the proper V shaped morphology. As compared with the next unassisted beat, the horizontal dotted line indicates proper inflation 1 little box or 40 msec before the midpoint of the unassisted beat's dicrotic notch.

Since the delay for waveform propagation to the femoral artery is 120 msec, step 2 of the previously outlined procedure would require moving 3 little boxes to the left. Inflation from the femoral artery, allowing for this 120 msec delay, would appear to be very early. Therefore femoral artery timing is not recommended.[8-10]

Landmarks of proper IAB deflation

Ratio of IAB assist should be set at 1:2. All IAB consoles have the capability of decreasing frequency of assist from every cardiac cycle (1:1 ratio of assist) to 1:2, 1:3, 1:4, and some manufacturers provide a 1:8 option. Recall from Chapter 6 that as the IAB inflates it displaces stroke volume out of the aorta, both proximally and distally. Therefore at the time of IAB deflation during isovolumetric contraction, a hypothetical void exists; aortic end-diastolic pressure is lowered from stroke volume displacement, which occurred with inflation. Point 1 of proper deflation is that balloon-assisted aortic end-diastolic pressure (BAEDP) should be lower than the unassisted aortic end-diastolic pressure (Fig. 16-7). Secondly, lowering of aortic end-diastolic pressure during isovolumetric contraction reduces the work that the left ventricle must do to eject the next systole's stroke volume. Therefore point 2 of proper deflation is that assisted systole (the systole that occurs after the balloon counterpulsated) should be ideally lower than but at least not higher than the unassisted systole (Fig. 16-7).[8-10] The term *assisted* is used to describe events that occur after an IABC cycle. The box summarizes points of correct inflation and deflation.

POINTS OF CORRECT INFLATION AND DEFLATION

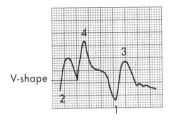

With proper IAB inflation, the dicrotic notch assumes a V shaped morphology. With proper deflation, BAEDP (1) is lower than UAEDP (2) and assisted systole (3) is lower, or at least equal to, unassisted systole (2). Balloon inflation raises diastolic pressure (4).

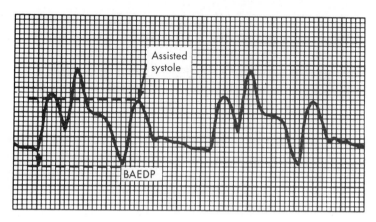

Fig. 16-7. Landmarks of proper IAB deflation. BAEDP should be lower than UAEDP. Point 2 assisted systole should ideally be lower than, but definitely not higher than, patient systole.

CONVENTIONAL TIMING

Conventional timing encompasses both a hemodynamic component and a computer logistic component. The impact of counterpulsation on the arterial pressure waveform, as described, is conventional, or put forth with the origin of IABC.[11] *Conventional timing* is also an operational term that describes the balloon pump console's logistics for coordinating IAB inflation-deflation with an ECG or arterial pressure "signal."

Clinicians are more focused on the hemodynamic aspects. The arterial pressure waveform is the reference for adjusting inflation and deflation. The patient always must have an arterial line in place to properly time IABC. When the clinician moves inflation and deflation controls earlier or later, using the arterial pressure waveform to achieve proper inflation-deflation morphological landmarks, the console logistics system also recognizes where inflation-deflation controls have been set but relates them to either R-to-R intervals from the ECG or intervals between each arterial pressure cycle. Balloon-pump consoles therefore need either an ECG or arterial pressure waveform, which is used as a "trigger signal."

Conventional timing from a console operational logistics point means that the pump "learns the signal interval" (i.e., the milliseconds between each R-to-R interval or arterial pressure interval). Fig. 16-8 illustrates two sinus rhythm ECG beats. The interval between the R waves is 100 msec. Inflation occurs 200 msec into this R-to-R cycle, based on where the clinician set the inflation control. Deflation occurs 800 msec into the R-to-R interval; again the computer received this command based on where the clinician positioned the deflation control.

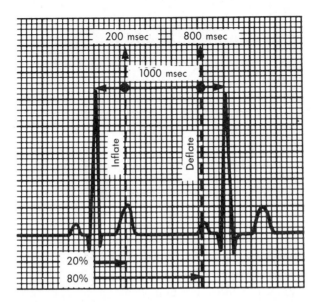

Fig. 16-8. Conventional timing requires regular R-to-R interval that serves as trigger signal sent to system's logistics center. Clinician adjusts inflation-deflation controls based on established standards, using arterial pressure waveform, which also sends message to logistics system as to how many msec into R-to-R trigger signal inflation and deflation should be initiated. In this example, of 1000 msec between R wave signals, inflation will occur 200 msec into R-to-R interval, and deflation will occur 800 msec after first R wave signal is recognized.

Obviously, conventional timing is maximized if the patient has a regular R-to-R rhythm. Irregular R-to-R intervals, as with atrial fibrillation, make it more difficult for the balloon pump's logistics system to track its trigger signal. Newer advances have, however, afforded improvements in the pump's ability to continue counterpulsating with irregular heart rates as high as 140 beats per minute. Efficiency is lost, however, as heart rates increase and become irregular.

FUNCTIONAL RANGE OF "SAFE TIMING"

There is probably no such thing as absolutely perfect IABC timing. Rather, timing can perhaps best be thought of in terms of the following three descriptive ranges: A, safe; B, unsafe; and C, optimal effectiveness (Fig. 16-9). "Safe" range is that segment of the cardiac cycle where the IAB can be inflated and deflated without competing with systolic ejection. This period extends from closure of the aortic valve until it reopens (diastole). Inflation during this phase will not harm the patient. Late and early inflation, however, will reduce optimal effective hemodynamic response.

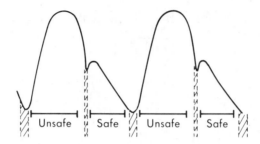

Fig. 16-9. Functional ranges of safe timing.

Deflation could occur before the onset of systole or "unsafe" portion of the cardiac cycle but still be less than optimal because it is early. Late deflation can be detrimental, since the balloon may still be inflated when systolic ejection begins, which would increase myocardial work and oxygen requirements.

The "unsafe" range of balloon inflation is during systole or that period between opening and closing of the aortic valve. Balloon pumps are engineered with a safety mechanism that prevents inflation during peak systole.

Optimal effectiveness occurs when maximal diastolic augmentation and afterload reduction are achieved for the patient's given hemodynamic state.

RECOGNIZING INCORRECT CONVENTIONAL TIMING INFLATION AND DEFLATION
Early IAB inflation

Early inflation is identified by IAB inflation that appears to be encroaching on the previous systole (Fig. 16-10). The dicrotic notch landmark is no longer visible

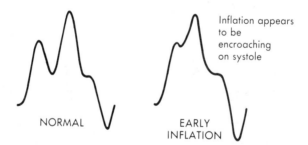

Fig. 16-10. Early inflation. Augmented diastolic pressure (IAB inflation) appears to be encroaching on previous systole. Dicrotic notch landmark is almost completely obliterated by early inflation.

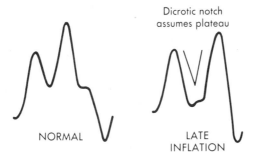

Fig. 16-11. Late inflation. Dicrotic notch is widened to plateau shape, rather than V shape, which occurs with proper inflation.

because of this premature rise in diastolic augmentation, which obliterates the notch. Potential consequences of early IAB inflation include the following:

1. Pressure in aorta is raised, which prematurely closes the aortic valve, thus the left ventricle does not completely empty.
2. Can cause regurgitation of blood into the left ventricle.
3. Stroke volume and cardiac output decrease.
4. Left ventricular volume and pressure (preload) increase.

Late inflation

Late inflation describes inflation that occurs well after aortic valve closures (Fig. 16-11). Potential consequences include the following:

1. Reduced diastolic augmentation.
2. Decreased coronary and systemic perfusion.

Early deflation

Early deflation is recognized by an assisted systole, which is higher than unassisted systole (Fig. 16-12). The anticipated drop in BAEDP does occur, but this occurs too early in the cardiac cycle. BAEDP equalizes to the patient's UAEDP. Assisted systole rises as the impedance to ejection is not timed to occur, when needed, during isovolumetric contraction. It is too early and therefore does not assist or unload the left ventricle. Retrograde flow may also occur from arterial vessels that have a higher pressure (coronaries, renals, carotids, and so on) into the lower pressure aorta. Evidence of retrograde flow is recognized as a slight plateau, which projects on the rising limb of assisted systole (Fig. 16-12). Potential consequences of early IAB deflation include the following:

1. Assisted systole rises in comparison with unassisted systole. Therefore the workload of systole ejection is not reduced.

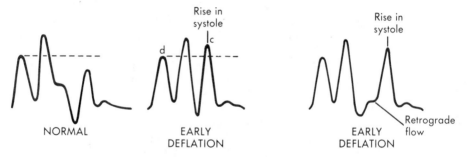

Fig. 16-12. Early deflation. Lowering of BAEDP occurs too soon to benefit next systole. Assisted systole (*c*) rises in comparison with unassisted systole (*d*). Decrease in intraaortic pressure occurs prematurely. Blood may flow retrogradely from higher pressure areas backward into aorta. Retrograde flow is recognized by plateau that occurs in ascending limb of assisted systole.

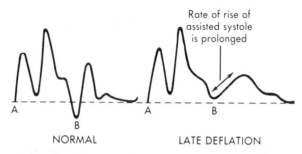

Fig. 16-13. Late deflation. Assisted BAEDP (*b*) is increased. Because of this increased impedance to left ventricular ejection, rate of rise of assisted systole (*dp/dt*) may be prolonged.

2. BAEDP equilibrates to UAEDP following early deflation. Retrograde flow may occur from other arteries back into the aorta (if from higher pressure vessel to lower pressure vessel). If retrograde flow occurs from the coronary arteries, the patient may develop angina. If it occurs from the cerebrals, the patient may experience a transient ischemia attack and so on.
3. Afterload reduction (IAB deflation) does not occur in synchrony with isovolumetric contraction, therefore myocardial work and oxygen demands are not reduced.

Late deflation

The balloon inflates in competition with the beginning of the next systolic ejection. Late inflation is recognized by a BAEDP that is as high as or higher than UAEDP (Fig. 16-13). The left ventricle has to work harder to try and eject against the impedance of the inflated balloon. Therefore rate of systolic pressure rise (*dp/dt*) may be prolonged. Potential consequences of late deflation include:

1. Myocardial work and oxygen consumption are increased.
2. Rather than receiving hemodynamic benefits from IABC, the patient suffers hemodynamic penalties. Indices of myocardial performance deteriorate (PACP increases, DO_2 decreases, cardiac output decreases, and MVO_2 increases).

REAL TIMING

Since IABC patients do develop irregular R-to-R rhythms, an alternative timing method exists that is termed *real timing*. This method no longer uses the R-to-R interval to designate deflation. Rather, deflation automatically occurs whenever the computer senses an R wave. Real timing is further described in Chapter 18.

SUMMARY

No single timing setting can be expected to provide optimal hemodynamics for various modalities of heart failure, such as biochemical, structural, and viral. As the molecular biologists establish antecedents and attributes of various models of heart failure, clinicians can begin a program of research that examines various "models of timing" and their efficacy for each of these underlying causes of heart failure. It is possible that the patient suffering heart failure because of a viral myocarditis may benefit from IABC inflation-deflation settings that are different from the acute myocardial infarction failure patient or the postextracorporeal circulation patient. Observations of effects of earlier-later inflation-deflation models and their impact on various heart failure entities is needed for future therapeutic algorithms and protocols to be established.

REFERENCES

1. Kantrowitz A: Percutaneous intra-aortic balloon counterpulsation, *Crit Care Clin* 8:819, 1992.
2. Gould KA: Perspectives in intra-aortic balloon pumping timing, *Crit Care Nurs Clin North Am* 1:469, 1989.
3. Burton AC: *Physiology and biophysics of the circulation*, ed 2, Chicago, 1972, Year Book Medical Publishers.
4. Maccioli GA, Lucas WJ, Norfleet EA: The intra-aortic balloon pump: a review, *J Cardiothor Anes* 2:365, 1988.
5. Craver JM, Hatcher CN: The percutaneous intraaortic balloon pump. In Hurst JW, Schlant RC, Rackly CE et al, eds: *The heart*, ed 7, New York, 1990, McGraw-Hill.
6. Rushmer RF: Systemic arterial pressure. In *Cardiovascular dynamics*, ed 4, Philadelphia, 1976, WB Saunders.
7. Little RC: Hemodynamics. In *Physiology of the heart and circulation*, ed 4, St. Louis, 1988, Mosby-Year Book.
8. Ford PI, Weintraub R: *Intra-aortic balloon pumping manual*, Boston, 1975, Beth Israel Hospital Department of Nursing.
9. Kontron Instruments: *Elements of timing in physiology and principles of counterpulsation*, Salt Lake City, 1992, Course Syllabus Advanced IABP Workshop.
10. Clinical Education Services Department: *Case studies in intra-aortic balloon pumping*, Montvale, NJ, 1990, Datascope Corp.

CHAPTER 17

Conventional timing practice exercises

Susan J. Quaal

The following exercises are intended to provide practical experience in recognizing improperly timed (early or late inflation-deflation) arterial waveform tracings. All tracings are examples of the balloon inflating on every other beat. Each strip is accompanied by a blank space for comments on inflation and deflation (early or late). A line is also provided for additional comments (e.g., hemodynamic consequences of the representative timing error and/or corrective action). The strips are reproduced beginning on page 271 with answers and discussions. Key:

A, Unassisted aortic end-diastolic pressure (UAEDP)
B, Balloon assisted aortic end-diastolic pressure (BAEDP)
C, Unassisted systole
D, Balloon assisted systole

No. 1

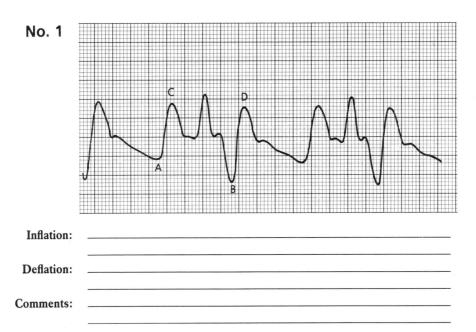

Inflation: _____

_____

Deflation: _____

_____

Comments: _____

_____

No. 2

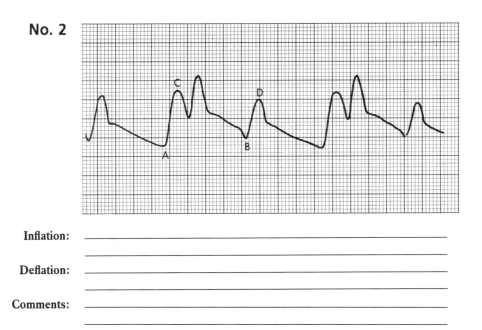

Inflation: _____

_____

Deflation: _____

_____

Comments: _____

_____

No. 3

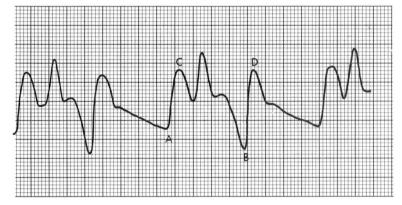

Inflation: _____

Deflation: _____

Comments: _____

No. 4

Inflation: _____

Deflation: _____

Comments: _____

No. 5

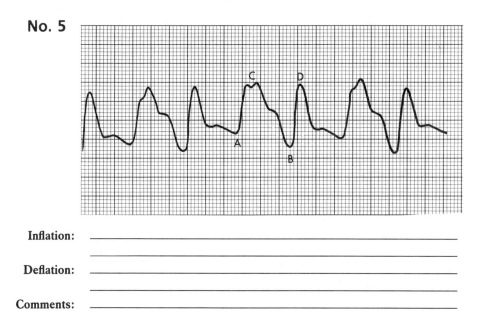

Inflation: _____
_____

Deflation: _____
_____

Comments: _____
_____

No. 6

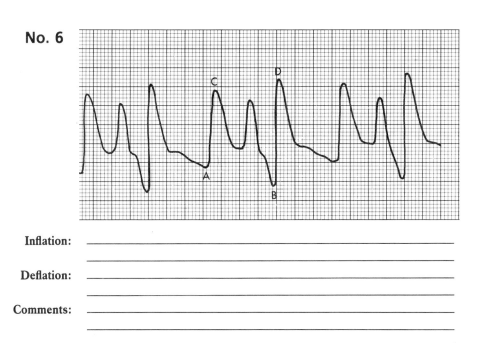

Inflation: _____
_____

Deflation: _____
_____

Comments: _____
_____

No. 7

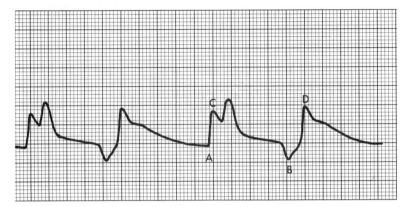

Inflation: _____

_____

Deflation: _____

_____

Comments: _____

_____

No. 8

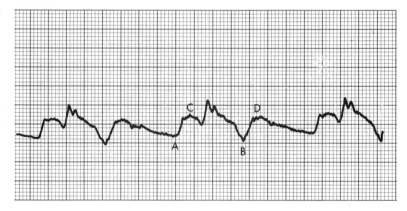

Inflation: _____

_____

Deflation: _____

_____

Comments: _____

_____

No. 9

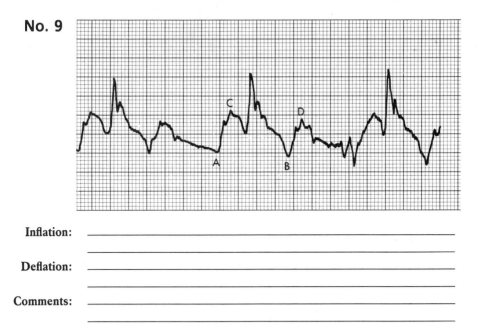

Inflation: _____

_____

Deflation: _____

_____

Comments: _____

_____

No. 10

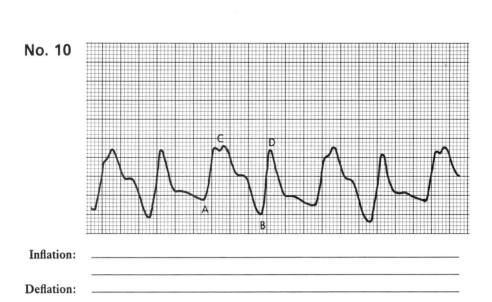

Inflation: _____

_____

Deflation: _____

_____

Comments: _____

_____

No. 11

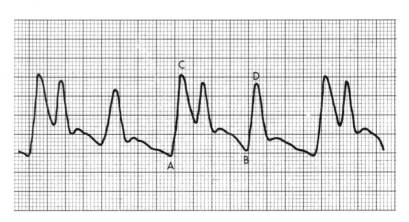

Inflation: _____

_____

Deflation: _____

_____

Comments: _____

_____

No. 12

Inflation: _____

_____

Deflation: _____

_____

Comments: _____

_____

No. 13

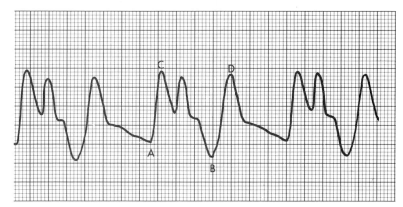

Inflation: _____

_____

Deflation: _____

_____

Comments: _____

_____

No. 14

Inflation: _____

_____

Deflation: _____

_____

Comments: _____

_____

No. 15

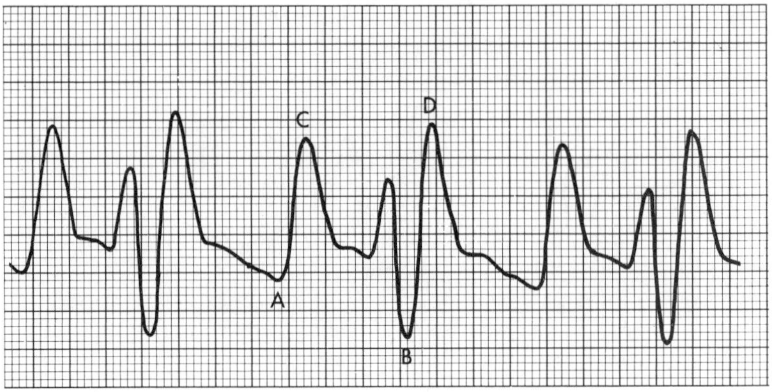

Inflation: _____

_____

Deflation: _____

_____

Comments: _____

_____

No. 16

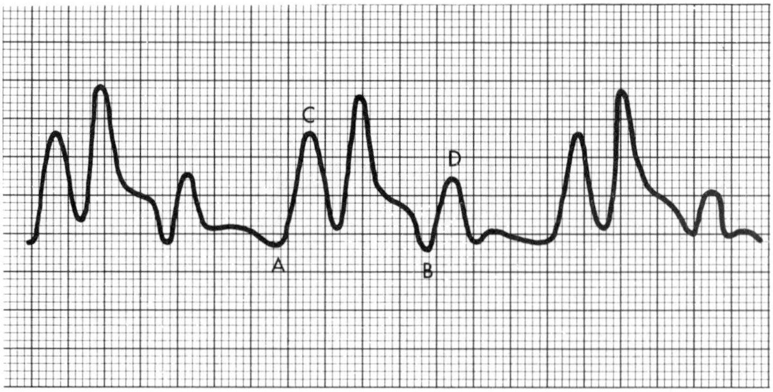

Inflation: _____

_____

Deflation: _____

_____

Comments: _____

_____

No. 17

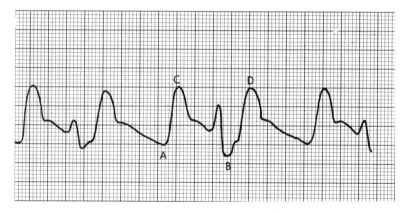

Inflation: _____

_____

Deflation: _____

_____

Comments: _____

_____

No. 18

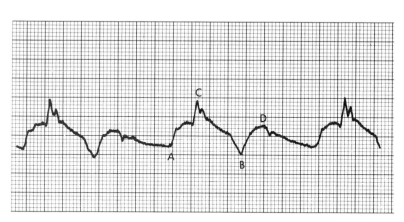

Inflation: _____

_____

Deflation: _____

_____

Comments: _____

_____

No. 19

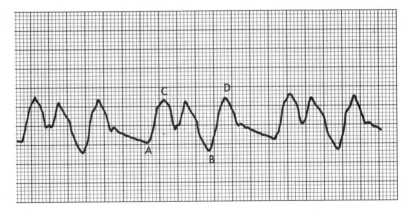

Inflation: _____

Deflation: _____

Comments: _____

No. 20

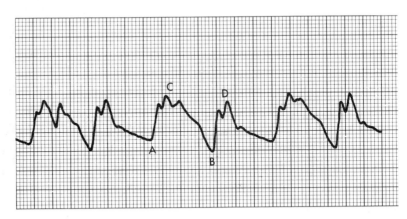

Inflation: _____

Deflation: _____

Comments: _____

Answers and discussion on timing arterial pressure tracings

No. 1

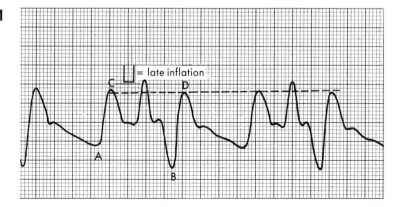

Inflation: Very late. Note square wave of dicrotic notch rather than V appearance.

Deflation: Okay. Assisted systole (D) is however not appreciably lower than unassisted systole (C).

Comments: Try adjusting deflation to occur slightly later in an attempt to further reduce assisted systole. However, you may find that BAEDP (B) elevates with later deflation. Thus this is the best that can be attained.

No. 2

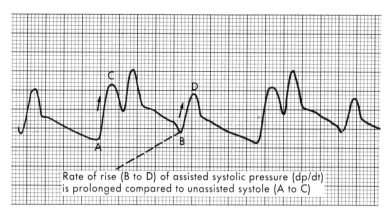

Inflation: Okay. Nice V appearance to dicrotic notch.

Deflation: Very late. BAEDP (B) is greater than UAEDP (A).

Comments: The left ventricle must eject against a greater resistance. Afterload is increased, isometric contraction is prolonged, and the rate of rise of systolic pressure (dp/dt) is prolonged.

No. 3

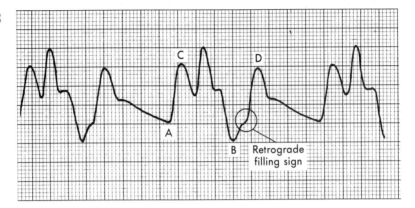

Inflation:	Okay. Nice V appearance to dicrotic notch.
Deflation:	Okay.
Comments:	BAEDP (B) is lower than patient UAEDP (A); balloon assisted systole (D) is lower than patient systole (C). Note the slight plateau on the anacrotic limb of assisted systole, which may indicate early inflation, despite point D appearing to be lower than point C.

No. 4

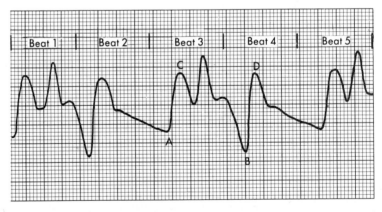

Inflation:	First beat is late; timing is then adjusted for proper inflation (dicrotic notch assumes a V shape by beat 5).
Deflation:	Okay. D < C; B < A.
Comments:	Examine several beats when assessing timing. An isolated beat can appear improperly timed, when the other beats are actually properly timed. A premature ECG beat can throw off the timing for that one cycle.

No. 5

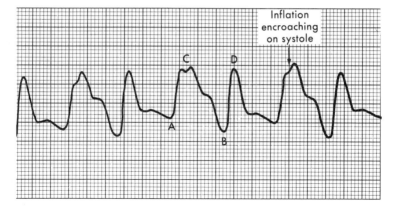

Inflation: Extremely early. Inflation appears to be encroaching on systole; the dicrotic notch is absent.

Deflation: Slightly early. Only the last beat appears to demonstrate a slight decrease in assisted systole D.

Comments: First adjust inflation to occur later, then reassess deflation.

No. 6

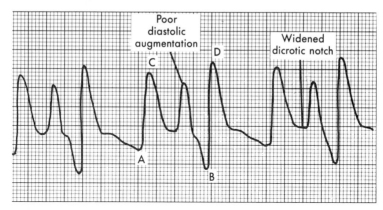

Inflation: Very late. Note plateau at area of dicrotic notch.

Deflation: Very early. Assisted systole (D) is greater than patient systole (C).

Comments: Early reduction of aortic pressure has no effect on reducing the work of the next systole (afterload reduction comes too early). More work is required for the next systole D > C. With early deflation the BAEDP equilibrates. Retrograde filling could occur from the coronary arteries, and the patient could develop angina. Balloon counterpulsation is not helping this patient. Note the very poor augmentation in diastole caused by late inflation and early deflation.

No. 7

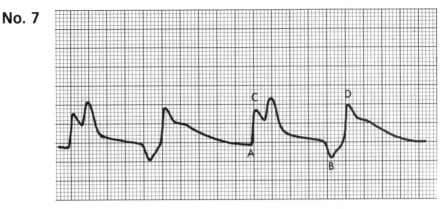

Inflation:	Okay.
Deflation:	Early. Assisted systole (D) is greater than patient systole (C).
Comments:	Go back to strip 6, and review the consequences of early deflation. Perform a dynamic response test (Chapter 15) to ensure that this line is not damped.

No. 8

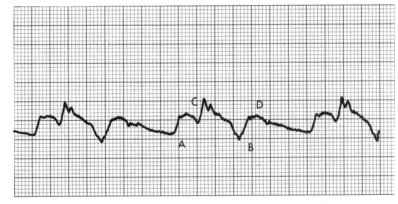

Inflation:	Okay.
Deflation:	Slightly late. BAEDP (B) is equal to or only slightly lower than UAEDP (A).
Comments:	Try deflating a bit earlier, and observe if balloon assisted AoEDP (B) is further reduced. Perform a dynamic response test (Chapter 15). This line may be underdamped. Note waveform distortion.

No. 9

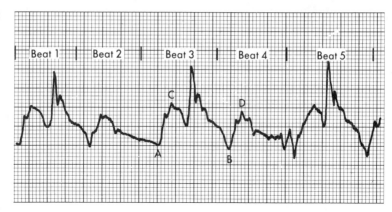

Inflation:	Progressively adjusted to occur earlier. (Compare beat 1 to beat 5.)
Deflation:	Late. There is no decrease in BAEDP (B).
Comments:	The left ventricle must eject against a greater impedance. Myocardial oxygen consumption is increased.

No. 10

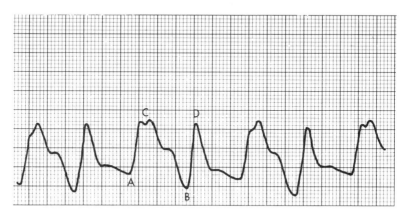

Inflation:	Very early. Inflation is encroaching on systole.
Deflation:	May be slightly early. Point D = Point C. Try deflating slightly later.
Comments:	The very early inflation may raise the pressure in the aorta and close the aortic valve prematurely. This action would limit the complete ejection of the intended stroke volume.

No. 11

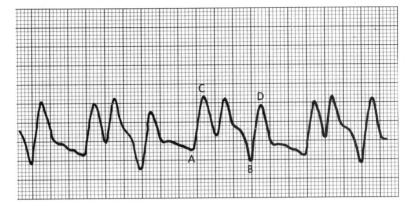

Inflation: Okay. Dicrotic notch assumes a V shape.
Deflation: Okay. B < A; D < C.
Comments: Proper timing.

No. 12

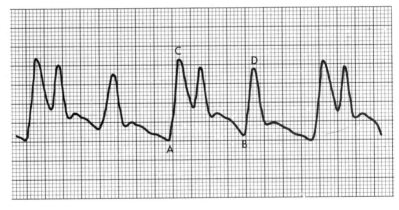

Inflation: Okay.
Deflation: Late. B > A, rather than B < A.
Comments: No afterload reduction is occurring. The work load of the myocardium is actually increased with late deflation. Correct by deflating earlier. Note poor diastolic augmentation. Review list of reasons for poor diastolic augmentation (Chapter 7).

No. 13

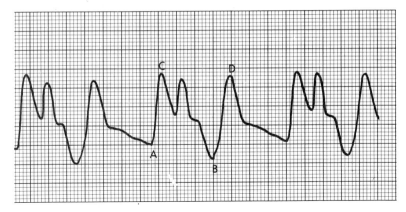

Inflation: Okay.

Deflation: B < A; D is slightly lower than C.

Comments: Deflation appears good, but try deflating a bit *later* in an attempt to further reduce assisted systole (D).

No. 14

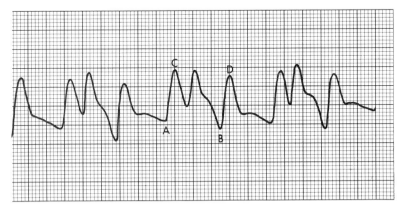

Inflation: Okay.

Deflation: B < A, and D < C.

Comments: Try deflating a bit *earlier* to determine if the assisted BAEDP can be lowered further.

No. 15

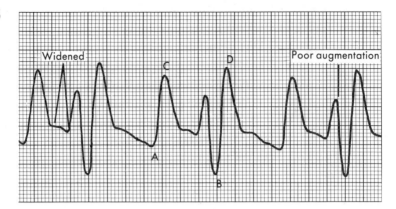

Inflation:	Very late.
Deflation:	Very early. D > C. The drop in BAEDF occurs too early to effectively reduce the ensuing systole.
Comments:	Note very poor diastolic augmentation. When the balloon is timed to inflate very late and deflate very early, there is little time available in the cycle for augmentation. Note that assisted systole (D) is actually higher than unassisted systole (C). The patient would probably be better off without the balloon than with this poorly timed counterpulsation.

No. 16

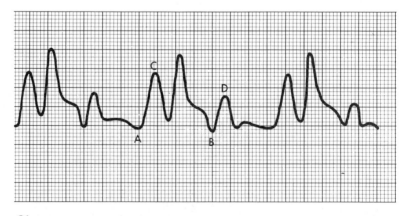

Inflation:	Okay.
Deflation:	BAEDP (B) = UAEDP (A). Balloon is deflating too late.
Comments:	There is increased impedance to ejection because the balloon is deflating at the point that systole occurs, rather than before systole begins. Myocardial oxygen consumption is increased.

No. 17

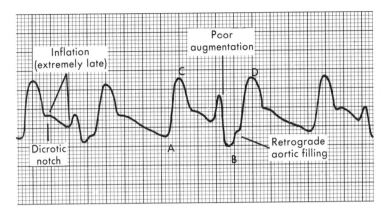

Inflation:	Extremely late. A long trough is present after the dicrotic notch.
Deflation:	Early. Note retrograde filling sign of ascending limb of assisted systole.
Comments:	The retrograde filling that occurs may be from the coronary, renal, cerebral, or any artery with pressure higher than aortic pressure at this moment. Because deflation occurs early, it does not reduce the work of the next systole (D). Late inflation and early deflation produce a very poor diastolic augmentation.

No. 18

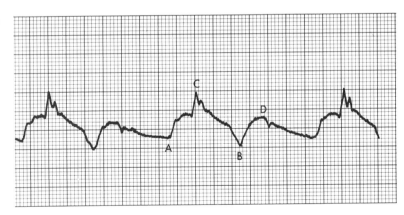

Inflation:	Early.
Deflation:	Late. BAEDP (B) is not effectively decreased.
Comments:	The patient has poor perfusion pressure to begin with in addition to some artifact. Perform a dynamic response test and attempt to improve fidelity of this arterial pressure waveform.

No. 19

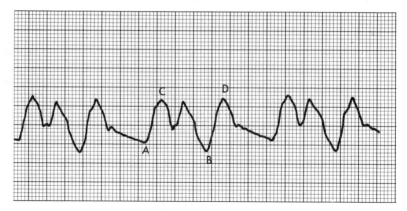

Inflation:	First beat, late inflation. Remainder are okay.
Deflation:	Assisted systole (D) = unassisted systole (C).
Comments:	Try deflating slightly *later* in an effort to lower assisted systole (D). However, even slightly later deflation may increase (B) or BAEDP. Therefore this may be the best timing that can be achieved.

No. 20

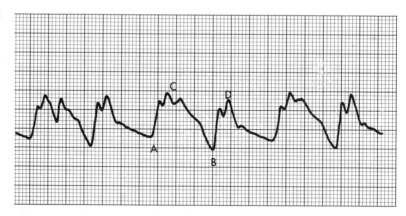

Inflation:	Very early. Inflation is encroaching on the preceding systole.
Deflation:	Assisted systole (D) is equal to or only slightly lower than patient systole (C).
Comments:	The early inflation of the balloon may raise aortic pressure to a point that closes the aortic valve prematurely. The notching of the systolic peaks may be caused by catheter fling. Perform a dynamic response test to assess line fidelity.

CHAPTER 18

Real timing

Cynthia A. Cadwell and **George Tyson**

Intraaortic balloon counterpulsation (IABC) timing requires balloon inflation-deflation synchronization to the cardiac systolic and diastolic phases. Appropriate intraaortic balloon (IAB) timing reduces left ventricular work and augments diastolic perfusion pressure.[11,12] IAB timing effectiveness is assessed by examining counterpulsation impact on left ventricular hemodynamics and the arterial pressure waveform.

RELATIONSHIP OF CARDIAC CYCLE ELECTRICAL AND MECHANICAL EVENTS

The delay between cardiac electrical and mechanical events (QRS complex and aortic valve opening) is labeled "preejection period" (PEP) (Fig. 18-1). This interval remains relatively fixed despite rate and rhythm variations.[2,7] PEPs have been measured from 40 to 130 msec (average 75 msec).[2,7] Ejection time (ET) occurs from aortic valve opening to aortic valve closure and also remains relatively constant throughout varying rates and rhythms. Ventricular diastole begins with aortic valve closure and continues until the next QRS complex. This phase does vary considerably with rate and rhythm changes. Ventricular diastole can therefore be used as a relative constant time frame in *regular rhythms only*. It is critically important to understand relationships among these cardiac cycle events to properly assess timing, using the arterial pressure waveform.

CONVENTIONAL TIMING

IAB consoles utilize a trigger event (usually QRS complex) to locate each cardiac cycle. *Conventional timing is based on duration of inflation during diastole.* The IAB is timed to inflate at the dicrotic notch and remains inflated throughout diastole. This approach to timing depends on regular, repeating diastolic intervals. Arrhythmias and irregular diastolic intervals therefore pose a problem for conventional timing.

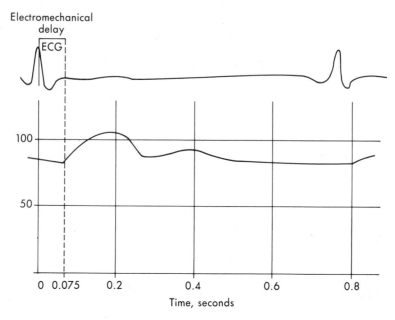

Fig. 18-1. ECG and arterial pressure sequence demonstrating the electromechanical delay between ventricular depolarization (QRS) and aortic valve opening (initiation of systolic upstroke on arterial wave).

Hemodynamic indicators used to validate adequate timing include lowering of assisted systole and assisted aortic end-diastolic pressure (see Chapter 6).

Early intraaortic balloon pump (IABP) technology was restricted to conventional timing because of console inefficiency. As long as 120 msec was required from the time a console recognized a deflation landmark until it actually evacuated balloon gas volume. To compensate for this mechanical delay, balloon-end deflation had to be approximated to occur concomitant with "isovolumetric contraction," thus assuring complete balloon emptying at the time of systolic ejection. Variables affecting balloon deflation included dead space, type of gas utilized, tubing diameter and length between balloon and console, signal interpretation, and console pneumatics rate of response. Because of IABP console technological limitations, conventional timing was the only feasible approach.

Studies conducted in 1972 and 1974 by Weber and Janicki[11,12] demonstrated that extending inflation past end diastole into early isovolumetric contraction offered a greater reduction in assisted systolic pressure (systolic unloading) and increased mean arterial pressure. Further studies replicated these findings.[5,13]

PRINCIPLES OF REAL TIMING

The basic principle underlying *real timing is duration of balloon deflation corresponding to cardiac systole.* As with conventional timing, a QRS complex is again used by the IABC console to locate each cardiac cycle. Real timing however differs from conventional timing because the IAB is "timed" to deflate at the onset of each QRS complex and remains deflated throughout systole. A constant diastolic interval is not required for real timing, since the mechanism of timing action corresponds to systole (PEP and ET), which remains relatively constant during changing rates and rhythms. Thus an advantage of real timing over conventional timing is its ability to foster desirable hemodynamic outcomes, even with arrhythmias and irregular diastolic cycles.

Modern IABC research and development have engineered balloon instrumentation with more rapid balloon gas evacuation times. Microprocessor technology and modification of previously mentioned variables affecting deflation have brought about a current generation of IAB consoles that can effectively implement real timing. Current consoles also have fail-safe mechanisms, which automatically trigger R wave deflation should a cardiac cycle be shorter than anticipated.

Despite this advanced technology, IAB gas evacuation time has not decreased in all consoles. Optimal real timing will occur only if balloon deflation can be synchronized to PEP. The evacuating IAB dv/dt must be greater than or equal to that of left ventricular ejection.[3,12]

BENEFITS OF REAL TIMING ON CARDIAC DYNAMICS

Diastolic augmentation

Real timing thus increases duration of balloon inflation to extend throughout diastole, compared with balloon deflation occurring during isovolumetric contraction with conventional timing. Diastolic augmentation is therefore optimized. Diastolic augmentation pressure and perfusion are potentially increased.[9,12]

Tyson[10] demonstrated an increase in mean *aortic diastolic pressure* associated with real timing (Fig. 18-2). This effect was attributed to the extended balloon inflation duration achieved with real timing.

Arrhythmias

One of the most outstanding benefits of real timing is its effectiveness in irregular cardiac rhythms. Both diastolic augmentation and systolic unloading are achieved, using real timing during an irregular rhythm. Since the duration of diastole varies in irregular rhythms, estimating diastolic intervals is impossible. Real timing utilizes each QRS complex, not duration of diastole, as the reference for deflation. Duration of inflation can therefore adjust to changing R-to-R intervals. The need for estimating duration of diastole is thus eliminated. Diastolic augmentation

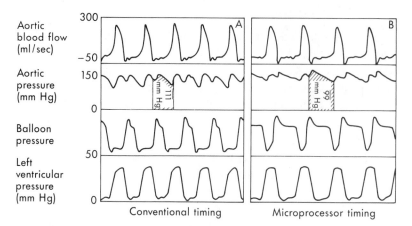

Fig. 18-2. Effects of IABC during conventional and microprocessor timing on aortic flow, aortic pressure, balloon pressure, and left ventricular pressure. Longer balloon pressure duration generates greater augmented diastolic pressure in microprocessor timing.

can therefore be maintained even in the presence of arrhythmias. Systolic unloading consistently occurs since deflation is initiated with each QRS complex regardless of rhythm.

Fig. 18-3 compares real timing (microprocessor) and conventional timing in various rhythms. Both real and conventional timing methods prove effective on diastolic balloon inflation and systolic balloon deflation in sinus rhythm. Diastolic balloon inflation and systolic balloon deflation remain accurate only in real timing during irregular R-to-R intervals generated by atrial fibrillation and frequent ectopy. These results suggest hazardous effects of conventional timing in irregular rhythms. Counterpulsation appears effective during arrhythmias only when real timing is employed.

Systolic unloading

Rapid balloon deflation in the PEP provides optimal systolic unloading.[5,12] Earlier deflation, as in conventional timing, reduces balloon deflation's effect on left ventricular ejection pressure. (The deflating balloon may assist left ventricular ejection through active energy transfer to the ascending aortic blood column in real timing.[10])

Fig. 18-4 compares real timing (microprocessor) and conventional timing in a left ventricular pressure volume loop. No significant differences are appreciated during diastolic filling, isovolumetric contraction, or isovolumetric relaxation. Ventricular ejection pressure, however, is greater in conventional timing than in real time. This result demonstrates greater enhancement of left ventricular ejection with real timing.

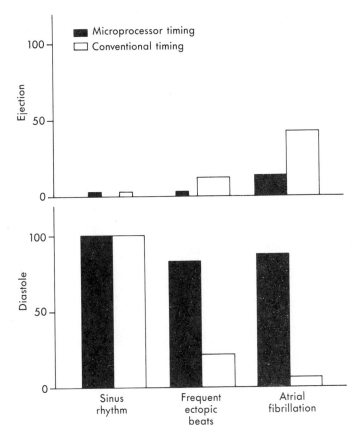

Fig. 18-3. Balloon inflation represented in percent of cardiac cycle during left ventricular ejection and in diastole in various rhythms. Microprocessor timing demonstrates greater accuracy than conventional timing during rhythm disturbance.

Afterload reduction

Afterload is typically measured using mean arterial pressure (MAP) and calculated systemic vascular resistance (SVR). Both parameters offer information regarding resistance to ventricular ejection.[6]

Presystolic or end-diastolic pressure decrease is commonly used to determine afterload reduction during counterpulsation. Balloon deflation before ejection produces this effect. Actual representation of decreased left ventricular workload is a reduction in peak systolic pressure. Later deflation, during PEP, produces lower peak systolic pressures and no drop in presystolic or end-diastolic pressure.[5,10]

Balloon-induced reduction of aortic end-diastolic pressure has disadvantages.[8,12]

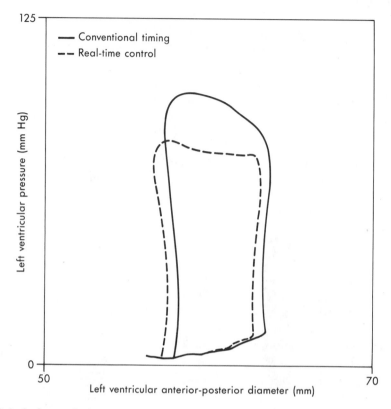

Fig. 18-4. Left ventricular pressure–volume loop during IABP assist with microprocessor and conventional timing. Less ejection pressure is required during microprocessor timing.

Retrograde flow occurs in varying degrees.[11] MAP and SVR artificially altered by balloon deflation are not demonstrative of vascular tone. Operator evaluation of counterpulsation effectiveness is confounded by unreliable parameters.

Fig. 18-5 illustrates real timing effects on the arterial waveform. Balloon-assisted reduction in peak systolic pressure is appreciated on both aortic and left ventricular pressures. Balloon deflation is timed for PEP. No reduction in aortic end-diastolic pressure is recognized. Aortic end-diastolic pressure drop does not necessarily represent afterload reduction and may reduce systolic unloading.

THE TIMING PROCESS IN REAL TIME

IABC timing requires familiarity with both ECG and arterial pressure waveforms. Assessment should include hemodynamic parameters and physical findings to best optimize counterpulsation effects.[1] Fig. 18-6 illustrates arterial waveform points of reference for timing.

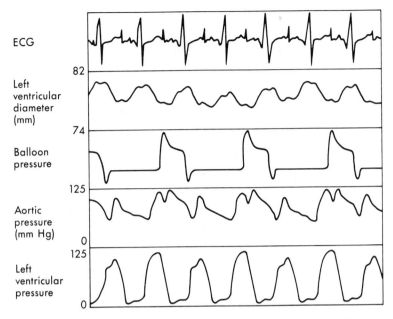

Fig. 18-5. Regular rhythm on 50% IABC assist, microprocessor timing. Effects seen on left ventricular diameter, balloon pressure, aortic pressure, and left ventricular pressure. Systolic unloading evident on aortic and left ventricular pressure following balloon assist.

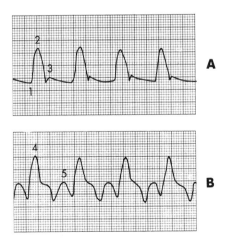

Fig. 18-6. **A,** Normal arterial waveform demonstrating *(1)* end diastole, *(2)* peak systole, and *(3)* dicrotic notch. **B,** IAB-assisted arterial waveform demonstrating *(4)* peak diastolic augmentation and *(5)* reduced systolic peak pressure.

Real timing deflation occurs on identification of a QRS complex. Relatively constant PEPs indicate aortic valve opening time is unaffected by balloon activity. Changing PEPs should be evaluated for possible late deflation. Balloon deflation ends with aortic valve closure (dicrotic notch), which signals onset of inflation. Relatively constant ET indicates aortic valve closure is unchanged by balloon activity. Changing ET should be evaluated as possible early inflation.

Comparing arterial waveforms both on and off balloon assist is used to evaluate timing. Fifty percent assist can be used for comparison or 100% assist vs. balloon off. Fuchs et al.[4] report negligible effects in 1:2 assist, which suggests measuring counterpulsation benefits might best be observed in 1:1 ratio.

Proper timing of deflation

Deflation should coincide with each QRS complex to generate reduction in peak systolic pressure (afterload reduction effect). Note, irregular rhythms have varying diastolic filling times and consequent varying stroke volumes.[2] Systolic unloading therefore cannot be measured from arterial pressure. The time from QRS to aortic valve opening (PEP) should be consistent with balloon assist on and off. Preload should be decreased as afterload reduction occurs.

Proper timing of inflation

Inflation should occur just before aortic valve closure (dicrotic notch) to generate upstroke on the diastolic arterial wave. This creates a V-like pattern at aortic valve closure. Time from aortic valve opening to aortic valve closure should be consistent with balloon assist on and off. MAP should increase with diastolic pressure augmentation. Peak balloon-augmented diastolic pressure should be higher than peak systolic pressure. Note that several variables affect this parameter, i.e., balloon size and position, stroke volume, vascular resistance, aortic compliance, and gas exchange time.[12]

Improper timing—late deflation

Only late deflation is discussed in this chapter regarding improper timing in real time. All other improper timing situations are no different from conventional control. However, early deflation in real timing is current practice in conventional timing.

The balloon remains partially inflated after the aortic valve opens in late deflation. Partial aortic obstruction causes an increase in left ventricular work altering ejection progress. Late deflation assessment includes inconsistent PEP, altered ET, prolonged ejection upstroke, or elevated peak systolic pressure in regular rhythms. Important parameters for evaluation of late deflation are increased filling pressures (PCWP, LAP) or heart rate and decreased cardiac index. Note aortic end-diastolic pressure will *not* determine late deflation. Aortic end-diastolic pressure may be elevated and left ventricular work still reduced with real timing because of rapid balloon deflation.

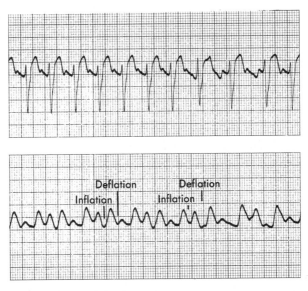

Fig. 18-7. Conventional control in 50% assist during slightly irregular rhythm. Inflation is late; poor diastolic augmentation and V-like pattern of inflating balloon is not sharp. Deflation is inconsistent secondary to changing R-R intervals and is early. Early deflation causes lack of systolic unloading. Hemodynamically, no improvement in MAP or reduction in PCWP was obtained with this conventional timing.

PRACTICE TIMING EXERCISES

Figs. 18-7 through 18-15 are offered as additional tutorial exercises.

SUMMARY

Clinically, assessment of timing is based on evaluation of multiple factors influencing patient hemodynamic status.[11] In most cases, patients receiving counterpulsation are fairly unstable and require various interventions to assist in their recovery. Most therapeutic measures also affect patient hemodynamics besides the IABC. Various cardiac disease processes may require different effects from counterpulsation therapy.[8] These variables may cause some patients to require real timing and some conventional control. It is best to evaluate each individual case for optimal results of IABC timing by respecting the overall picture. Real timing will prove beneficial in most instances. To evaluate timing effectiveness, arterial waveform, hemodynamic parameters, and physical findings should be assessed in each patient.

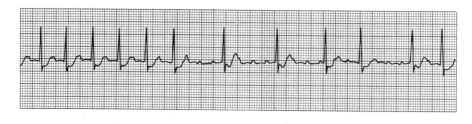

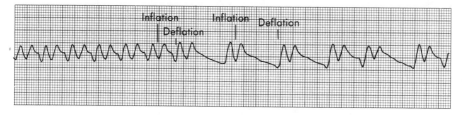

Fig. 18-8. Real time control in 100% assist during irregular rhythm. Inflation is accurate; diastolic augmentation is present with a sharp V-like pattern indicating proper inflation. Deflation is consistent regardless of R-R interval. PCWP is reduced, and MAP is increased with balloon assist in this mode.

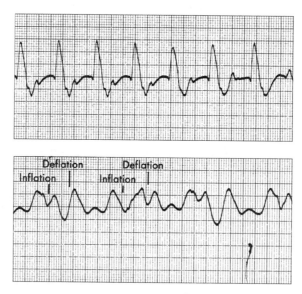

Fig. 18-9. Conventional control in 50% assist with slightly irregular ECG rhythm. R wave deflation is fail safe. The irregular R-R intervals are averaged. Inflation is inconsistent, occurring late and early. Deflation is inconsistent, late and early. Hemodynamic deterioration, PCWP increase, and no MAP increase were found with this timing modality.

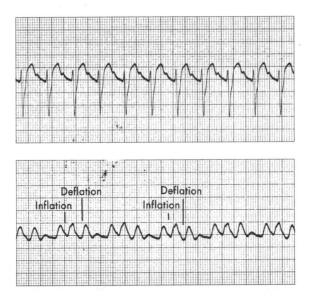

Fig. 18-10. Conventional control in 50% with a regular ECG rhythm. Inflation is adequate but could be slightly earlier to appreciate greater diastolic augmentation effect. Deflation is adequate for conventional timing but early for real timing. Note slight presystolic drop in pressure but minimal systolic unloading. Some hemodynamic improvement is afforded in this mode.

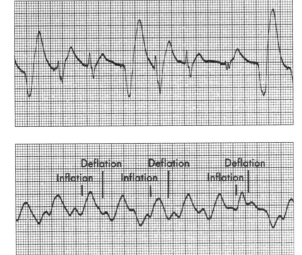

Fig. 18-11. Real time control in 100% assist during an arrhythmia. Inflation and deflation are consistently accurate. Note systolic wave barely evident at times, secondary to the arrhythmia. There is no change in systolic ejection time, however, indicating accurate timing. Considerable hemodynamic improvement was appreciated with this method of assist. When assist was momentarily withheld in this patient, no systolic ejection was ascertainable on the arterial pressure waveform and PCWP increased.

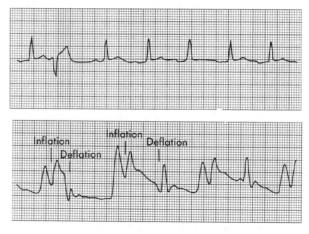

Fig. 18-12. Real timing in 50% assist during slightly irregular ECG rhythm. Inflation is accurate. Deflation is consistent but late. PEP following balloon assist is prolonged approximately 40 msec to reduce ejection time. There is no systolic unloading and PCWP increased.

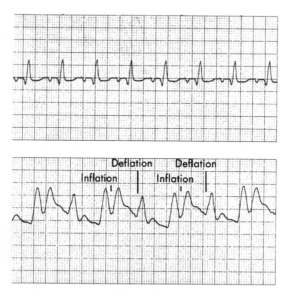

Fig. 18-13. Real timing in 50% assist during regular rhythm. Inflation is slightly late; V-like pattern of balloon inflation is not sharp. Deflation is accurate; systolic unloading is appreciable and there is no change in ejection time. Mean arterial pressure improved and PCWP decreased with this method of timing.

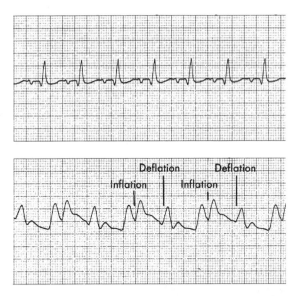

Fig. 18-14. Real timing in 50% assist during regular rhythm. Inflation is accurate; diastolic augmentation achieved, and a sharp V validates proper inflation. Deflation is accurate; ejection time is consistent, and systolic unloading is achieved. Hemodynamics improved during this timing mode.

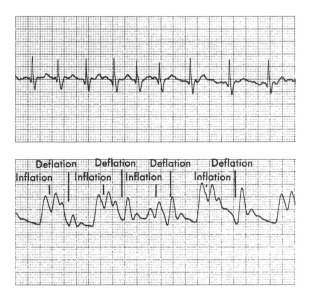

Fig. 18-15. Real timing in 50% assist during arrhythmia. Inflation is accurate; diastolic augmentation and a sharp V verifies accurate inflation. Deflation is consistent and accurate; ejection time remains accurate. Systolic unloading cannot be appreciated secondary to arrhythmias. With this timing mode, the patient's MAP increased and PCWP decreased.

REFERENCES

1. Ahern Gould K: Perspectives on intra-aortic balloon pump timing, *Crit Care Nurs Clin North Am* 3, September 1989.
2. Braunwald E et al: Time relationship of dynamic events in the cardiac chambers, pulmonary artery and aorta in man, *Circ Res* 4:100, 1956.
3. Burton AC: *Physiology and biophysics of the circulation*, ed 2 Chicago, 1972, Year Book Medical Publishers.
4. Fuchs RM et al: Augmentation of regional coronary blood flow by intra-aortic balloon counterpulsation in patients with unstable angina, *Circulation* 68:1, July 1983.
5. Jaron D, Moore TW, He P: Control of intra-aortic balloon pumping: theory and guidelines for clinical applications, *Ann Biomed Eng* 13:155, 1985.
6. Lang RM et al: Systemic vascular resistance: an unreliable index of left ventricular afterload, *Circulation* 74:5, November 1986.
7. Miura DS, Dangman K: Systolic time intervals: non-invasive measurement of left ventricular performance, *Cardiovasc Rev Rep* 7:12, December 1985.
8. Thoma H: Drive and management of circulation support systems. In Unger F, ed: *Assisted circulation* ed 2, New York, 1986, Springer-Verlag.
9. Tyson GS et al: Improved performance of the intra-aortic balloon pump using real time analysis of electromechanical variables, *Surg Forum* 34:339, 1983.
10. Tyson GS, Davis JW, Rankin JS: Improved performance of the intra-aortic balloon pump in man, *Surg Forum* 37:214, 1986.
11. Weber KT, Janicki JS: Intra-aortic balloon counterpulsation, *Ann Thorac Surg* 17:6, June 1974.
12. Weber KT, Janicki JS, Walker AA: Intra-aortic balloon pumping: an analysis of several variables affecting balloon performance, *Trans Amer Soc Artif Int Organs* 28:486, 1972.
13. Welkowitz W, Li JKJ: Modeling and optimization of assisted circulation, *IEEE Trans Biomed Eng* 31:12, December 1984.

CHAPTER 19

Use of the balloon pressure waveform in conjunction with the augmented arterial pressure waveform

Janet Kalina

During an inflation/deflation cycle, helium is moved rapidly in and out of the balloon catheter. Optimal balloon performance is influenced by both internal and external balloon environments. Counterpulsation involves changes in the aortic pressure environment. There is also a predictable pattern of helium gas pressure observed with balloon inflation and deflation. Helium gas pressure characteristics can be delineated by a waveform that is sensitive to gas behavior. This transduced waveform, or *balloon pressure waveform*, affords the operator direct information about the internal balloon environment. Information from both internal and surrounding balloon environments can be correlated for troubleshooting in a variety of clinical situations.

Some balloon pump consoles display a balloon pressure waveform. Distinct differences in pneumatic, alarm, and display system designs of the various manufacturers' consoles exist. See Chapters 26 to 30 for more detailed information concerning specific products.

NORMAL MORPHOLOGY

The balloon pressure waveform has a normal shape as well as variations that are considered normal in particular clinical situations. Understanding a normal waveform is necessary in order to identify abnormal waveforms, unsafe operating conditions, and to optimize the troubleshooting process.

A simplified pneumatics system diagram is presented in Fig. 19-1 **A,** which illustrates propagation of the balloon pressure waveform. To initiate counterpulsation, the pneumatics system must be filled with helium gas. Helium exerts a small posi-

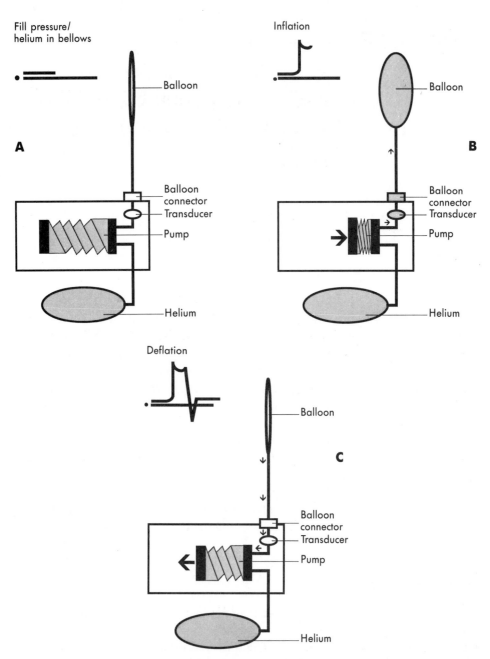

Fig. 19-1. A, Simplified pneumatics system diagram illustrates propagation of the balloon pressure waveform. **B,** Gas waveform generated during inflation as system is filled with helium. **C,** Gas waveform generated during deflation with an undershoot artifact below the baseline.

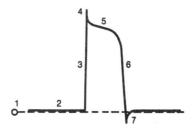

Fig. 19-2. Normal balloon gas waveform. 1, zero baseline; 2, fill pressure; 3, rapid inflation; 4, peak inflation artifact; 5, plateau pressure or inflation plateau pressure; 6, rapid deflation; 7, peak deflation pressure and return to fill pressure. (Courtesy Kontron Cardiovascular, Everett, Mass.)

tive pressure on an internal transducer that is located between the helium gas tank and balloon. This "fill pressure" registers as the balloon baseline. Fig. 19-1 **A**, contrasts balloon baseline with zero baseline. Fig. 19-1 **B**, demonstrates the inflation portion of a counterpulsation cycle. As inflation begins, a rapid upstroke is created as helium is compressed and propelled into the catheter. At peak inflation, there is an overshoot pressure artifact that is caused by gas pressure in the pneumatic line. The waveform then settles to a plateau, which indicates helium pressure required to maintain inflation throughout diastole. In Fig. 19-1 **C**, the diastolic waveform component is added. Deflation is marked by rapid waveform descent and undershoot artifact as helium gas rapidly returns to the pump. Balloon pressure baseline then returns demonstrating complete gas return to the pump. One complete inflate/deflate cycle is labeled and presented in Fig. 19-2.

CORRELATION WITH AUGMENTED ARTERIAL PRESSURE

It is important to consider the following points when determining normal relationships between balloon pressure waveform and the augmented arterial pressure waveform (Fig. 19-3 **A** and **B**):

1. The balloon pressure waveform width is approximately the duration of diastole, during which the balloon is active.
2. Assuming a transmembrane pressure of zero, the balloon plateau pressure reflects the aortic arterial pressure and the gas pressure required to maintain inflation throughout diastole. Therefore balloon pressure waveform plateau pressure should be within a few mm Hg of the peak augmented arterial diastolic pressure. It is suggested that a variance of plus or minus 20 to 25 mm Hg is acceptable for adult patients[1,3] and plus or minus 10 mm Hg is acceptable for pediatric patients.[2] Monitoring of the balloon pressure waveform inflation plateau and peak augmented diastolic arterial pressure, as described,

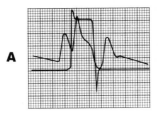

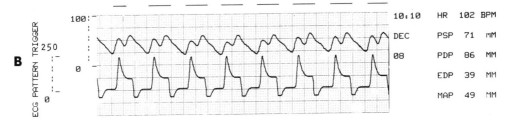

Fig. 19-3. A, Balloon pressure waveform superimposed on the arterial pressure waveform. **B,** Actual recording of an arterial pressure waveform (*top*) and balloon gas waveform (*bottom*) from a balloon-pumped patient. (**A,** Courtesy Kontron Cardiovascular, Everett, Mass.)

will facilitate complete assessment of the relationship between intraaortic balloon size and aortic diameter.

VARIATIONS OF NORMAL[4]

The most common alterations observed in balloon pressure waveforms are related to variations in length of cardiac cycles and aortic pressure. Assuming appropriate timing and balloon gas volume, these variations may indicate that current patient treatment regimen modification is necessary.

Variations due to heart rate

Fig. 19-4 illustrates varying balloon pressure waveform widths, corresponding with varying heart rates. Since balloon inflation occurs only during diastole, tachycardias (short diastolic phase, Fig. 19-4 **A**) will produce a narrow balloon pressure waveform. Bradycardias (longer diastolic phase, Fig. 19-4 **B**) produce a wider balloon pressure waveform.

If the heart rate is irregular, such as occurs with atrial fibrillation or frequent premature complexes, balloon pressure curves will vary in width (Fig. 19-5). Irregular balloon pressure curves generated despite a regular ECG rhythm indicate irregular triggering possibly related to motion or artifact.

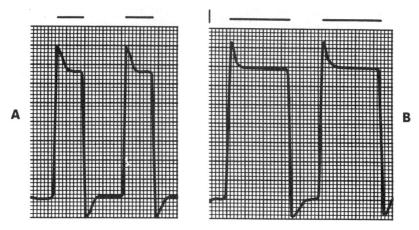

Fig. 19-4. A, Balloon gas waveform generated from a patient with a tachycardia. **B,** Balloon gas waveform generated from a patient with a bradycardia.

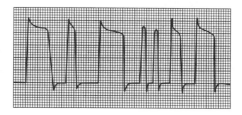

Fig. 19-5. Balloon gas waveform generated from a patient with an irregular heart rate.

Variations due to aortic pressure

Balloon pressure curve height reflects the driving pressure necessary to achieve and maintain full inflation in the aortic environment. If aortic pressure is relatively low (Fig. 19-6 **A**), resistance to inflation is low and therefore balloon pressure is also low. The converse is true with a hypertensive or centrally vasoconstricted patient (Fig. 19-6 **B**). Occasionally, balloon pressure curves generated from a hypertensive patient will demonstrate a very small or absent peak deflation artifact. There is no absolute pressure at which the artifact is lost, but as the hypertension is controlled and reduced the artifact reappears. An appropriately sized balloon should demonstrate a normal correlation to augmented arterial pressure in both the hypotensive and hypertensive patient.

Variations of normal for the pediatric patient

The balloon pressure waveform is likely to remain squared off or slightly rounded (especially in the 4 cc or smaller balloons—Fig. 19-7) because of elasticity

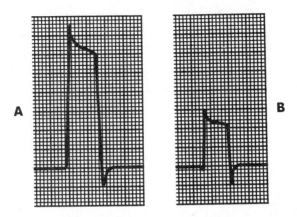

Fig. 19-6. A, Balloon gas waveform illustrates low plateau pressure. **B,** Balloon gas waveform illustrates high plateau pressure. (Courtesy Kontron Cardiovascular, Everett, Mass.)

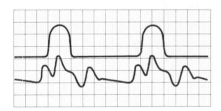

Fig. 19-7. Balloon gas waveform illustrates a rounded plateau. (Courtesy Kontron Cardiovascular, Everett, Mass.)

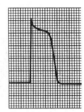

Fig. 19-8. Balloon gas waveform illustrates absent peak deflation artifact. (Courtesy Kontron Cardiovascular, Everett, Mass.)

of the child's aorta. This should pose no significant risk to aortic integrity. If vasoconstrictors are added, it is important to reevaluate both balloon pressure waveform and peak augmented diastolic pressure to determine if a volume adjustment is required.[2] The peak deflation artifact may also be very small or absent as a normal variation in the pediatric patient (Fig. 19-8).

ABNORMAL MORPHOLOGY

Alterations in balloon pressure waveform or baseline may indicate problems with the console, balloon, or reflect certain patient conditions. Most effective troubleshooting utilizes knowledge of normal balloon waveform morphology to recognize

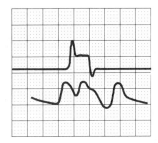

Fig. 19-9. *Top,* Balloon gas waveform illustrates low plateau pressure. *Bottom,* Arterial pressure.

abnormal variations. Correlation with the augmented arterial pressure is also very helpful. Certain intraaortic balloon pump consoles monitor balloon-fill pressure. On these consoles, some of the abnormal balloon pressure waveforms may initiate one or more console alarms to alert the clinician to potentially unsafe conditions.

Low balloon plateau pressure

Low balloon plateau pressure is illustrated in Fig. 19-9. As discussed earlier, a low plateau pressure may be observed in the clinical presentation of hypotension and hypovolemia. It may also be observed if:
- Balloon size is too small for the patient
- Volume setting is too low
- Balloon position is too low in the aorta
- Low systemic vascular resistance exists

In these cases, reduction in arterial diastolic augmentation pressure coincides with the normal waveform relationships.

If balloon pressure morphology appears normal with an augmented diastolic pressure greater than the balloon plateau pressure, consider the possibility of overshoot artifact on the arterial pressure waveform.

High balloon plateau pressure

An abnormally high plateau pressure changes the actual waveform shape. At times, the waveform will demonstrate loss of peak inflation and deflation artifacts as well as a squared or rounded top.

Fig. 19-10 demonstrates a very high balloon plateau pressure and absence of arterial pressure diastolic augmentation observed immediately after balloon insertion when counterpulsation was initiated. This situation is most likely to have been caused by a kink in the system.

Potential sources of restrictions or kinks include the following:

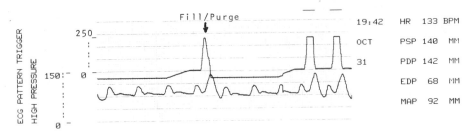

Fig. 19-10. This strip was recorded when the "high pressure" alarm sounded immediately after balloon insertion. *Top,* Balloon gas waveform is "squared off." *Bottom,* Arterial pressure waveform.

- External—plastic connecting tubing
            —sutures too tight around gas lumen
- Internal—balloon positioned too high or too low
            —balloon in aortic intimal wall
            —balloon has not fully exited insertion sheath
            —balloon has not fully unwrapped

If a high pressure waveform or alert is noted immediately after insertion, one should first suspect that the prewrapped, percutaneous balloon may not have fully unwrapped.

Nursing interventions might include visualizing the balloon silhouette under fluoroscopy. In the absence of fluoroscopy, one should again attempt to initiate console pumping. If unsuccessful, one option is to decrease pumping volume for a short time allowing the balloon membrane to reach body temperature. Returning to full balloon volume after 15 to 30 minutes may reveal normal arterial augmented pressures and balloon pressure waveforms.

Another option is to manually inflate and deflate the balloon rapidly with an appropriate volume of air via syringe after aspiration of the gas lumen to check for absence of blood return.*

It is also possible that the balloon is too large for the aorta.† Assuming previous interventions have failed, decrease helium inflation volume 1 to 2 cc at a time (Fig. 19-11 **A, B, C,** and **D**). After each increment of helium decrease, reattempt to initiate counterpulsation. Observe the relationship between the augmented diastolic pressure and the emerging balloon pressure. Continue to decrease balloon volume until this relationship is within normal limits.‡

---

*Consult specific manufacturer's operations manual for clarification of recommendations for this procedure.
†See Chapter 14 for more information on balloon sizing.
‡It is recommended *not* to decrease inflation volume to less than two-thirds capacity of the balloon.

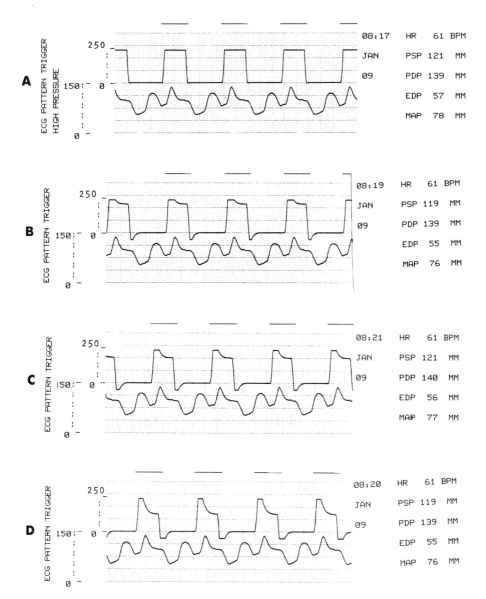

Fig. 19-11. A, This strip was recorded after the "high pressure" alarm sounded. Balloon volume is at full capacity (40 cc). Balloon gas waveform *(top)* is "squared-off." Normal arterial pressure waveform *(bottom).* **B,** Same patient after decreasing balloon volume by 2 cc. Balloon gas waveform *(top).* Arterial pressure waveform *(bottom).* **C,** Same patient after decreasing balloon volume by 4 cc. Balloon gas waveform *(top).* Arterial pressure waveform *(bottom).* **D,** Same patient after decreasing balloon volume by 6 cc. Balloon gas waveform *(top).* Arterial pressure waveform *(bottom).* Note normal relationship between balloon pressure plateau and augmented diastolic arterial pressure.

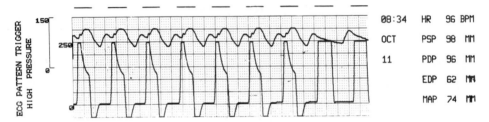

Fig. 19-12. *Top*, Arterial pressure. *Bottom*, Balloon gas waveform. High balloon pressure plateau secondary to a restriction of gas shuttle through the catheter.

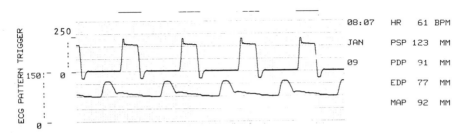

Fig. 19-13. *Top*, Normal balloon gas waveform. *Bottom*, Arterial waveform. No augmentation is demonstrated. Balloon may not be placed in the aorta.

Fig. 19-12 depicts effective counterpulsation followed by 2 cycles of high balloon pressure plateau without diastolic augmentation. This scenario is most likely related to an abrupt obstruction in the gas delivery system, as might be observed if the connecting tubing or catheter is kinked.

Rarely, the clinician might observe a tracing such as that in Fig. 19-13. In this tracing, the balloon appears to be inflating and deflating in a normal pattern; however, no diastolic augmentation is observable in the arterial pressure trace. This condition indicates the balloon may not be within the arterial system but may have exited the aorta or been placed in the venous system.

Balloon pressure baseline elevation

If baseline balloon pressure is greater than the prescribed positive pressure for helium at rest in the console pneumatics, the balloon pressure baseline will be elevated as in Fig. 19-14.

A kink in the catheter or a partially wrapped balloon can cause this alteration. This alteration may also be a result of gas system overpressurization or internal transducer drift. In both of these cases, a service engineer should examine the console.

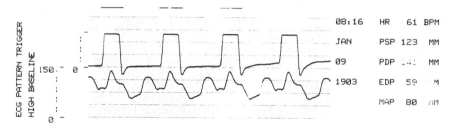

Fig. 19-14. *Top*, Balloon gas waveform. *Bottom*, Arterial pressure waveform. Note balloon waveform baseline is gradually elevating (compare baseline of first cycle to fourth cycle).

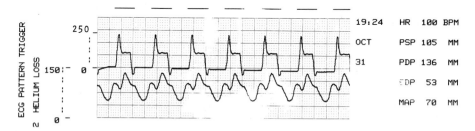

Fig. 19-15. *Top*, Balloon gas waveform. *Bottom*, Arterial pressure waveform. Note falling balloon gas waveform baseline occurred due to an accidental needle-stick of the connecting tubing, creating a leak (compare first cycle to last cycle).

Balloon pressure baseline depression

Return of the balloon pressure baseline to the fill pressure after an inflate/deflate cycle indicates a patent closed-loop system of gas delivery. A baseline pressure falling below minimum limits (Fig. 19-15) indicates there may be a leak in the gas circuit. It is possible for a leak to be either external or internal. If a leak is suspected, nursing interventions should include a leak test (see box on p. 306).

Other conditions that will prevent the gas and hence the balloon pressure baseline from returning to the fill pressure include:

- Extremely late deflation
- Rapid ECG irregularities (in certain trigger modes)

A possible auto-fill failure or an initial underfill with a manual system may also be responsible for a low or falling balloon pressure baseline. If a console is operating in the manual mode, the system does not automatically refill to compensate for gas diffusion over time. Therefore operating in the manual mode for prolonged periods will also demonstrate a falling balloon pressure baseline. If conditions dictate the use of manual mode, routine manual fills are necessary.

THE LEAK TEST

A leak test is performed to make a definitive diagnosis of helium loss and isolate both location and cause of the loss. Begin by observing balloon connecting tubing at proximal end of the catheter bifurcation. As helium is a clear, colorless gas, any red or brownish discolorations inside this tubing indicate a hole in the balloon bladder itself.* If blood is observed in the tubing, nursing interventions should include notifying the physician immediately and probable console shutdown. The balloon should be removed or replaced within ½ hour.

If no blood is visible in the tubing, proceed with the leak test as follows:

1. Collect the following items: a pair of rubber-shod hemostats, a pair of scissors, and a spare balloon connector plug (if applicable).
2. Turn the pump off and decrease balloon volume to approximately one half the balloon capacity.
3. Turn alarms off if required.
4. Clamp the clear plastic tubing with a hemostat, just proximal to the hard plastic bifurcation of the lumens.†
5. Turn console on, assure adequate trigger, and begin pumping in the manual mode.

Observe the balloon pressure waveform for a drop in baseline over a 1 to 2 minute period. Plateau pressure of the waveform will be distorted by the clamp. It is only important to observe the baseline pressure when troubleshooting in this manner. If the baseline remains stable (Fig. 19-16), the leak is either in the balloon catheter or at the junction of the balloon connecting tubing to the bifurcation. You may want to check all connections and repeat this step. Pouring betadine over the plastic bifurcation after removing the clamp and attempting to resume counterpulsation may reveal small bubbles at the site of a leak. Bone wax or adhesive tape may be used to stop an external leak.

If the baseline falls (Fig. 19-17), there is probably no leak in the balloon or at this connection; however, a leak may exist somewhere between the clamp and the console's internal pneumatics. Next, place the clamp on the clear plastic tubing as it exits the console connection. Turn console on, assure adequate trigger and begin pumping in the manual mode. Observe the balloon pressure baseline. If the baseline remains stable, the leak has been isolated to somewhere in the connecting tubing. All tubing connections should be carefully inspected. Submerging portions of the tubing in a basin of water, while pumping, may reveal bubbles at the site of a leak. Small tubing portions may be isolated with the clamp (working from patient toward console) until the exact leak site is determined.

However, it the baseline falls, the leak must be either at the console connection or within the console pneumatics. Replacing the balloon connector or cutting approximately ½-inch off the tubing end and replacing the connector may remedy small leaks at this junction.

After isolating and repairing an external leak, the shuttle gas volume should be returned to full capacity and pumping should be initiated with alarms engaged in the automatic mode. If leak alarms continue, or if the pump is unable to fill, disconnect balloon from the pump and occlude the gas exit from the pump with your finger. Assuring adequate trigger, begin to pump in the manual mode with alarms off. If the pump is unable to fill or balloon pressure baseline continues to fall, it can be assumed a leak exists somewhere inside the console pneumatics. This would require the operator to switch consoles and identify the malfunctioning pump to a service engineer.

---

*Make certain to clean any betadine or blood from the external surface of the tubing.
†*Never* clamp the double lumen of the catheter.

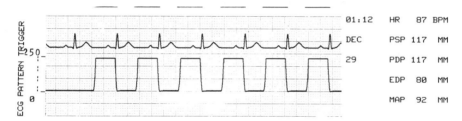

Fig. 19-16. *Top,* ECG. *Bottom,* Balloon gas waveform. Note stable baseline during a leak test.

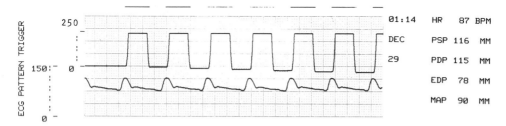

Fig. 19-17. *Top,* Balloon gas waveform. *Bottom,* Arterial pressure waveform. Note falling balloon gas waveform baseline during a leak test.

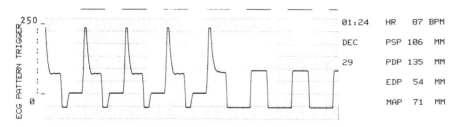

Fig. 19-18. Balloon gas waveform recorded from a kinked catheter, which may initially appear to be a loss of helium.

If a kink interrupts the gas movement during the deflation (vacuum) artifact, the waveform will demonstrate a drop in balloon pressure baseline followed by a high squared plateau pressure characteristic of a kink as presented in Fig. 19-18. Note that augmentation was normal until the kink prohibited helium from re-entering the balloon.*

---

*Note that augmentation would have been normal until the kink prohibited helium from re-entering the balloon. (See Fig. 19-12.)

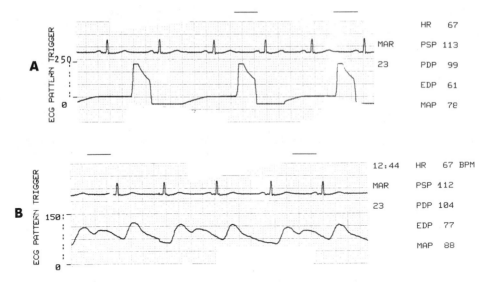

Fig. 19-19. A, ECG *(top).* Balloon gas waveform *(bottom)* from a patient with a kinked catheter. Note widening of peak inflation and deflation artifact on balloon gas waveform. **B,** ECG *(top).* Arterial pressure waveform *(bottom)* from the same patient. Note reduced diastolic augmentation and late deflation.

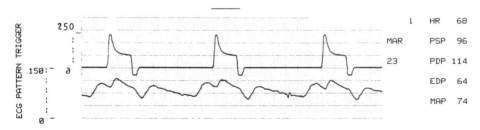

Fig. 19-20. *Top,* Balloon gas waveform. *Bottom,* Arterial pressure waveform from the same patient. Normal relationship noted after releasing gas obstruction.

Partial obstructions to gas shuttle may cause distorted balloon pressure plateaus and baseline changes. The widened peak inflation and deflation artifacts demonstrate slow gas transition, which is responsible for the reduced diastolic augmentation and afterload reduction depicted in Fig. 19-19 **A** and **B.** Two possible sources of partial obstruction include:
- Suture material tied too tightly around the gas lumen
- Proximal portion of balloon bladder caught in the insertion sheath

The patient in Fig. 19-19 had the intraaortic balloon placed emergently following coronary artery bypass surgery. Upon close inspection it appeared that the 11-inch introducer sheath may not have been pulled back. Fig. 19-20 represents results of releasing this partial obstruction. Notice the return to normal morphology waveforms with customary correlations. Duration of the partial obstruction along with the amount of balloon stretching will determine the balloon's ability to perform optimally once the obstruction is released.

SUMMARY

Waveform assessment is a critical step in the care of intraaortic balloon counterpulsation patients. Assessment of the balloon pressure waveform in conjunction with the arterial waveform provides the clinician with information on which to base treatment strategies and maintain optimal patient support.

REFERENCES

1. Aires: *Model 700 Control System Quick Reference Guide*, Rev A, May 1986.
2. Hanlon P: *Intra-aortic balloon pumping in children: a primer*, 1985.
3. Kontron: *Operators manual K2000*, Rev G, Feb 1990.
4. Kontron: *Physiology and principles of counterpulsation*.

PART FOUR

PATIENT MANAGEMENT

CHAPTER 20

Nursing care of the IABC patient

Susan J. Quaal

DOCUMENTATION

Fig. 20-1 **A** illustrates a suggested flowsheet for documentation of intraaortic balloon counterpulsation (IABC) patient assessment. Each hospital needs to customize a flowsheet to include specific balloon pump manufacturer recommended points of assessment. The flowsheet in Fig. 20-1 **A** can serve as a supplement to the patient's general flowsheet. Parameters included in Fig. 20-1 are specific to pressure documentation, peripheral vascular assessment, and balloon pump function. Chapter 23 includes suggestions regarding documentation of balloon demographic data.

PLAN OF CARE

A detailed generic care plan is presented as a guideline for nursing care of the IABC patient. The nurse must modify this plan of care to (1) meet individual patient care needs, (2) be in compliance with balloon pump manufacturer specific recommendations, and (3) adhere to hospital policies and procedures.

The care plan is presented in a nursing diagnosis conceptual framework, which defines the body of knowledge nursing is held accountable for to provide the highest standard of care. Additional information is provided to further elaborate on the nursing diagnosis and present nursing related research. An extensive list of potential nursing diagnoses is included with the intent that nurses will use only those that are relevant to each individual patient.

Most common nursing diagnoses anticipated for the IABC are Decreased Cardiac Output, Potential Alteration in Cardiac Output, High Risk for Vascular Complications, High Risk for Injury, Potential Alteration in Tissue Perfusion, High Risk for Decreased Renal Function, High Risk for Impaired Gas Exchange, Alteration in Comfort, High Risk for Balloon Pump Malfunction, High Risk for Alteration in Bowel Elimination, High Risk for Alteration in Nutritional Status, Potential Alteration in Skin or Muscle Integrity, Potential Alteration in Immunological Defense System, Potential Alteration in Level of Consciousness, Potential Alteration in

BALLOON PUMP PATIENT FLOWSHEET (DATE _5-2-93_)

NAME _Mr. Jones_ ID# _5374_ AGE _57_ WT _76_ BSA _2.0_

DATE AND TIME INSERTED _5-1-93 15:00_ INSERTION SITE _R femoral_

IS THIS   ((ORIGINAL))   OR   (REPLACEMENT)   BALLOON (Circle One)

NUMBER OF DAYS IAB HAS BEEN IN PLACE AT PRESENT INSERTION SITE _1_

TIME	0800											
TRIGGER SOURCE	Peak											
RATIO OF ASSIST	1:2											
BALLOON VOLUME (cc)	4.0											
HELIUM LEVEL (psi)	400											

Trigger Source   PE = Peak; P = Pattern; AF = Atrial Fib; AP = Atrial Pace; VP = Vent Pace
Codes: Art = Arterial; Int = Internal

A

ASSESSMENT OF PRESSURES WITH 1:2 RATIO OF ASSIST

TIME	0800											
PDP	108											
BAEDP	64											
UAEDP	69											
ASSISTED SYSTOLE	90											
UNASSISTED SYSTOLE	96											
MEAN PRESSURE	78											

CODES (Pressures in mm Hg)

1 = PDP (Peak Diastolic Augmented Pressure)
2 = BAEDP (Balloon Assisted Aortic End Diastolic Pressure)
3 = UAEDP (Unassisted Aortic End Diastolic Pressure)
4 = Assisted Systole
5 = Unassisted Systole

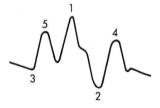

Fig. 20-1. A, Front of IABC patient flowsheet. Sample data is provided.

TIME	0800																									
	R	L	R	L	R	L	R	L	R	L	R	L	R	L	R	L	R	L	R	L	R	L	R	L	R	L
DORSALIS PEDALIS PULSE	1+	3+																								
POSTERIOR TIBIAL PULSE	1+	3+																								
ANKLE ARM INDEX	0910																									
CAPILLARY REFILL	I	I																								
THIGH MEASUREMENT (cm)																										
CALF MEASUREMENT (cm)																										

Pulses: 3+ =Bounding; 2+ = Normal; 1+ = Weak; D = Doppler -
Capillary Refill: (1) = Immediate (D) = Delayed

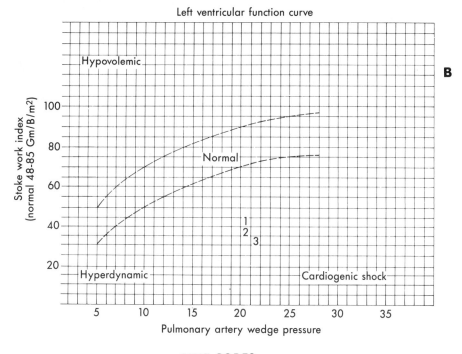

B

Left ventricular function curve

TIME CODES

1 0800   3 1000   5_____   7_____   9_____   11_____

2 0900   4_____   6_____   8_____   10_____   12_____

Fig. 20-1, cont'd. B, Back of IABC patient flowsheet.

Thought Process, High Risk for Anxiety and Knowledge Deficit, High Risk for Alteration in Family Process, and Powerlessness. These nursing diagnoses are a composite of the author's personal experience, the Datascope Corporation's "Plan of Care for the Patient/Family Requiring Intraaortic Balloon Counterpulsation Therapy in a Nursing Diagnosis Framework," and Chapter 23.

These nursing diagnoses, patient outcomes, interventions, and evaluation criteria are outlined with expanded information that supports the plan of care.

Discussion

Since hemodynamic indices are critically important in assessment of the IABC patient's left ventricular failure (LVF), the nurse must ensure a high standard of quality assurance before using these parameters to modulate therapy. Proper zeroing, balancing, and dynamic response testing must be executed before any direct pressure measurements can be made (see Chapter 15).

NURSING DIAGNOSIS 1: decreased cardiac output

Related to	Patient outcomes	Interventions	Evaluation
LVF that necessitated IABC	Signs and symptoms of LVF resolving as evidenced by: Normalization of CI, PACP, SWI, Do_2, SVR	Nurse will assess indicators of LVF: CI, PACP SWI, Do_2 and SVR according to unit procedure Utilize LVFC to track left ventricular performance Administer IV fluids, vasodilator and inotropic agents as indicated to maximize left ventricular performance	Patient demonstrated improvement in LVF
	Adequate urine output	Monitor urine output hourly	
	Skin warm and dry	Monitor skin temperature hourly	
	Patient alert and oriented	Monitor sensorium	
	Absence of chest pain	Ask patient to rate any chest pain on a scale of 1-10	
	Chest auscultation free of rales	Auscultate chest for presence of rales; may require an assistant to logroll patient, keeping IAB insertion leg straight	

A left ventricular function curve (LVFC) is illustrated in Fig. 20-1 **B**. Numbers are used to chronologically plot the bisection of stroke work index and pulmonary artery capillary pressure. Each number corresponds to a specific time code, listed at the bottom of the page. Left ventricular function is a most useful parameter to track in the IABC patient. Some hospitals also use an LVFC that is silk-screened on erasable plexiglass, which can be mounted on a wall in the patient's room. Another option for documenting LVFC is a computer print-out.

Documenting blood pressure in the IABC patient

Blood pressure components are greatly impacted by IABC. Note Fig. 20-2 **A**. Normally, systole is the highest pressure generated. Bedside monitors recognize this pressure point and digitalize to a numeric display as "systolic pressure." Likewise, the first Korotkoff sound heard when taking a cuff blood pressure is also systolic pressure.[2]

As the balloon inflates, peak diastolic pressure becomes the highest pressure generated (Fig. 20-2 **B**). What is actually balloon inflated "peak diastolic augmented pressure" will be registered as "systole" by the bedside monitor. The first Korotkoff sound auscultated, when measuring an indirect cuff blood pressure in the IABC patient, is produced by peak diastolic augmented pressure not systole.

When counterpulsation is engaged at a 1:2 ratio of assist, "blood pressure" now is expanded into five components (Fig. 20-3). Peak diastolic augmented pressure is usually the highest pressure reference point generated. The other references points are balloon-assisted aortic end-diastolic pressure (BAEDP), unassisted-aortic end-diastolic pressure (UAEDP), assisted systole, and unassisted systole. (Review timing in Chapter 16.) Expansion of blood pressure from the standard two components of systole and diastole in the non-IABC to the five reference points in the IABC (1:2 ratio of assist) must be understood by all members of the patient's health care team. It is impossible to attempt to use a 2-component blood pressure reference system in the IABC patient. The IABC patient's blood pressure reference points become especially critical when computing mean arterial pressure and titrating vasopressor and vasoactive medications.

Calculating mean arterial pressure in the balloon-pumped patient. Mean arterial pressure (MAP) is an average pressure or calculated value that does not exist except during an instantaneous measurement during the rise and fall of patient's pulse.[2] Arithmetic and integration procedures exist for computing MAP (Figs. 20-4 and 20-5). Arithmetic MAP is computed by the sum of the systolic pressure + 2 diastolic pressures/3.[2] With a systolic pressure of 120 mm Hg and a diastolic pressure of 80 mm Hg, the calculated arithmetic MAP is 93 mm Hg. This would represent the true average pressure only if the pressure waves were symmetrical.[3]

A true functional mean divides the area of the pressure waveform by length of the sample (time), which is described as the integration method of calculating MAP.

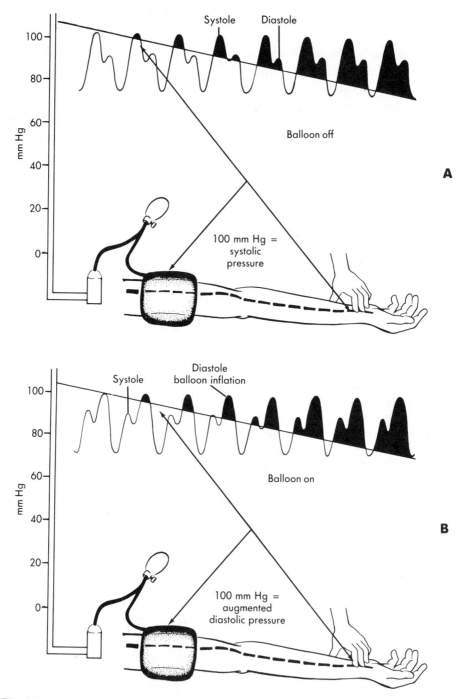

Fig. 20-2. A, Arterial blood pressure from a non-IABC patient. Systole is the highest pressure generated from the invasive line pressure. Likewise, when recording an indirect or cuff pressure, the first Korotkoff sound auscultated is the systolic sound. **B,** Arterial blood pressure from an IABC patient. The highest pressure wave generated is now the peak diastolic augmented pressure. The first Korotkoff sound heard is that produced by balloon inflation, or peak diastolic augmented pressure, rather than systole.

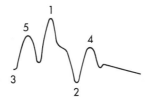

Fig. 20-3. The blood pressure from an IABC patient at a 1:2 ratio of assist has five reference points: *(1)* peak diastolic augmented pressure; *(2)* balloon-assisted aortic end-diastolic pressure; *(3)* unassisted aortic end-diastolic pressure; *(4)* assisted systole; and *(5)* patient systole.

Instrumentation usually uses the integration method. However, it is crucial that clinicians investigate which method is used by each piece of instrumentation employed, i.e., bedside monitor, balloon pump, portable transport monitor, anesthesia monitor, or catheterization laboratory monitoring equipment. The potential for error exists when changing from one instrument to another.

The integration method seems most appropriate for the IABC patient when peak and trough pressures are changing from beat to beat. These changes may further be accentuated by ectopic beats. If the clinical MAP is from a system that uses an arithmetic method of computation, it is imperative to investigate just how this computation is performed for an IABC patient on a 1:1 ratio of assist, as compared with 1:2, 1:3, and so on. The most important point of MAP monitoring for the IABC patient is to use the same instrumentation source, i.e., if MAP is recorded from the balloon pump console, then each nurse should consistently use that digital value, which is recorded on the patient's flowsheet and used in calculating derived indices, such as systemic vascular resistance and stroke work index.

Pressure reference point for titration of vasopressor or vasoactive drugs. Since blood pressure in the IABC patient at a 1:2 ratio of assist has 5 components, it can be confusing for both physician and nurse trying to use an arbitrary number as a guide for titration of vasoactive or vasopressor drugs. Each pressure reference point must be assessed with regard to the potential impact of various pharmacological agents used in conjunction with IABC. Refer again to Fig. 20-3.

Dobutamine exerts primarily beta-adrenergic effects. Therefore the intended pharmacological action is inotropic with an increase in contraction. As the heart empties more efficiently and completely, a greater stroke volume should also be ejected. As stroke volume increases, a greater volume displacement effect should be appreciated during balloon inflation, hence an increase in peak diastolic augmented pressure.

Dopamine exhibits alpha-adrenergic effects at infusion rates >10 µg/kg/min, which produces peripheral vasoconstriction. As systemic vascular resistance rises, systolic pressure also increases. Therefore concomitant with dopamine infusions, the clinician should expect a possible increase in both assisted and unassisted systole. Assisted systole should remain comparatively lower than patient systole, reflecting the reduction in ventricular work secondary to balloon deflation during isovolumetric contraction.

With mild vasoconstriction, stroke volume may actually be increased. Therefore as the balloon inflates and displaces an increased stroke volume, peak diastolic augmented pressure will rise. As the patient's aorta further vasoconstricts with higher doses of alpha-adrenergic pharmacological agents, less stroke volume can be accommodated and potential volume displacement (and concomitant elevation of peak diastolic augmented pressure with balloon inflation) is minimized. Thus as the dosage of a vasoconstricting agent increases, the clinician may also note a decrease in peak diastolic augmented pressure.

A vasodilator drug, such as nitroprusside or nitroglycerin, could potentially impact several aspects of the IABC patient's arterial pressure waveform. Since these

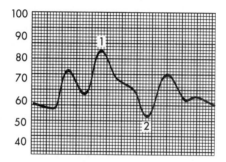

Fig. 20-4. Arithmetic method of computing a MAP in the IABC patient. In this example the monitoring system substitutes peak diastolic augmented pressure (1) as systole and balloon assisted aortic end-diastolic pressure (2) as diastole. This patient's MAP would be computed as:

$$\frac{84 + 2\,(54)}{3} = 64 \text{ mm Hg}$$

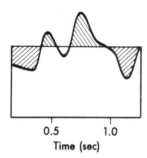

Fig. 20-5. Integration method of computing a MAP. The area outside the rectangle should equal the area inside the rectangle.

NURSING DIAGNOSIS 2: potential alteration in cardiac output

Related to	Expected outcomes	Nursing interventions	Evaluation
Impaired myocardial contractility, secondary to myocardial ischemia	Absence of myocardial ischemia, as evidenced by: No chest pain Normal isoenzymes No ST segment changes	Assess patient for chest pain, having patient rate any pain on a scale of 1-10 Monitor isoenzymes Record daily 12-lead ECG Continuous bedside ST-segment monitoring, when available	Patient has no evidence of myocardial ischemia
Incorrectly "timed" IABC	Optimal timing observed as evidenced by peak diastolic augmented pressure; highest pressure point and BAEDP are lower than UAEDP; assisted systole is ≤ unassisted systole unless patient's physiological status accounts for deviance from standard timing	Assess timing minimally every 4 hours and whenever patient's heart rate changes by ± 10 beats, or a significant change in hemodynamic status is noted Establish a "clean" ECG signal for triggering or artifact-free arterial pressure signal Choose trigger mode according to manufacturer's recommendations	IABC will be properly timed
Arrhythmias	Arrhythmia will be restored to patient's baseline	Select monitoring leads that will provide maximum information on arrhythmia[4] Assess hemodynamic tolerance of arrhythmia Utilize manufacturer recommended trigger mode during arrhythmia Administer antiarrhythmic agents as ordered	Patient maintains hemodynamically stable rhythm

drugs are afterload-reducing agents, it is possible that both BAEDP and UAEDP may be lowered. Vasodilation can decrease stroke volume. With this decrease in stroke volume peak diastolic augmented pressure may be lowered, as stroke volume exceeds the balloon's displacement capabilities.

The important principle of infusing vasoactive, vasodilating, or inotropic drugs in conjunction with IABC is to assess the entire hemodynamic profile. Review Chapter 15 and use of flow parameters, such as oxygen delivery, utilization, and venous reserve, which are more comprehensive indicators of combined pharmacological and IABC therapy rather than an isolated arterial pressure reference point.

If the nurse is confronted with an order that reads "titrate dopamine to maintain a pressure of 90," it is crucial to clarify with the physician as to what this means for the IABC patient. Deleterious outcomes can arise if one nurse assumes this refers to MAP, another assumes the order refers to peak diastolic augmented pressure, and another assumes this order refers to the patient's natural systole. Communication between physician and nurse with regard to titrating pharmacological therapy in the IABC patient is a most important aspect of patient care.

Discussion

When assessing chest pain, it is important that the nurse offer the patient a scale of 1 to 10 with which to quantify and track the severity of pain. Continuous ST-segment monitoring analysis is now available via bedside monitoring microcomputer-assisted multichannel ECG monitoring systems. It has been demonstrated that painless ST-segment ischemic changes occur about twice as often as those associated with pain.[5]

An artifact free ECG signal is sent to the IABC console for the purpose of triggering. Skin prep must be done according to electrode manufacturer recommendations. Use of diaphoretic or karaya adherence electrodes is suggested to ensure good skin contact and prevention of trigger loss. It is recommended that the balloon pump ECG leads be used to establish a "trigger ECG" in any configuration (not necessarily a conventional lead) that affords a clear tracing, with at least a 2 mV QRS amplitude. Consult with manufacturer regarding the option of triggering of a positive or negative complex. The bedside ECG cable should be used to establish diagnostic monitoring leads.

The clinician must be aware of the physical and biological factors that can alter diastolic augmentation. A change in peak diastolic augmented pressure may be invoked by factors other than incorrect timing (see Chapter 7).

Much new information is now available regarding ECG monitoring lead selection based on actual or potential threatening arrhythmias.[4] The clinician should therefore customize the IABC's monitoring leads in compliance with this new standard of care.

NURSING DIAGNOSIS 3: high risk for vascular complications

Related to	Expected outcomes	Nursing interventions	Evaluation
Traumatic IAB insertion or removal	Patient will exhibit signs of adequate peripheral vascular perfusion as evidenced by:	Assess peripheral vascular status per unit's standard of care	Patient maintained baseline peripheral vascular perfusion status during and after removal of IAB
IAB is a foreign body in a potentially atherosclerotic vessel, producing peripheral ischemia	$\geq$2+ dorsalis pedalis and posterior tibial pulses (Fig. 20-6) Normal capillary refill Normal peripheral skin color and temperature Ankle-arm index 0.8-1.2	Assess ankle-arm index minimum of every 4 hours	
Compartment syndrome	No throbbing sensation in calf of leg with IAB insertion No calf pain with dorsal foot flexion No loss of lower leg sensation When feet are elevated 45 degrees there is no sign of pallor	Assess for compartment syndrome by: Checking for throbbing sensation in calf Calf pain with foot dorsal flexion Pallor in feet when feet are elevated 45 degrees	
Excessive bleeding at insertion site	Minimal bleeding at insertion site Coagulation counts maintained within a therapeutic range	Notify physician of any bleeding at insertion site or change in peripheral vascular status	Patient did not experience excessive bleeding at IAB insertion site

Discussion

Assessment of peripheral vascular complications is an important component of IABC nursing care. Review Chapter 10 for peripheral vascular complications and their signs/symptoms. The ankle-arm index is an objective monitor of peripheral vascular perfusion.[6] A decreasing ankle-arm index suggests decreasing peripheral

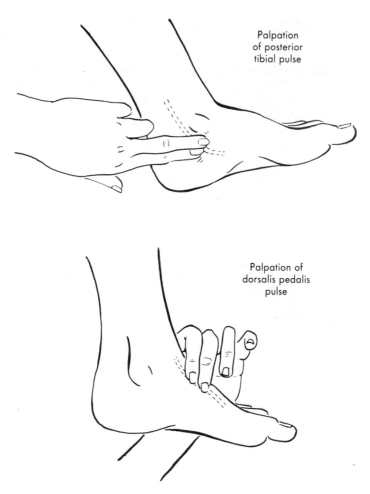

Fig. 20-6. Location of posterior tibial and dorsalis pedalis pulses.

PROCEDURE FOR PERFORMING THE ANKLE-ARM INDEX★

1. Locate posterior tibial or dorsalis pedalis pulse with a Doppler.
2. Apply blood pressure cuff around the ankle above the malleolus.
3. Inflate cuff to 20 mm Hg above the current brachial systolic pressure.
4. Note the reappearance of Doppler signal as cuff deflates.
5. Divide the ankle systolic pressure by the brachial systolic pressure to determine ankle-arm ratio.

From Flewelling-Goran S: *Crit Care Nurs Clin North Am* 1:459, 1989.
★Normal value is 0.8 to 1.2.

vascular perfusion. This procedure is outlined in the box on p. 324. Vascular complication rates are higher in patients with difficult insertion and removal, hence the nurse should be alerted to this potential.

IABC patients are also susceptible to compartment syndrome because of prolonged immobilization, loss of capillary blood flow, preexisting peripheral vascular disease, and difficult insertion. Compartment syndrome may be suspected, if on elevation of the feet by 45 degrees, pallor is noted. It is important to consult with specific IAB manufacturer before implementing this intervention. Some IAB catheters have a metal component within the catheter interior; the manufacturer may therefore advise against raising the feet 45 degrees. A CPK level may reach as high as 5000 IU in a patient with compartment syndrome. Pressure measurements may also be made by inserting a catheter connected to a transducer directly into the compartment. This test is inconclusive unless the pressure is over 30 mm Hg, however.

NURSING DIAGNOSIS 4: high risk for injury

Related to	Expected outcomes	Nursing interventions	Evaluation
Anemia and thrombocytopenia secondary to mechanical trauma to blood produced by IABC	Patient will not experience anemia, thrombocytopenia, and decrease in RBC	Assess daily laboratory values for signs of anemia and thrombocytopenia	Patient maintained baseline nematocrit, RBC, and platelet counts
Infection secondary to invasive lines combined with patient's debilitated state	Absence of infection as evidenced by: Patient afebrile Normal white blood count IAB insertion site and other invasive lines insertion sites are free from redness, swelling, tenderness, and drainage	Use aseptic technique when changing dressings Inspect IAB insertion site and all invasive line insertion sites for redness, swelling, and drainage Monitor WBC and temperature Use meticulous handwashing technique Culture any drainage from line insertion sites	Patient will remain free of infections
Gastric bleeding secondary to stress ulcers	Patient will not experience stress ulcers or GI bleeding	Guaiac all stools, emesis, and nasogastric tube returns, if present Administer H_2 antagonists according to unit policy	Patient will not experience GI bleeding

NURSING DIAGNOSIS 5: potential alteration in tissue perfusion

Related to	Expected outcomes	Interventions	Evaluation
Arterial obstruction of subclavian, carotid, renal, or femoral artery Transient arterial spasm Inadequate limb perfusion related to invasive lines or IAB Embolus dislodged during IAB insertion, while counterpulsating or during removal Balloon dissection through intima, media, or adventitia of aorta.	Adequate tissue perfusion as evidenced by: No signs of arm, neurological, renal, or peripheral vascular ischemia Absence of mesenteric and back pain Good capillary refill of hands and feet	Assess for possible obstruction to subclavian, carotid, renal, or femoral artery; checking color, temperature, and pulses of brachial, radial, and leg Assess capillary refill Assess neurological status Monitor urine output Assess for back and flank pain Perform Allen test on hand that contains indwelling radial artery catheter	Patient will not exhibit signs of inadequate tissue perfusion

Discussion

The patient is prone to alteration in tissue perfusion because both IAB and radial arterial lines are foreign bodies. Also embolization may occur during IAB insertion, while counterpulsating, and during removal. Therefore assessment of tissue and organ perfusion is a high priority of the nursing care plan. An Allen test should be undertaken at least every 4 hours to ensure adequate perfusion through the radial arterial lines.[7] This procedure is illustrated in Fig. 20-7.

Aortic dissection can occur during insertion or ongoing counterpulsation. Arterial wall dissection that produces an intimal flap opening in the direction of blood flow promptly seals itself and is of little clinical consequence. In contrast, an intimal tear facing into the direction of circulation may cause a more serious dissection and may lead to occlusion of aortic branches.[8] A summary of reported aortic dissections[8] placed the incidence at 0.94% to 3.4%. Areas of dissection reported include the aortoiliac region, abdominal aorta or distal portion of the descending thoracic aorta, and midthoracic aorta.

Clinical presentations of dissections have varied from no symptoms (dissection discovered only at autopsy) to sudden onset of back pain during insertion associated with difficulty in passing the balloon beyond the distal portion of the descending thoracic aorta or proximal segment of the abdominal aorta.[8] An autopsy finding of aortia dissection by an IAB is found in Fig. 20-8.

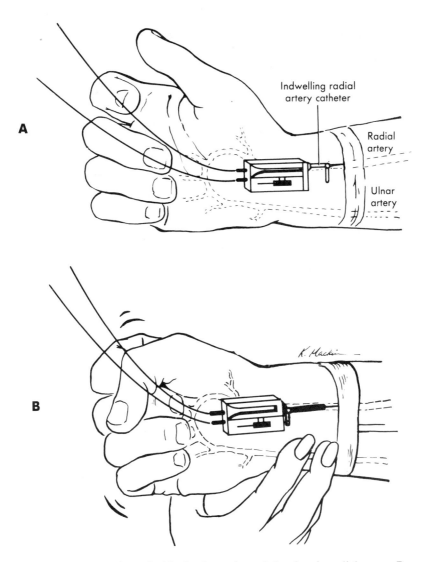

Labels in figure:
Indwelling radial artery catheter
Radial artery
Ulnar artery

A

B

Fig. 20-7. Allen test procedure. **A,** Monitoring catheter is in place in radial artery; **B,** patient makes a fist while examiner manually compresses ulnar artery. If patient is unable to make a fist, the examiner can manually position the hand in a fist position.   *Continued.*

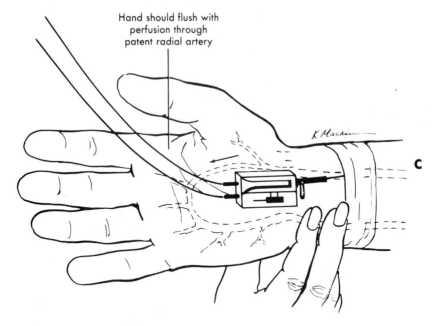

Hand should flush with
perfusion through
patent radial artery

K Mackin

C

Fig. 20-7, cont'd. C, Examiner maintains compression on ulnar artery while patient opens fist. The hand should flush and resume pink color immediately if blood perfusion through the radial artery is adequate.

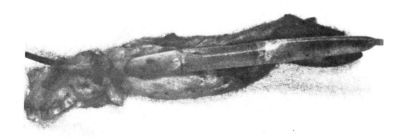

Fig. 20-8. Aorta that has been dissected by an IAB.

Discussion

Swartz et al.[9] examined the impact of positioning IABs adjacent to the renal arteries on renal blood flow. Left and right renal blood flows were measured in 14 dogs; IAB position was randomized so that it was initially placed in either the thoracic (control) or at the level of the renal artery (experimental) position. IABC was performed for 4 hours in each position. Fifty-seven percent of the dogs demonstrated at least partial renal artery occlusion (23% to 98%) and decreased renal flow

NURSING DIAGNOSIS 6: high risk for decreased renal function

Related to	Expected outcomes	Nursing interventions	Evaluation
Occlusion of the renal arteries by IAB catheter Hypotension or cardiogenic shock	Patient will exhibit optimum renal function as evidenced by: Urine output 30 ml/hr Balanced intake and output BUN and creatinine values remain at patient's baseline	Measure urine output hourly Accurate fluid intake and output documentation Serum K^+, creatinine, and BUN laboratory values daily Daily weight Check position of IAB on daily chest x-ray film	Patient has no signs of renal failure

NURSING DIAGNOSIS 7: high risk for impaired gas exchange

Related to	Expected outcomes	Nursing interventions	Evaluation
Bedrest and immobility Extended intubation Inadequate pulmonary status	Patient will exhibit respiratory status as evidenced by: Adequate spontaneous or mechanically controlled ventilation Arterial blood gases and mixed venous saturation optimized Lungs clear on auscultation and absence of cough or secretions	Assess respiratory status via: Auscultation of lung fields Assessment of respiratory rate and pattern Monitoring of arterial and mixed venous blood gases every 8 hours and PRN Daily chest x-ray Provide log-rolled position changes every 2 hours Suction intubated patient every 2 hours and PRN Provide moisture to loosen secretions Encourage nonintubated patient to deep breathe and cough	Patient will not exhibit respiratory failure, atelectasis, pneumonia, or pleural effusions

while the IAB was in the renal position. Decreased renal blood flow was not apparent by conventional hemodynamic monitoring indices. Assessment of IAB placement by daily chest x-ray is therefore suggested in an effort to preclude distal migration to a position that might compromise renal artery flow.[9]

NURSING DIAGNOSIS 8: alteration in comfort

Related to	Expected outcomes	Nursing interventions	Evaluation
IAB catheter insertion, movement within femoral artery or removal	Patient discomfort will be minimized	Immobolize leg with long-leg knee brace to prevent movement of IAB catheter within femoral artery and nerve irritation	Patient complained of minimal discomfort
		Inspect IAB insertion site for any signs of infection	
		Apply ice to insertion site to minimize discomfort	
General musculoskeletal pain from immobility		Log roll and offer back rubs every 2 hours	
		Utilize therapeutic beds to facilitate circulation and promote general musculoskeletal comfort	
Environmental stress from noise, overstimulation		Protect "quiet time" when patient is guaranteed an uninterrupted time period to facilitate sleep	
		Make conscious effort to reduce conversational noise	
		Close glass doors, when possible, to shield patient from noise and allow view of patient	

Discussion

Quaal[10] undertook a qualitative study, conducting interactive interviews with patients who had undergone an IABC experience. Patients described the physical discomfort caused by IABC as "knifelike pain" at the insertion site to actually feeling counterpulsation within their aorta. Comments recorded included " . . . that blasted thing (IAB) moved around inside my groin and was so sore and stabbed me. It was just like a knife in there" and " . . . it burned so much, right at the groin." These patients also endured environmental discomforts through overstimulation by

Related to	Expected outcomes	Nursing interventions	Evaluation
Loss of trigger signal secondary to inappropriate trigger selection, poor ECG signal, inadequate arterial pressure (when using arterial pressure trigger)	Trigger signal will be effective for providing ongoing IABC	ECG lead used for trigger should be designated to meet pump console's trigger requirements rather than a diagnostic lead; a redundant set of electrodes from the bedside monitor can be used to obtain needed arrhythmia diagnostic leads, such as MCL_1 and MCL_6 Troubleshoot loss of trigger according to manufacturer's guidelines, i.e., appropriate use of pacemaker and arterial pressure waveforms as trigger signals; be aware of minimum arterial pressure required to be sensed as a trigger signal	Absence of balloon pump malfunction
Kink in IAB system	System free of kinks	An envelope opening in the bedding allows for continuous visualization of IAB connecting tubing and inspection for kinks Be familiar with console's criteria for sensing a kink and sounding an alarm	
Balloon leak or catheter disconnect	System free of leaks	When helium leak alarm is activated, institute manufacturer-recommended procedure for leak test Check all balloon connections from insertion sight to pump connector for possible loose connections When transporting patient, one attendant should ensure pump catheter and patient are intact so that IAB does not become disconnected or dislodged	

NURSING DIAGNOSIS 10: high risk for alteration in bowel elimination

Related to	Expected outcomes	Nursing interventions	Evaluation
Antegrade IAB placement in mesenteric artery	Optimal bowel function as evidenced by:	Check IAB placement with daily chest x-ray	Patient will exhibit optimal bowel function
Bowel infarction	Active bowel sounds	Assess bowel sounds with each shift nursing assessment (may need to briefly turn IABC to standby to hear bowel sounds)	
Immobility and decreased gastrointestinal motility	Abdomen soft and nontender		
	Absence of constipation, impaction, and ileus		
Tube feedings	Absence of diarrhea	Assess abdomen for tenderness and rigidity	
		Measure abdominal girth every shift	
		Administer stool softener as ordered	
		Minimize risk of diarrhea by slowly increasing rate and concentration of tube feeding	
		Guaiac all stools	

equipment sounds and alarms. These findings suggest that the IABC patient's plan of care must include measures to reduce discomfort that arises at the IAB insertion site. Long-leg knee braces have been employed as a pilot project. Preliminary observations suggest that this device provides leg immobilization controlled by the patient with Velcro straps and yet effectively restricts catheter movement within the femoral artery insertion site, thereby minimizing local discomfort. Comfort has also been provided by placing an ice pack at the insertion site.

IABC patients complain of general musculoskeletal aching, most likely imposed by long periods of bedrest and inactivity. The patient should be log rolled every 2 hours with back rubs and pillow positioning in an effort to provide comfort. The patient should also be evaluated for a therapeutic bed, which promotes circulation and gentle continuous controlled mobility.

Discussion

Each manufacturer has specific "trigger signal" options. Various criteria exist for recognizing an ECG and for using an atrial or ventricular pacemaker spike or arterial pressure to trigger. "Trigger" refers to the console's ability to reference systole or diastole to a biological signal (electrical or mechanical) and to counterpulse the IAB

NURSING DIAGNOSIS 11: high risk for alteration in nutritional status

Related to	Expected outcomes	Nursing interventions	Evaluation
Decreased appetite due to severity of illness Prolonged intubation and failure to take oral nourishment Lack of total nutritional assessment and parenteral administration of adequate calories and nutritional supplements Low serum albumin	Patient will demonstrate optimal nutritional status to meet caloric needs associated with the illness	Explore the possibility of oral nutritional intake in the intubated patient Make sure endotracheal cuff is inflated and throat is locally mildly anesthesized to minimize discomfort associated with swallowing Involve nutritional support team with complete assessment of caloric, protein and mineral/vitamin needs; reassess these needs daily Monitor serum albumin and electrolytes daily When patient is able to take oral nourishment, consult a dietitian in an effort to offer appetizing foods within dietary plan	Patient will demonstrate optimal nutritional status

with helium, based on this trigger signal reference. The nurse must therefore be knowledgeable in individual manufacturer's trigger signal criteria and ensure that they are met. The operator must also be familiar with situations that require alternative triggers, such as IABC in the operating room where an electrical bovie may interfere with the ECG signal, therefore the operator must be prepared to switch to arterial pressure trigger when the bovie is used. Different manufacturers' consoles respond differently to atrial and ventricular pacemaker signals. Balloon console operators therefore must thoroughly orient themselves to correct trigger choices for atrial, ventricular, and A-V sequential pacemakers.

Discussion

During antegrade IAB insertion, the potential exists for inadvertent catheterization of the superior mesenteric artery (Fig. 20-9).[11] This potential risk supports the

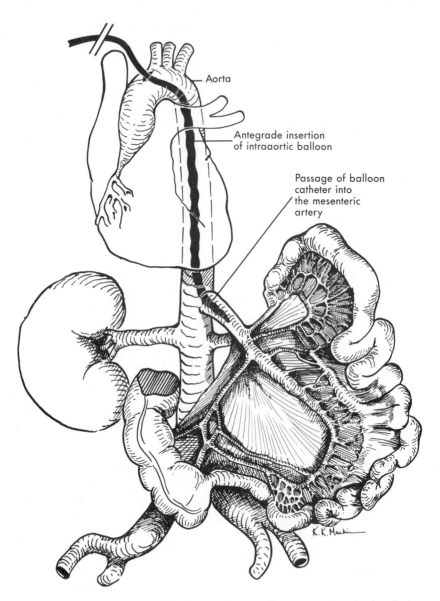

Fig. 20-9. Schematic illustration of inadvertent mesenteric artery catheterization during antegrade IAB insertion.

NURSING DIAGNOSIS 12: high risk for potential alteration in skin or muscle integrity

Related to	Expected outcomes	Nursing interventions	Evaluation
Immobilization and inadequate tissue perfusion Poor nutrition	Patient will exhibit normal skin and muscle integrity as evidenced by: Lack of decubiti Good skin turgor; skin is pink and warm to touch Absence of muscle wasting	Assess patient with each log-roll turn for evidence of skin breakdown Use preventive measures, i.e., frequent turning and repositioning (keeping IAB insertion site straight) Keep skin dry Prompt cleansing and drying of affected area if patient is incontinent of urine or stool Evaluate patient for use of therapeutic bed to promote circulation and prevent skin breakdown Use high-top tennis shoes or foot board to prevent footdrop Complete nutritional assessment with correction of any identified caloric, protein, vitamin, and or mineral deficiencies	Patient exhibits healthy skin and muscle integrity with healing of any skin wounds

need for fluoroscopic verification of balloon placement and ongoing assessment for loss of bowel sounds and abdominal distension.

Discussion

Nutritional assessment has developed into a sophisticated science. Dietitians are now trained to compute total caloric, protein, and vitamin/mineral needs for the patient's given state. It is imperative that nutritional energy requirements be met with daily reassessment to prevent a catabolic state.

Discussion

Flewelling-Goran[12] surveyed spouses, siblings, and children of patients who had undergone IABC. She found that most spouses obtained their information on IABC from the attending physician or resident. Siblings usually were informed by other

NURSING DIAGNOSIS 13: high risk for alteration in immunological defense system

Related to	Expected outcomes	Nursing interventions	Evaluation
Debilitated state secondary to stress of illness and poor nutritional state Loss of normal immunological defense mechanisms Nosocomial infections Indwelling lines Wound infections	Patients will demonstrate absence of any infectious process	Assessment of nutritional status (see Nursing diagnosis 11) Monitor T-cell, B-cell, total WBC, and differential counts Administer antibiotics as ordered for specific infections Daily care of all invasive lines according to unit developed protocol utilizing aseptic technique Inspect all invasive lines for redness, swelling, and drainage Monitor temperature	Patient did not develop infectious process

family members. Adult children of patients (ages 19-46) were usually provided information by the patient's nurse. Respondents confused IABC with angioplasty. All seemed to understand that IABC "helped the heart." All participants requested additional information. Most frequently asked questions were: (1) How long must the IABC be left in place? (2) How will it come out? (3) Does the patient feel it pumping? (4) Can the patient go home with it in? (5) What are the complications? and (6) Can we do anything to help? A consistent comment was "I would like to know more but don't even know what to ask." All family members indicated that they preferred the individual method of instruction, rather than receiving information from a videotape or brochure.

Discussion

Quaal interviewed patients after an IABC experience. She utilized an ethnographic qualitative approach of interactive interviews. Patients also rated themselves on a powerlessness Likert-like scale. Patients rated themselves as having felt "powerless" during the experience that was confirmed by analysis of the interactive interview data. The following three themes emerged: (1) physiological powerlessness; (2) contextual powerlessness; and (3) environmental powerlessness (Fig. 20-10).

Physiological powerlessness emerged by collapsing three selective categories of hurting, internal feeling, and suffering, which conceptualized physical sensations

Text continued on p. 341.

NURSING DIAGNOSIS 14: high risk for alteration in level of consciousness

Related to	Expected outcomes	Nursing interventions	Evaluation
Intensive care unit psychosis Carotid artery obstruction from IAB catheter misplacement or migration Decreased cerebral perfusion secondary to decreased cardiac output Oversedation	Unaltered level of consciousness as evidenced by: Orientation to person, place, and time Normal neurological assessment Appropriate response to verbal and nonverbal stimuli	Protect periods of uninterrupted rest in an attempt to afford much needed sleep Facilitate orientation by placing clock in patient's sight Offer television, music, and talking books if patient is interested When possible, arrange bed with view to outside Verify catheter placement with daily chest x-ray Neurological assessment every shift should include pupil reaction, speech response, hand grasp quality, peripheral motor movement, appropriate response to verbal and nonverbal commands, and demonstration of orientation to person, place, and time	Patient will demonstrate a normal level of consciousness

NURSING DIAGNOSIS 15: high risk for anxiety and knowledge deficit

Related to	Expected outcomes	Nursing interventions	Evaluation
Lack of understanding of intended therapeutic action of IABC Misperception that heart will stop if IABC stops Fear of unknown Fear of dying Unfamiliar environment and treatments	Patient anxiety will be decreased as evidenced by: Patient verbalization Relaxed appearance Longer sleep intervals	Offer brief explanations about IABC on initiation, explain that patient's heart will not stop if counterpulsation stops Offer to expand explanation as patient indicates increasing interest; show patient diagram of IAB placement within the aorta and an actual IAB If IAB insertion is nonemergency, prepare patient ahead of time by allowing IAB and diagram of insertion to be seen Always inform patient if pain and pressure will be felt during insertion Explain to patient that balloon counterpulsating may be felt Ask patient what is contributing to anxious feeling to determine appropriate interventions	Patient will verbally validate that anxiety has been eliminated

NURSING DIAGNOSIS 16: high risk for alteration in family process

Related to	Expected outcomes	Nursing interventions	Evaluation
Lack of understanding about the process Intensive care unit is a foreign and frightening environment Loss of control Feeling of helplessness and hopelessness Fear of loved one dying	Family members will demonstrate: Expression of factors contributing to fears, feelings of helplessness, hopelessness, and loss of control A basic understanding of IABC after good teaching from the nurse	Offer simple but consistent explanations of IABC Show family members an actual IAB and an arterial pressure waveform of IAB diastolic augmentation Show family members the pump and offer reassurance of ongoing pump monitoring that nursing staff is providing Reassure family that if IABC ceases, patient's heart can continue to beat Encourage family members to express their fears and concerns, and to ask questions regarding aspects they do not understand	Family members will demonstrate successful coping mechanisms, an understanding of IABC, and will feel free to express their fears, concerns, and pose questions to the medical and nursing staff

NURSING DIAGNOSIS 17: powerlessness

Related to	Expected outcomes	Nursing interventions	Evaluation
Physiological, contextual, and environmental factors Physiological conceptualization of physical discomforts, such as pain at insertion site and feeling balloon counterpulsating inside their chest Environmental conceptualization of feeling powerless because patient is unable to move freely within their limited physical space, confused about surroundings, overstimulated by equipment and alarms, and sometimes lacks confidence in their doctors and nurses Contextual conceptualization of patient's feeling that ability to exercise authority, direct, and regulate was taken away; lack of understanding about IABC; and feeling overwhelmed by the experience	Patient's feelings of powerlessness will be minimized	Use long-leg knee brace to mobilize IAB insertion leg. Allow patient to "control" tightness of Velcro straps and when brace is used. Explain to patient that when he/she is awake and wants to be responsible for keeping the involved leg straight, he/she need not wear the brace Orient patient to surroundings, sounds of the balloon pump, and other equipment. Make sure immediate items (water, tissue, call light) are within patient's reach); empower patient to summon a nurse immediately; explain concepts of IABC and physiological parameters are continuously monitored at central station even when nurse is not in patient's room; explain that there is an alarm system which also monitors balloon pump function Ask directly if patient has questions and what the nurse could do to make the patient feel more in control	Following the IABC experience, patient will not feel that he/she was totally powerless during the experience

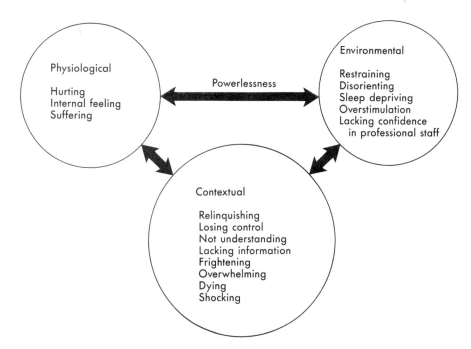

Fig. 20-10. Conceptual model of "powerlessness" from interactive interview analysis of patients who had undergone IABC.

the patient experienced as a result of having an IAB inserted into their femoral artery and counterpulsed. Power reserves were depleted by having to endure unpleasant physical sensations caused by IABC. Pain experienced at the femoral artery insertion site ranged from "knifelike" to a tingling or burning sensation. Some patients also experienced internal sensations such as balloon catheter movement within their groin or actual IAB "expansion."

Environmental powerlessness was abstracted from selective categories of restraining, disorienting, sleep depriving, overstimulating, and lacking confidence in professional staff. This theme represented the patient's feeling unable to move freely within the limited physical environment (bed), confusion about IABC and intensive care environment and procedures, overstimulation by lights and sounds, and how he/she viewed the professional staff.

Contextual powerlessness arose from subcategories of relinquishing, losing control, not understanding, lacking information, frightening, overwhelming, and dying. These categories all related to patients' attitudes, feelings, beliefs, concerns, perceptions, and misperceptions about the IABC experience.

REFERENCES

1. Carpenito LJ: *Nursing diagnosis: application to clinical practice*, ed 5, Philadelphia, 1993, JB Lippincott.

2. Little RC: Regulation of systolic, diastolic, and mean arterial blood pressure. In *Physiology of the heart and circulation*, ed 4, Chicago, 1988, Mosby-Year Book.

3. Hewlett-Packard: *A guide to physiological pressure monitoring*, Waltham, Mass, 1977, Hewlett Packard.

4. Conover M: Diagnostic monitoring leads. In *Understanding electrocardiology*, ed 6, St. Louis, 1992, Mosby-Year Book.

5. Clochesy JM: Continuous ST-segment analysis. In Dracup K, editor: *Advanced technology in critical care nursing*, Rockville Md, 1989, Apsen Publications.

6. Flewelling-Goran S: Vascular complications of the patient undergoing intra-aortic balloon pumping, *Crit Care Nurs Clin North Am* 1:459, 1989.

7. Allen EJ: Thromboangiitis obliterans: methods of diagnosis of chronic occlusive arterial lesions distal to the wrist with illustrated cases, *Am J Med Sci* 177:237, 1929.

8. Yuen JC, Riggs OE: Aortoiliac dissection after percutaneous insertion of an intra-aortic balloon pump, *South Med J* 84:1135, 1991.

9. Swartz MT, Sakamoto T, Hirokuni A et al: Effects of intraaortic balloon position on renal artery blood flow, *Ann Thorac Surg* 53:604, 1992.

10. Quaal SJ: An exploratory descriptive study of physiological variables and the nursing diagnosis powerlessness in a population of intra-aortic balloon pumped patients, Unpublished doctorate dissertation, 1992, University of Utah.

11. Jurmolowski CR, Poitier RL: Small bowel infarction complicating intra-aortic balloon counterpulsation via the ascending aorta, *J Thorac Cardiovasc Surg* 79:735, 1980.

12. Flewelling-Goran S: Family perceptions of the intra-aortic balloon pumping experience, *Crit Care Nurs Clin North Am* 1:475, 1989.

CHAPTER 21

IABC patient case studies

Susan J. Quaal

CASE STUDY 1

A 52-year-old male was admitted with sharp stabbing chest pain. His admission ECG demonstrated the hyperacute phase of inferior infarction. B/P 92/64, HR 112 (sinus tachycardia with occasional unifocal left PVCs), RR 30, heart sounds normal S_1 and S_2; S_3 also present. Pulmonary artery catheter inserted and the following pressures were obtained: P/A 41/26, PACP 28, RA 6, CO 2.8 L/min, pH 7.29, $PaCO_2$ 50 mm Hg, PaO_2 42 mm Hg, SaO_2 76%, SvO_2 52%. BSA is m². Hemoglobin was 15 g. Dopamine was started at 10 µg/kg/min and dobutamine at 5 µg/kg/min. The patient was also treated with tissue-type plasminogen activator thrombolytic therapy.

1. Calculate left ventricular stroke work index (LVSWI) and plot LVSWI and PCWP on the left ventricular function graph on p. 344.
2. Calculate his systemic vascular resistance.
3. Calculate his oxygen delivery (DO_2), oxygen utilization (VO_2), and mixed venous reserve.
4. Discuss the intended therapeutic effect of dopamine and dobutamine.
5. After 30 minutes, the dobutamine was increased to 10 µg/kg/min; no improvement in hemodynamic status was noted. Review this patient's hemodynamic profile and discuss potential therapeutic benefits associated with intraaortic balloon counterpulsation (IABC). Is the fact that the patient has just received thrombolytic therapy a contraindication to IABC?
6. What specific components of nursing history and physical assessment are important before implementing IABC?
7. How are you going to prepare this awake and alert man for IABC?

A 40 cc 9 Fr IAB was inserted by percutaneous technique without difficulty.

8. On p. 345 is a tracing of balloon gas waveform and arterial pressure waveform with an assist ratio of 1:2. Troubleshoot the potential causes of the "squared-off" balloon gas waveform.

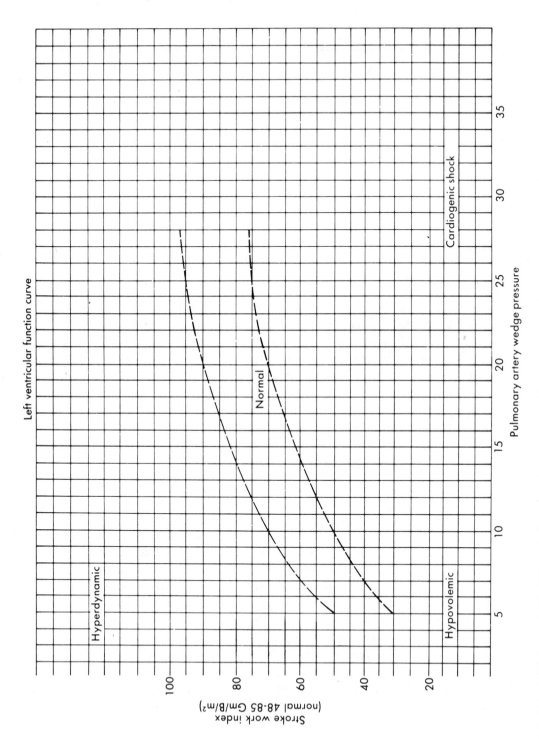

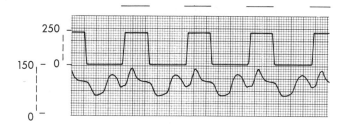

9. Calculate appropriate IAB gas volume for this patient's current hemodynamic status.
10. The balloon gas waveform and arterial pressure waveform were recorded after the nurse assessed the first tracing and intervened. What intervention do
   you think occurred?
11. Two hours after commencing IABC, his parameters are CO 3.0, Sao_2 88%,
   Svo_2 60%, and PACP 16. Recalculate DO_2, VO_2, and mixed venous reserve.

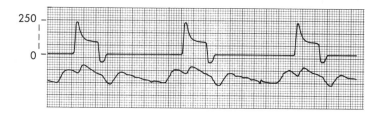

CASE STUDY 2

A 35-year-old female diabetic was admitted with the hyperacute phase of anterior
infarction. Hemodynamic parameters were: B/P 118/92, HR 160 (sinus tachycardia),
a pulmonary artery catheter was inserted with an initial P/A of 38/22, PACP of 20,
RA of 7, CO 3.0, pH 7.48, PCO_2 30, PO_2 68, Sao_2 95%, Svo_2 45%, Hgb 10, and
BSA 1.8 m^2.

1. She is uncomfortable with the head of bed (HOB) flat. Can her P/A and
   PACP be taken with the HOB elevated?
2. Calculate her SWI, SVI, SVR, DO_2, VO_2, and mixed venous reserve.
3. Discuss pros and cons of IABC for this patient.
4. Calculate theoretical ideal balloon volume for this patient if her cardiac index
   was normal (2.5 L/min/m^2) with a heart rate of 70 and what her ideal balloon
   volume should be, given her current hemodynamics.
   A 30 cc 8 Fr IAB was inserted.
5. Label the following components of the patient's arterial pressure waveform at
   1:2 ratio of assist: (A) unassisted aortic end-diastolic pressure; (B) assisted

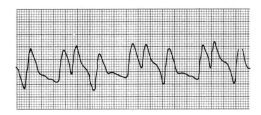

aortic end-diastolic pressure; (C) unassisted systole; (D) assisted systole; (E) peak diastolic augmented pressure. (Scale: each large box = 20 mm Hg.) Assess timing. Are inflation and deflation correct?

6. What are the potential causes of the patient's poor diastolic augmentation.
7. Discuss compartment syndrome and specific signs and symptoms you will monitor in this patient.

CASE STUDY 3

The patient is a 69-year-old male who underwent redo mitral valve replacement with a St. Jude prosthesis and an internal mammary to left anterior descending coronary artery bypass graft. He received a porcine valve 11 years ago that served him well. Approximately 6 months ago he began developing symptoms of heart failure and aortic valve regurgitation. His preoperative ejection fraction was 45%. The surgeon initiated IABC before coming off extracorporeal circulation in anticipation that the patient would require hemodynamic support. The IAB was easily inserted but when attempting to initiate IABC, the console continuously shut down and displayed a "large helium leak" alarm. No blood was seen in the external IAB catheter or connecting tubing.

1. Troubleshoot the probable cause of this "large helium leak" alarm.
2. After corrective action was taken, the following tracing was recorded. Troubleshoot this problem.

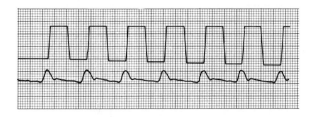

The patient successfully came off extracorporeal circulation and was returned to the SICU. A 40 cc 9.5 Fr IAB had been inserted in the operating room.

3. Note the tracing below. The operator is not adjusting the inflation control. Patient is on a 1:2 ratio of assist. Note the fourth IABC arterial pressure waveform cycle that displays "early inflation." Troubleshoot this tracing.

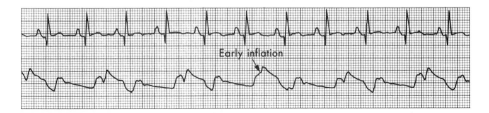

The thoracic surgical resident wrote an order to "titrate dopamine to maintain a mean arterial pressure (MAP) of 90 mm Hg." He is now on an assist ratio of 1:1.

4. What pressure points should be used to compute a MAP?
5. This patient was a redo open heart surgery patient. Therefore he has a good appreciation as to what to expect. However, the first time around, he did not require IABC. What are you going to tell this patient, who is intubated, when he first starts regaining consciousness after anesthesia?

The patient did well overnight. The next morning, his cardiac output is 6.5 L/min and his heart rate is 78. Note the following tracing. Discuss the most likely cause for poor diastolic augmentation.

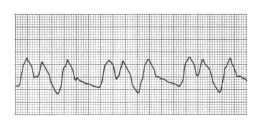

The physician suggests that the patient should be weaned from IABC.

7. Discuss two methods for weaning and pros and cons of each method.

ANSWERS TO CASE STUDIES
Case study 1

1. LVSWI is a measurement of the amount of work the left ventricle performs per beat, when ejecting its stroke volume. It is derived from the calculation of work, which is pressure generated × volume of blood pumped[1]:

$$LVSWI = (MAP - PACP) \times SVI \times 0.0136 \quad \text{Normal value} = 38\text{-}62 \ Gm/B/m^2$$

The patient's MAP is 73.5 − a PACP of 28 × SVI of 12.5 × 0.0135

$$\textbf{SWI} = \textbf{7.7 Gm/B/m}^2$$

Derivation of SVI is

$$\frac{\text{Cardiac index (ml/min)}}{\text{Heart rate}}$$

This patient's SVI is 1400/112 = 12.5. A PACP of 28 and a LVSWI of 7.7 disclosed severely depressed left ventricular function, as was plotted on the left ventricular function curve on the next page.

2. The formula for systemic vascular resistance is

$$\frac{\text{MAP} - \text{RA}}{\text{CO}}$$

where MAP is 73.5, RA is 6, and CO is 2.8, therefore

$$\text{SVR} = \frac{(73.5 - 6)}{2.8} = \textbf{24 Wood units}$$

To convert the above Wood units to dynes/sec/cm^{-5}, multiply × 80.

$$24 \times 80 = \textbf{1920 dynes/sec/cm}^{-5}$$

3. $DO_2 = CO \times Cao_2 \times 10$
   $Cao_2 = 1.34 \times Hgb \times Sao_2$, therefore
   $DO_2 = CO \times (1.34 \times Hgb \times Sao_2) \times 10$ (normal = 900-1000 ml/min)[4]
   $DO_2 = 2.8 \times (1.34 \times 15 \times .76) \times 10 = 428$ ml/min
   $VO_2 = CO \times 1.34 \times Hgb \times (Sao_2 - Svo_2) \times 10$ (normal = 250 ml/min)
   $VO_2 = 2.8 \times 1.34 \times 15 \times (.76 - .52) \times 10$
   $\textbf{VO}_2 = \textbf{135 ml/min}$

Venous reserve = $CO \times (1.34 \times Hgb \times Svo_2) \times 10$ (normal = 750 ml/min)
Venous reserve = $2.8 \times (1.34 \times 15 \times .52) \times 10 = \textbf{293 ml/min}$

Oxygen delivery is obviously inadequate. Look at the oxygen delivery components. Hemogolobin is adequate, but cardiac output and arterial saturation are low. Cardiac output is the product of heart rate × stroke volume, which is governed by preload, afterload, and contractility. Dobutamine is administered to achieve inotropic effects and improve myocardial contraction. IABC should improve oxygen delivery by augmentation of perfusion provided by IAB inflation in diastole and afterload reduction, which occurs with IAB deflation. Fortunately, this patient is quiet and using very little oxygen. With increased oxygen utilization demands, such as may occur if the patient becomes restless, is weighed, given a bedbath or other procedure, experiences pain, and so on, his mixed venous reserve will further decrease.

4. Dopamine at 10 μg/kg/min affords a dopaminergic effect and a mild alpha-adrenergic effect. Alpha receptors are located in the peripheral arterioles. Stimula-

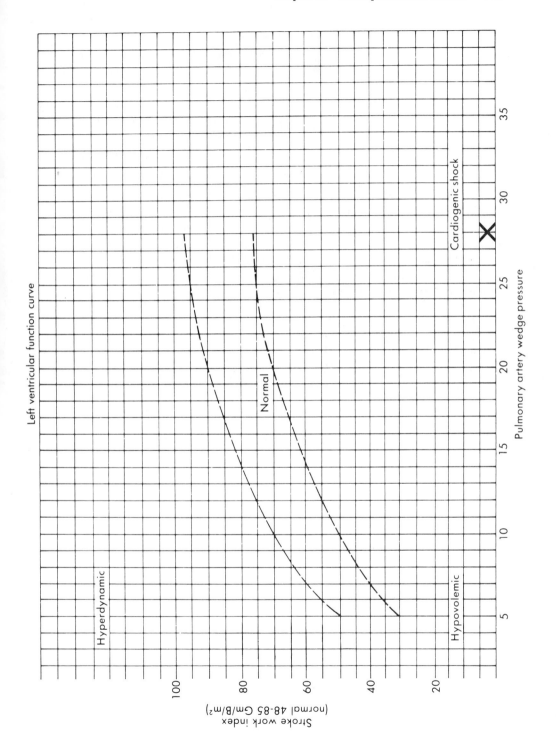

tion causes peripheral vasoconstriction that should result in an elevation of blood pressure. Dobutamine is administered to effect a beta-adrenergic response, resulting in improved myocardial contraction (review dopamine and dobutamine in Chapter 5).

5. Potential hemodynamic benefits from IABC include enhancement of the intrinsic *"Windkessel effect,"* therefore augmenting proximal and distal perfusion and afterload reduction with IAB deflation. Afterload reduction lowers the impedance to systolic ejection, thereby reducing left ventricular work and oxygen demands. Thrombolytic therapy is not a contraindication to IABC. George[2] summarized IABC in conjunction with thrombolytic therapy:

Far from regarding thrombolytic therapy as a contraindication to IABC, patients who fail to respond to thrombolytics may, in fact, be in the greatest need of IABC assistance. As the most seriously ill patients, their most urgent need is the restoration of hemodynamic stability, which can be most expeditiously accomplished by IABC. The balloon pump has proven effective prior to initiation of more definitive measures—such as opening the artery by either pharmacologic or mechanical means (with balloon angioplasty), or even in some cases with emergency bypass surgery.

6. Any past history which suggests peripheral vascular disease is important to solicit. Sample questions should include: How is circulation to your feet? Do you ever have pain in your hips, legs, or feet when exercising or walking? Have you ever had any treatment for poor circulation to your legs and feet?

Physical assessment should include specific emphasis on peripheral vascular assessment. Does the patient exhibit loss of hair on his feet and ankles, thickened toenails, feet cool to touch, a pale, dusky, or rubra red color? Perform a baseline ankle-arm index on both ankles (see box).

7. The patient should be given simple explanations about what he will see, hear, and feel, such as

The doctor is going to insert a small balloon through the artery in your groin and pass this up into the large blood vessel called the aorta that comes off your heart. The balloon will

---

PROCEDURE FOR PERFORMING THE ANKLE-ARM INDEX*

1. Locate posterior tibial or dorsalis pedis pulse with a Doppler.
2. Apply blood pressure cuff around the ankle above the malleolus.
3. Inflate cuff to 20 mm Hg above the current brachial systolic pressure.
4. Note the reappearance of Doppler signal as cuff deflates.
5. Divide the ankle systolic pressure by the brachial systolic pressure to determine ankle-arm ratio.

From Flewelling-Goran S: *Crit Care Nurs Clin North Am* 1:459, 1989.
*Normal value is 0.8 to 1.2.

connect to a machine which pumps about an ounce of helium gas into the balloon when your heart is at rest. This helps the circulation and makes your own heart work downhill instead of uphill. You will feel a couple of needlesticks in your groin as the doctor numbs the area with novacaine, just like the dentist does before having a tooth drilled. You may feel the balloon moving inside your chest. Sometimes if you move around a little, the pump will stop, but your heart will continue to function just fine without the pump. The nurse just will need to push a switch to restart the pump. It is important that you do not bend your groin once the balloon is inserted. You need to tell us how much more information you would like to have. We can show you an old balloon and pictures, if you are interested. We want you to feel free to ask questions at any time.

8. Troubleshooting should begin by assessing for the most common technical problems: (1) a kink in the catheter; (2) sutures placed too tightly around the catheter; (3) balloon has not exited the sheath; (4) balloon is not fully unwrapped; (5) balloon is too large for the patient's aorta; or (6) balloon is positioned too high in the aorta. Note late inflation on the arterial pressure waveform.

9. Review balloon volume sizing in Chapter 14. Formula is

$$\frac{CI \times BSA}{HR} \times 0.5 = \frac{1400 \times 2}{112} \times 0.5 = 12.5$$

However, it is recommended that IAB volume not be decreased more than two thirds of the total capacity. Two thirds of 40 cc is 27 cc. Kantrowitz et al[3] determined that "the balloon is limited by the volume of blood contained within the aorta just prior to inflation. Further increases in pumping volume result only in distention of the aorta and not in the effective pumping of blood."

10. The nurse decreased IAB gas volume by 5 cc. Note the resumption of a more normal balloon gas waveform with presence of peak overshoot and undershoot artifacts. Balloon gas volume needs to be reduced to 27 cc total according to the calculations in question 8. **Check with manufacturer regarding specific recommendations for periodically inflating the balloon to full gas volume capacity as a prophylaxis to prevent clot formation in balloon folds.** Note arterial pressure waveform. Diastolic augmentation is less after balloon gas volume was decreased.

11. DO_2 2 hours after commencing IABC:
$DO_2 = 3 \times 1.34 \times 15 \times .88 \times 10 =$ **530 ml/min**
$VO_2 = 3 \times 1.34 \times 15 \times (.88 - .60) \times 10 =$ **169 ml/min**
MRV $= 3 \times 1.34 \times 15 \times .60 \times 10 =$ **361 ml/min**

It appears that IABC has improved oxygen delivery by approximately 100 ml/min.

Case study 2

1. Several studies[5-7] have now demonstrated that P/A and PACP can be taken with the patient's HOB elevated 60 degrees without a clinically significant change in

pressures, provided that the system is rezeroed after each position change. However, all studies had isolated outlyers, therefore the recommendation is to perform repeated measures with each patient as his own control, that is, record the P/A and PACP with the patient in a supine position and then remeasure these pressures with the patient's HOB elevated to the level of comfort.

    2. SVI (normal is 41-51 ml/beat/m^2) is

$$\frac{\text{Cardiac Index}}{\text{HR}}$$

Her cardiac output is 3.0 L/min. Her BSA is 1.8 m^2. Her cardiac index is

$$\frac{\text{CO}}{\text{BSA}} \text{ which is } \frac{3}{1.8} = \textbf{1.67 ml/beat/m}^2$$

$$\text{Her SVI is } \frac{1670}{116} = \textbf{14 ml/beat/m}^2$$

$$\text{SWI} = (\text{MAP} - \text{PACP}) \times \text{SVI} \times 0.0136$$

$$\text{SWI} = (100 - 7) \times 14 \times 0.0136 = \textbf{17 Gm/B/m}^2$$

    Use the left ventricular function curve graph in the first study from Case Study 1 and plot her SWI of 17 and PACP of 20. Note her poor left ventricular function.

$$\text{SVR} = \frac{(\text{MAP} - \text{RA})}{\text{CO}} = \frac{(100 - 7)}{3} = \textbf{31 Wood units}$$

$$31 \times 80 = \textbf{2480 dynes/sec/cm}^{-5}$$

    This patient is maintaining a blood pressure but at the expense of a high systemic vascular resistance. Remember mean arterial pressure is the product of cardiac output and systemic vascular resistance

$$(\text{MAP} = \text{CO} \times \text{SVR})$$

    Now let's look at the impact on her oxygen delivery.

$DO_2 = \text{CO} \times 1.34 \times \text{Hgb} \times Sao2 \times 10$ (normal $= 900 - 1100$ ml/min)

$DO_2 = 3 \times (1.34 \times 10 \times .95) \times 10 = \textbf{382 ml/min}$

$VO_2 = \text{CO} \times 1.34 \times \text{Hgb} \times (Sao_2 - Svo2) \times 10$

$VO_2 = 3 \times 1.34 \times 10 \times (.95 - .45) \times 10$

$VO_2 = \textbf{201 ml/min}$

Venous reserve $= \text{CO} \times 1.34 \times \text{Hgb} \times Svo_2 \times 10$

Venous reserve $= 3 \times 1.34 \times 10 .45 \times 10$

Venous reserve $= \textbf{168 ml/min}$

    Factors influencing oxygen delivery are cardiac output (heart rate $\times$ stroke volume), hemoglobin, and arterial oxygen saturation. This patient has a low cardiac output. Her SVI is only 14 ml/min. Note her low Hgb of 10 (etiology unknown at time of admission; she was not actively bleeding). Her heart is beating 160 times per minute to try to compensate. Her SVR is 31 Wood Units in an effort to maintain a blood pressure. Therefore interventions must be undertaken to improve her oxygen delivery. Improving myocardial contractility will improve stroke volume. The low Hgb of 10 is also limiting her oxygen delivery. Decreasing systemic vascular resistance will lower the impedance to systolic ejection, improve stroke volume, and lower myocardial oxygen needs. IABC will potentially achieve these desired therapeutic outcomes.

3. IABC will potentially lower afterload and improve perfusion, thereby increasing oxygen delivery. However, this is a female diabetic patient who has a high risk of peripheral vascular complications. The IAB catheter occupies a greater internal diameter in women than in men, thus increasing the chance of thrombus formation. Women have a 1.66 to 1.8 times greater risk of developing limb ischemia and vascular complications.[8] Peripheral vascular complications have been observed to be as high as 34% in diabetics who undergo IABC[9] (see Chapter 10). These risks must be explained to the patient and her family. Sheathless insertion technique should be considered for this patient to reduce the area of femoral/iliac artery occlusion and thus decrease the potential for peripheral flow obstruction.

4. With a normal CI of 2.5 L/min/m^2 and heart rate of 70, ideal balloon volume would be:

$$\frac{CI \times BSA}{HR} \times 0.5 = \frac{2500 \times 1.8}{70} \times 0.5 = \textbf{32 cc}$$

With her given hemodynamics:

$$\frac{1670 \times 1.8}{160} \times 0.5 = \textbf{10 cc}$$

A 30 cc IAB should be inserted in this patient. Currently her calculated theoretical volume capacity is 10 cc, but it is recommended that IAB volume not be decreased more than ⅔ of maximum capacity (20 cc). IAB volume will increase as her heart rate decreases and SVI increases. Because of her small BSA and current low CI and high heart rate, a larger IAB volume would place her at a higher risk for balloon tear, thrombocytopenia, and obstruction to peripheral vascular flow (see Chapter 10).

5. The Figure on p. 354 shows the correct labeling for the patient's arterial pressure waveform at 1:2 ratio of assist. Timing assessment: Inflation: Good, there is a "V-shape" to the dicrotic notch. Deflation: Assisted systole (D) is lower than Unassisted systole (C) and BAEDP (B) is lower than UAEDP (A). Timing is satisfactory. Her poor diastolic augmentation is most likely due to <30 cc helium gas volume inflating the balloon and low SVI (14 ml/B/m^2).

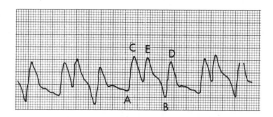

6. Recall that the thighs, buttocks, and lower legs are made up of bone, muscle, nerves, and blood vessels (compartments) surrounded by a fibrous membrane (fascia). When pressure increases within this closed nondistensible fascial space, capillary blood flow is reduced, which compromises the enclosed tissues. Symptoms of compartment syndrome include (1) deep throbbing feeling of pressure; (2) calf pain with foot dorsal flexion; (3) loss of lower leg sensations or function; or (4) pallor when feet are raised 45 degrees. Direct compartment pressure measurement can also be made (normal is 0 to 12 mm Hg). A compartment pressure >30 mm Hg is highly diagnostic for compartment syndrome.[10] **Before elevating the patient's feet 45 degrees, check with manufacturer recommendations if the IAB catheter contains a metal component.**

Case study 3

1. Check all IAB connections between catheter, tubing, and balloon connector. With this patient, a loose connection was found between tubing and balloon connector. Corrective action consisted of tightening this connecting point and reinforcing with a suture. After corrective action was taken, the following tracing occurred.

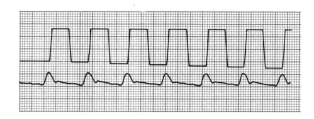

This tracing illustrates a "squared off" helium gas waveform (*top*) and arterial pressure waveform with no sign of IABC. The "squared off" gas waveform occurred because the suture which was placed to reinforce the site of tubing and balloon connector was placed too tightly. Helium was totally obstructed from flowing into the balloon catheter. The suture was removed and a normal helium gas and IABC arterial pressure waveform resumed.

3. Ratio of assist is 1:2 on the strip on p. 355. Note the fourth IABC cycle which demonstrates very early inflation.

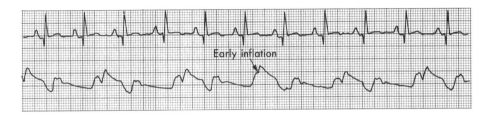

The operator did not adjust the inflation control. Most likely cause is the "biphasic" ECG. Note that the Q wave of the QRS complex preceding the early inflated arterial pressure wave beat is just a little more negative, or deeper than the others. The balloon pump probably recognized this negative signal as an R wave and used this as a reference point for adjusting inflation. Corrective action is to change ECG leads so that the patient has a monophasic ECG (complex is all positive or all negative).

4. Review Chapter 20. It is important to realize that biomedical instrumentation uses different techniques for achieving a MAP. The "arithmetic method" for an IABC patient consists of summing the peak diastolic augmented pressure (reference point *1* in Fig. 20-4), plus two BAEDP (labeled as reference point *2*), divided by 3. The "integration method" sums the area under the curves (Fig. 20-5). The nurse must understand methods used by balloon pump and bedside monitor instrumentation. If the methods used to calculate MAP from both bedside monitor and IABP are identical, then either source can be used. However, if methods are different between instrumentation, then it is important that one source be used for consistency. Also, nurses and physicians must discuss calculation of MAP in the IABC patient and how this differs from the non-IABC patient. This becomes very important when the MAP is used to guide titration of vasoactive or vasopressive drugs.

5. It is important to know the content of this patient's preoperative teaching and whether he was prepared for the possibility of IABC. If he was prepared, then the nurse can reinforce that IABC is in process, as well as reinforcing what the patient was taught regarding what he would hear, see, and feel. If the patient was not preoperatively prepared for the possibility of IABC, it is important that the nurse simply explain that the patient has one thing that is different from his first open heart surgery, such as

There is a catheter going into your (state *right* or *left*) groin artery, which attaches to a balloon in your aorta, the big blood vessel coming off your heart. This balloon is inflating and deflating to make your heart work easier. You may feel this balloon moving inside your chest and you may hear a machine making noise every time the balloon inflates. This movement may stop from time to time, but it doesn't mean your heart has stopped. When the breathing tube is removed and you can talk, you can ask me questions and I can explain this further.

6. The patient's cardiac output is 6500 ml/min and heart rate is 78. Therefore

$$SV = \frac{CO}{HR} = \textbf{83 cc.}$$

He has a 40 cc balloon in place. His stroke volume is double the IAB displacement capacity. Remember diastolic augmentation is maximized when stroke volume is closet to IAB volume (see Chapter 7). With a stroke volume of 83 cc, one would not expect high diastolic augmentation.

7. Review Chapter 24 on IAB weaning. Two methods of weaning are currently recommended: (1) frequency ratio and (2) volume weaning. Frequency weaning is accomplished by reducing the ratio of assisted to total number of heart beats from 1:1 to 1:3, 1:4, and so on. Kantrowitz et al. suggest that decreasing the ratio of assist exposes the patient's heart muscle to large changes in the amount of external work the myocardium is expected to perform. These authors propose that reduced assist ratios may not represent an intermediate level of balloon assistance but may be hemodynamically equivalent to turning the balloon off.

Volume weaning consists of gradually reducing the volume of gas used to inflate the balloon. Volume is reduced in 20% increments but never below 20% of the maximum capacity. Kantrowitz et al. (Chapter 24) suggest that this method entails no sudden significant increments on the heart's load.

Nurses and physicians must discuss these two methods of weaning and develop a procedure. It is important that heparin be discontinued a minimum of 4 hours before IAB removal. Also the nurse is cautioned to consult with the IAB manufacturer before initiating volume weaning. Since movement of IAB surface lessens with volume weaning, the potential for clot formation theoretically increases.

REFERENCES

1. Daily EK: Hemodynamic monitoring. In Guzzetta CG, Dossey BD, editors: *Cardiovascular nursing: holistic practice*, ed 2, St. Louis, 1992, Mosby-Year Book.
2. George BS: Thrombolysis and intra-aortic balloon pumping following acute myocardial infarction—experience in four TAMI studies, *Cardiac Assists* 4:1, 1988.
3. Kantrowitz A: *Cardiac assistance by the intra-aortic balloon pump*, Boston, 1969, Second Medical Physics Conference.
4. White K: *The delicate balance*, Mountain View, Calif, 1991, Abbott Critical Care Workshop Syllabus.
5. Laulive J: Pulmonary artery pressure and position changes in the critically ill adult, *Dimen Crit Care Nurs* 1:28, 1982.
6. Chulay M, Miller T: The effect of backrest position on pulmonary artery and pulmonary capillary wedge pressures in patients after cardiac surgery, *Heart Lung* 13:138, 1984.
7. Lambert CW, Cason CL: Backrest elevation and pulmonary artery pressures: A research analysis, *Dimen Crit Care Nurs* 9:327, 1990.
8. Funk M, Gleason J, Foell D: Lower limb eschemia related to use of the intra-aortic balloon pump, *Heart Lung* 18(6):542, 1989.
9. Wasfie T, Freed PS, Rubenfire M et al: Risks associated with intra-aortic balloon pumping in patients with and without diabetes mellitus, *Am J Cardiol* 61(8):558, 1988.
10. Conry K, Bies C: Compartment syndrome: a complication of IABP, *Dimens Crit Care Nurs* 4(5):274, 1985.

CHAPTER 22

IABC in the community hospital setting

As derived by Susan J. Quaal

Intraaortic balloon counterpulsation: an important component of community hospital care

FROM GOTTLIEB S: *CARDIAC ASSISTS* 5(3):1, 1990.

Major pharmacological and technological developments in recent years have revolutionized the treatment of patients with serious cardiovascular conditions, significantly improving survival rates and dramatically changing the face of cardiac care. As a result, it has become increasingly imperative that the community hospital with cardiac catheterization facilities have access to and employ intraaortic balloon counterpulsation (IABC) to provide mechanical cardiac assist in helping to stabilize the patient with compromised hemodynamics.

A growing number of community hospitals have begun to play an increasingly active role in the care of patients with both acute and chronic cardiac conditions. For example, the widespread availability of thrombolytic therapy for the treatment of acute myocardial infarction (MI) has made it imperative that patients with MI be assessed and treated as soon as possible in the community hospital setting.

Accordingly, thrombolytic agents are commonly administered in the emergency room or cardiac intensive care unit of many community hospitals. In those cases where thrombolytic agents alone prove insufficient and patients therefore remain hemodynamically unstable, IABC may well be a necessary adjunct to treatment before transporting the patient to a tertiary care center for more definitive management.

Another important developing trend for many community hospitals is the availability of cardiac catheterization for assessing cardiac function in patients with acute MI or more chronic conditions, such as atherosclerotic coronary artery disease and valvular lesions. Critically ill patients undergoing cardiac catheterization may also be candidates for IABC in the community hospital setting.

TECHNOLOGICAL DEVELOPMENTS

In view of the growing need for IABC within the community hospital, it is indeed timely that major technological advances have significantly facilitated the use of this treatment modality and simplified training requirements. Currently available percutaneous catheters, as small as 8.5 Fr in diameter, can be inserted by an experienced operator in little more than 3 minutes. Patient groups that were formerly at higher risk from vascular complications during IABC, particularly women and those with peripheral vascular disease, can now benefit from this treatment with fewer complications.

Miniaturization and simplification of the balloon pump console have also played a major role in the increased use of IABC in the community hospital setting. Technological advances in IABC instrumentation have directly led to the development of newer systems ideal for community hospital use. With a high degree of portability, modern IABC units are significantly lighter, smaller, and easier to maneuver than were earlier models. Portable IABC systems weigh approximately 100 pounds, are transported on their own small wheeled cart, or can be placed on a stretcher. They may be placed directly aboard an ambulance or helicopter.

CLINICAL APPLICATIONS OF IABC IN THE COMMUNITY HOSPITAL

Indications for the use of IABC in the community hospital include many cardiac conditions requiring temporary hemodynamic support. IABC should, however, be initiated with the ultimate objective of transporting the patient to a tertiary care center, because this treatment modality generally represents a commitment to more definitive interventions (e.g., angioplasty or coronary artery bypass surgery).

The conditions most likely to require IABC in the community hospital setting include severe refractory myocardial ischemia not responding to medical treatment, aortic stenosis or mitral regurgitation with hemodynamic compromise, and MI accompanied by cardiogenic shock and/or mechanical defects such as ventricular septal defect or severe mitral regurgitation.

The incidence of refractory myocardial ischemia is particularly high among those patients with left main coronary artery disease or high-grade triple-vessel disease. Because these patients generally exhibit hemodynamic impairment during ischemia, IABC can be of value in supporting diastolic coronary flow.

Patients with valvular lesions, particularly severe mitral valve regurgitation, may also require hemodynamic support for which the balloon pump is ideally suited. Indeed, IABC can provide potentially life-saving assistance in treating the hemodynamically impaired patient with mitral regurgitation and cardiogenic shock.

Finally, IABC is finding increased application in the community hospital in the management of acute MI complicated by cardiogenic shock, acute ventricular septal defect, or septal rupture. Aggressive treatment with the combination of thrombolytic therapy and IABC support until patency is achieved in the infarcted artery, or until angioplasty can be performed, may significantly improve survival rates in such patients.

This technique has proven especially useful in the unstable patient with a large anterior infarct who has sought treatment early in the course of the infarct. In such cases, IABC may be initiated along with thrombolytic therapy to provide hemodynamic support for the patient while thrombolysis proceeds. The balloon is then generally removed 1 or 2 days after patency has been restored in the infarcted artery and the patient has become hemodynamically stable.

The role of the community hospital in treatment of acute MI has expanded greatly with the initiation of therapy occurring before transporting the patient to a tertiary care center. This major evolutionary development is in recognition of the fact that the benefit of thrombolytic therapy is directly related to its immediate application during a precisely defined "window of opportunity." Thus thrombolysis generally takes place at the community hospital where the patient is first admitted; moreover, the patient with an uncomplicated MI who responds well to thrombolytic therapy may be treated entirely within the community hospital.

In more complicated cases, the community hospital must be prepared to provide hemodynamic support until the patient's condition is sufficiently stabilized to permit transport to a tertiary care center. It is in these cases that IABC plays a particularly important role.

GROUND TRANSPORT WITH IABC

Initiation of IABC in our institution, Francis Scott Key Medical Center, generally precedes transport to the Johns Hopkins Hospital for further treatment. The transport team—consisting of a nurse, or catheterization technician, experienced in IABC operation and a physician—employs a private ambulance equipped with defibrillation equipment, emergency cardiac medications, and intravenous administration supplies. An ambulance with a high roof is advantageous if resuscitation procedures must be performed en route.

During transport, the patient's IABC unit is operated on battery power. Because nearly 1 hour in total is required to accomplish the interhospital transfer, the battery is fully charged after each run.

An important factor to consider is the possibility of interference within a moving vehicle that may disrupt the electronically generated ECG signal. For this reason, we have occasionally found it useful to change the triggering of the pump from the ECG tracing (in this mode it is keyed to the R wave) to the upstroke of the arterial pressure waveform.

At the receiving hospital, the medical team transports the patient from the emergency room receiving area to the coronary care unit, where the change from battery operation of the IABC unit to electric power is made. Once this has been accomplished, the patient is then transferred to the receiving hospital's IABC system; of course, complete compatibility of the two systems—including length of the connecting tubing—must be ensured before transport. This includes determining in advance the need for any connectors or adapters that may be required.

This institution also acts as a provider of IABC transport services for other hospitals in emergency situations. This involves having our team travel to a community hospital without IABC capability to initiate IABC and then transporting the patient to the Johns Hopkins Hospital for coronary bypass surgery or angioplasty.

CASE HISTORIES

The following case histories represent the ways in which IABC is typically employed at Francis Scott Key Medical Center.

Case 1

A 70-year-old woman scheduled for elective bypass surgery and mitral valve replacement at another hospital was found to have triple-vessel disease and moderately severe mitral valve regurgitation on cardiac catheterization. Several days before the scheduled surgery, she developed pulmonary edema, hypotension, and cardiogenic shock with ischemia. The patient, who was already known to physicians at this hospital, was considered a good surgical candidate.

The Francis Scott Key medical IABC transport team was dispatched to the referring hospital, where IABC was initiated. This immediately restored the patient's blood pressure and stabilized her for transport to the Johns Hopkins Hospital. She underwent successful triple bypass surgery and mitral valve replacement, was discharged home, and has done extremely well.

Case 2

A 48-year-old patient with acute anterior MI infarction and cardiogenic shock sought treatment within 1 hour of the onset of chest pain. The intraaortic balloon was inserted at the same time that intravenous thrombolytic therapy was initiated. IABC restored adequate perfusion and, within 30 minutes of administration of the thrombolytic agent, the chest pain abated and ST segments normalized on the ECG. The patient was transferred to the Johns Hopkins Hospital where catheterization the following day revealed a patent 95% proximal LAD stenosis with adequate perfusion. The patient underwent successful angioplasty to this lesion, and the left ventricular ejection fraction was found to be 50% with mild anterior hypokinesis. This case illustrates the successful combination of thrombolytic therapy and IABC in which the balloon pump supported the patient during the early hours after MI but before reperfusion of the infarction artery.

OUTLOOK

Major technological advances in recent years have greatly simplified the operation of IABC devices and expanded their utility in the setting of the community hospital. These timely developments have coincided with the increasing role of the community hospital in the treatment of acute MI and the diagnosis of serious cardiovascular conditions. Thus there is a growing need for IABC capabilities in the community hospital environment. With the immediate availability of IABC and the early initiation of thrombolytic therapy, community hospitals can now provide effective—and often life-saving—therapy for acute MI before transporting the patient to a tertiary care center for further treatment. IABC also permits safer transport for the critically ill cardiac patient, resulting in the patient's arriving in better condition for the necessary surgery. As IABC becomes increasingly available in the community hospital, the outlook for survival for the critically ill cardiac patient will continue to improve.

IABC in the community hospital: the nursing perspective

FROM HUCKSTEP-REED C: *CARDIAC ASSISTS* 5(3):4, 1990.

In 1976, St. Francis Medical Center in Cape Girardeau, Missouri, became one of the first community hospitals to make use of the IABP device. The critical care nursing staff has long played a pivotal role in the successful implementation of balloon counterpulsation.

IABP: THE ST. FRANCIS EXPERIENCE

St. Francis Medical Center is a 272-bed community hospital with a cardiac catheterization laboratory and two intensive care units—a 10-bed cardiac intensive care unit and a 10-bed medical/surgical intensive care unit. St. Francis provides cardiac care for patients with acute MI or cardiogenic shock who are not candidates for surgery. Thus patients requiring open-heart surgery are transported to a tertiary care center.

Over the course of a year, this hospital's IABP system is employed approximately 25 times, with approximately one half of treated patients remaining at St. Francis for the entire period of hospitalization. The balance of this hospital's IABP patients are transported to institutions that offer open-heart surgery with the Datascope System 90T IABP system.

Critical care nurses are directly involved in all aspects of IABC from insertion of the balloon until the patient is either weaned from IABC or is transferred to another hospital for subsequent surgery.

IABC TRAINING FOR NURSES

When St. Francis first initiated IABC therapy, the critical care nurses that would compose the first IABC team were sent to another hospital where this instrumentation was already in place to observe the balloon pump in use. Because this technology was so new, the nurses observed in the clinical setting and also received first-hand instruction in a canine laboratory.

Today, those selected for the IABC team are experienced critical care nurses. Of the 58 critical care nurses currently on staff, 21 are qualified on the IABC team.

Initial training is undertaken at an in-service training program developed by Datascope, the instrument's manufacturer. The training includes set-up of the pump, interpretation of waveforms, and trouble-shooting. After attending the class, nurses complete a practical IABC orientation period during which they obtain hands-on experience using the balloon pump under the guidance of an experienced preceptor. In addition to the initial training session, Datascope conducts a periodic IABP review, at which time any changes in operation or equipment are discussed.

Because St. Francis—similar to most hospitals—uses the IABP system on a sporadic basis, the hospital uses the Datascope System Trainer, a patient simulator that simulates conditions that may arise in actual clinical use. Each IABC team member is required to use the System Trainer once each month. During the session, the nurse completes a checklist of items that includes set-up procedures, trouble-shooting techniques, and clinical problems. This listing is then retained in the personnel file to demonstrate the nurse's continued proficiency with IABC procedures.

IABC NURSING PROCEDURES

St. Francis maintains IABC team coverage 24 hours a day, with one IABC team member on duty at all times, and an IABC team captain on call. Thus at least one nurse is always available to initiate IABC when needed, while a second nurse is on hand to assist with the insertion or begin IABC treatment for a second patient if this should prove necessary.

At St. Francis, IABC is approved for use in patients with cardiogenic shock, intractable angina, or cardiac arrhythmias resistant to medical therapy; in unstable patients undergoing cardiac catheterization; or in patients with severe cardiac disease who require major, noncardiac surgery.

The IABC team nurses' responsibilities begin at the time of balloon catheter insertion with assisting the cardiologist and catheterization laboratory technician in preparing for the insertion procedure. While the balloon is being inserted, the IABC team nurse is responsible for initial set-up of the IABP unit. The ECG is generally the most reliable IABP trigger. Although arterial pressure triggering may also be used, this is not generally advisable in patients with cardiac arrhythmias.

During insertion of the balloon catheter, the nurse monitors bilateral pedal pulses to check for diminished circulation to the lower extremities and prepares the pressure monitoring system that connects to the central aortic monitoring lumen on the dual lumen IAB catheter and displays arterial waveform.

After insertion, the nurse connects the catheter to the IABP unit and sets the pump in accordance with the physicians' standing orders. The timing of balloon inflation and deflation may be controlled automatically or manually, and adjustments can be made in either mode. Major alterations to the IABP settings are made on the physicians' orders, but the nurse may adjust the timing if necessary to improve effectiveness of IABC.

A most important aspect of the IABC nursing responsibility is close and careful monitoring of the patient's condition, in addition to monitoring IABP performance. Because patients on IABC are often seriously ill, deterioration in vital signs or hemodynamic condition may indicate a worsening of the underlying condition or suboptimal operation of the IABP unit. By remaining alert to both possibilities, an experienced nurse is able to advise the physician of important changes and implement necessary actions.

When the IABP system is functioning properly and the patient's condition has stabilized, the cardiac index increases, blood pressure stabilizes, pulmonary wedge pressure decreases, urine output rises, and the level of consciousness improves.

IABC PATIENTS AT ST. FRANCIS

Among the 25 or so patients who require IABC each year, the typical patient is maintained on the pump for fewer than 4 days, although occasionally IABC will be required for up to 10 days. IABC patients in the community hospital setting generally fall into one of three categories:
1. A patient admitted to the cardiac catheterization laboratory for evaluation. On examination, a high-grade critical lesion is discovered in a coronary artery, and the balloon catheter is inserted to prevent occlusion in that artery before coronary artery bypass surgery.

   The patient is then immediately prepared for transport to a hospital at which open-heart surgery is performed. This type of patient is generally in good hemodynamic condition and can be easily maintained in IABC.
2. A patient admitted to the cardiac catherization laboratory for evaluation. During evaluation, the patient's condition rapidly deteriorates. The patient may have severe chest pain that does not respond to vasodilating agents or may develop a severe hypotensive episode.

   The balloon catheter is inserted, and the patient's hemodynamic condition is stabilized so that the catheterization may be completed. This patient generally requires short-term IABC support if the hemodynamic deterioration was the result of the catheterization procedure itself.
3. An acute MI patient in cardiogenic shock. The cardiac index is low, as is blood pressure and urinary output. Pulmonary congestion may be present. Mental status may be deteriorating. This patient is generally placed in IABC at 1:1 frequency. Vasoactive agents are typically administered along with IABC to stabilize blood pressure and normalize cardiac function.

After 4 to 6 hours of IABC therapy, the clinical picture may change quite dramatically. Urinary output rises, pulmonary congestion is relieved, and blood pressure increases. Dosages of vasoactive medications are gradually lowered, and the frequency of IABC assistance is reduced to 1:2 and later to 1:3.

After all vasoactive agents have been discontinued, pulmonary congestion has eased, urinary output is elevated, blood pressure is stable, and the patient is conscious and has no chest pain, the intraaortic balloon may be removed.

IABC TRANSPORT

Those patients on IABC in the community hospital who require open-heart surgery must be transported to a facility with this capability. The patient and the pump are taken by ambulance to the receiving hospital, accompanied by the IABC team nurse and a second critical care nurse. The IABP unit operates either on battery or electrical power, with battery power generally reserved for the loading and unloading phases. During transport, the unit is connected to the ambulance's portable generator. Once the patient has reached the receiving institution, transfer to the IABP unit in that hospital is made, and the transport unit is returned to the originating hospital.

CONCLUSION

Similar to the rapidly growing number of other community hospitals with IABC capability, St. Francis has found this long-term program to be of great value. IABC allows the community hospital to provide potentially life-saving treatment for patients with lethal cardiac problems requiring immediate support.

The simplification of both the IABP units and the balloon catheters has considerably expanded the availability of this technology in the community hospital. For the community hospital first initiating an IABC program, it may be helpful for staff members to be trained initially at another institution that already has an IABC program in place. Once the IABC program has been fully established, frequent refresher courses using the Datascope System Trainer and regular, in-service training will ensure that the team's IABC skills are maintained at a high level, even when the system is not in daily use.

Financial considerations in the use of IABC in the community hospital

FROM KELLY JP: *CARDIAC ASSISTS* 5(3):7, 1990.

In this era of the availability of fewer resources to meet ever-expanding healthcare needs, financial considerations in the purchase and use of costly—but important—new technology must be carefully evaluated within the local hospital setting.

Community Hospital in Lancaster, Pennsylvania, is a 218-bed facility that has just recently acquired an IABP system. Although the decision to initiate IABP service was based on careful clinical considerations, before the program could be instituted an in-depth financial analysis was performed to determine the cost effectiveness of this new capability. The financial considerations involved in the initiation of the IABP service at Community Hospital are reviewed here.

CLINICAL NEED

Before assessing the financial viability of any new service at Community Hospital, the clinical need for that capability must first be clearly established. In this case, both the cardiology and critical care staff strongly supported the clinical need for IABP, estimating that Community Hospital would use IABP at least 12 times annually. In addition, the absence of IABP capability would lead to the transfer of those patients requiring this service to several other area hospitals that had already acquired it. For these reasons, it was concluded that the clinical need for IABP in this hospital justified a financial evaluation of this capability.

FINANCIAL CONSIDERATIONS

In considering the institution of any new program, Community Hospital must assess whether the new service will be capable of generating sufficient revenue to be self-supporting, or preferably, income-producing. The following factors must be considered in such an analysis:

1. Capital costs associated with the new program
2. Operating costs (e.g., nursing time, training, supplies)
3. The charge structure for the service

Of course, a primary cost of instituting IABP involves the purchase of the balloon pump system itself. It was decided to purchase a Datascope Transport Intraaortic Balloon Pump System (Model 90T). For the purposes of analysis, it was assumed that the system would be amortized over a 5-year period, although it had been determined that other institutions had used an IABP unit for longer periods without the need for replacement.

Operating costs

Several operating costs were added into the assessment. Prominent among these was the additional nursing time required during the care of a patient on IABC. In Community Hospital's critical care units, a 1:2 nurse-to-patient ratio is normally maintained. By contrast, during the early hours after the initiation of IABC, one specially trained nurse would be required to monitor the patient and the unit at all times.

Training time was also included in the cost calculations. In addition to initial training, which was provided as an in-service program by the IABP manufacturer, the hospital purchased the Datascope System Trainer Patient Simulator for use as a refresher training course. Finally, the cost of supplies such as balloon catheters had to be calculated and taken into consideration in the process of financial analysis.

Charge structure

The charge structure for IABP service must take into account the patient mix. At Community Hospital, our patients fall into four distinct groups for billing purposes:
- Medicare patients (40% to 45%)
- Medical assistance patients (12% to 15%)
- Blue Cross patients (8% to 10%)
- Commercial insurance carriers or self-pay patients (30% to 40%)

Thus the calculations of charge structure had to take into account the amount of reimbursement that would be received from Medicare, medical assistance, and Blue Cross. Although patients on IABC are in a diagnosis-related group (DRG) with a higher reimbursement rate than those with similar diagnoses who are not receiving IABC, the approved Medicare reimbursement rate would not cover the entire charge for the service, even when capital cost reimbursement was included. Thus the patient mix was crucial, with the 100% reimbursement that would be received from patients with commercial insurance essential for the program to pay for itself. A summary of the IABC cost analysis made by Community Hospital is listed in the box.

As noted in this analysis, when all factors were considered, it was concluded that an IABP employed with a frequency of 12 times or more each year would not only pay for itself, but also would generate additional revenue for the hospital.

CONCLUSION

Although IABC is not expected to generate considerable revenue for Community Hospital, in our view the provision of this potentially life-saving clinical service is important to the future of this institution and its ability to function as a major provider of healthcare services within the community.

As other local hospitals do, we currently contract with two other facilities to provide those services not available at Community Hospital. Thus, before initiation of the IABC program at Community Hospital, a patient needing this form of treatment was transferred to another hospital, requiring us to reimburse them if that patient was then returned to Community Hospital for follow-up.

IABP COST ANALYSIS

Calculation of Impact

Anticipated Volume   12/Year

Anticipated Payor Mix   Medicare   6

                        Medicaid   1

                        Blue Cross   1

                        Commercial

                        Ins/Self-Pay 4

                        TOTAL   12

Expenses

A. Nursing Care
    (Assuming 1:1 nurse-to-patient ratio
    for first 16 hours after insertion)
    Estimated Average Hourly
    Rate × Benefits (approx. $13.00
    20%   × 120%
    Total Additional Salary Cost per
    hour × 12 Procedures $15.60
                                 × 12
                                 $187.20
    × Number of Hours   × 16
    Additional Annual Nursing
    Costs   ($ 2,995)

B. Equipment
    Approximate Cost of Equip-
    ment $40,000
    ÷ Estimated Life   ÷ 5
    Annual Depreciation   ($ 8,000)

C. Service Contract
    After year 1, warranty expires
    (Annual Estimate)   ($ 3,000)

D. Supplies
    Estimated Annual Supplies
    (including balloons and other
    supplies)   ($20,000)

E. Financing Cost   ($ 2,000)
    TOTAL ADDITIONAL
    EXPENSES/ANNUAL   ($35,995)

Reimbursement

    Increase in Medicare
    Reimbursement $7,000
    M/C Procedures   × 6
                                 $42,000
    Increase in Medicaid Reimbursement
    (Minimal)   -0-
    Increase in Blue Cross
    Reimbursement
    (under cost reimbursement) $2,800
    Increase in Commercial/Self-Pay
    Reimbursement (assuming 3-day
    stay, assuming 4 procedures) $5,000
    TOTAL INCREASE IN
    REIMBURSEMENT $49,800

Total Cost Impact of IABP Program

    TOTAL INCREASE IN
    REIMBURSEMENT $49,800
    TOTAL ADDITIONAL
    EXPENSES   ($35,995)
    POSITIVE IMPACT $13,805

This positive impact does not include
the additional reimbursement that
will be received from Medicare
under the capital cost provision of
the regulations.

Thus, given that we will meet the
projected volume, this acquisition is
appropriate for our hospital.

Even if additional revenue generated was expected to be relatively small, it was judged to be advantageous to be able to provide this important technological treatment modality to those patients in urgent need of cardiac support. It is through the provision of services such as IABC that a community hospital can maintain its occupancy rate while providing optimal clinical care to all of its patients.

CHAPTER 23

A total quality management IABC program

Susan G. Osguthorpe

Intraaortic balloon counterpulsation (IABC) has been used to provide temporary cardiac support for patients with left ventricular failure and to improve myocardial oxygen supply relative to demand since it was introduced in the early 1960s.[1] Clinical application of the IABC gained acceptance in the late 1960s and early 1970s,[2-4] and became widely used to manage left ventricular failure after cardiac surgery, unstable angina, postinfarction angina, and complications of acute myocardial infarction such as cardiogenic shock, papillary muscle dysfunction, ventricular septal defects, and refractory ventricular dysrhythmias.[5] In the 1980s, expanding indications for IABC included preoperative and operative support for high-risk surgical patients, procedural support during cardiac catheterization, intracoronary thrombolysis, percutaneous transluminal coronary angioplasty (PTCA), and providing a bridge to cardiac transplantation.[6]

Today, IABC has become a valuable therapeutic tool and the medical standard of care for management of the failing myocardium in rural, community, and referral hospital settings. Each setting provides unique challenges for successful implementation of an IABC program. IABC requires adequate administrative support, program structure, and resources regardless of the healthcare delivery setting to ensure appropriate medical and nursing program direction, competent IABC team personnel, sufficient number of IABC consoles, essential biomedical maintenance and support, and appropriate management of the IABC patient. **Total quality management** of an IABC program involves monitoring and evaluation of medical and nursing management of the IABC patient. Efforts to maintain appropriate education, credentialing, and privileging direct quality improvement activities by all providers.

Management of IABC patients requires collaborative multidisciplinary assessment and intervention to restore physiological stability, prevent complications, and achieve and maintain optimal responses.[7] Multidisciplinary problem solving and ethical decision making are essential considerations to ensure the preservation of patient rights, including the right to refuse treatment or the right to die.[7] As the one constant in a critical care environment, the critical care nurse is responsible for coordination of multidisciplinary delivery of care for IABC patients with life-threatening problems.[7]

This chapter describes the scope of IABC programs in rural, community, and referral hospital settings; identifies appropriate IABC guidelines for program direction and personnel; delineates basic and advanced nursing education programs; discusses medical and nursing IABC patient management issues; and, finally, explores the nurse manager role as a facilitator for a total quality management approach to IABC.

SCOPE OF AN IABC PROGRAM

The scope of a hospital IABC program is determined by available human, material, and financial resources. The mission statement of each healthcare organization defines the level of services provided by the hospital, which in turn drives allocation of scarce resources to meet the mission statement. Other essential considerations for an IABC program are listed in the box on p. 370.

Rural hospital setting

In a rural hospital setting, the focus of medical management and an IABC program should be directed toward early patient stabilization and timely transport of patients requiring IABC support to a referral facility for additional medical and surgical interventions such as cardiac catheterization, PTCA, and cardiac surgery for revascularization, repair of structural defects, or transplantation. In the rural setting, the balloon pump can be inserted in the emergency department (ED), intensive care unit (ICU), or monitored bed unit (MBU) by a qualified medical practitioner and managed by qualified nursing staff until ground or air transport to a referral facility can be accomplished. Intraaortic balloon (IAB) insertion, management, and patient transport may be provided by personnel from the referral hospital or transport team, depending on available resources and referral agreements.

Barriers to successful IABC management in the rural setting include lack of (1) a defined IABC program, (2) qualified medical practitioners to insert IAB catheters and manage IABC, (3) qualified nursing staff to assist with insertion and provide IABC patient management, (4) IABC console(s) and other critical care monitoring equipment, (5) defined referral system agreements, and (6) timely transport, as well as an infrequent need for IABC support.

Community hospital setting

In the community hospital setting, the IABC program is directed toward medical and surgical support for most IABC patients and transport of a select number of IABC patients requiring additional treatment modalities. Many community hospital

---

PLANNING CONSIDERATIONS AFFECTING IABC PROGRAM

Administrative considerations

Hospital mission statement
Level of service
Scope of IABC program
Intrahospital referral agreements
Intrahospital IABC resource sharing agreements
Critical care unit(s)
Personnel budget
   On-call system 24 hours per day
   Education and training time
Equipment budget
   IABC consoles
   IABC training simulator
   IAB catheters and supplies
   IABC service contract

Human resource considerations

IABC medical director
Physicians qualified to insert and remove the IAB catheter and manage IABC patients
IABC nursing director
Nurses qualified to assist with insertion and removal of the IAB catheter, manage the
IABC patient, and the IABC console
   IABC team first responders
   IABC direct bedside providers
Biomedical personnel qualified to troubleshoot and repair IABC consoles

Educational resource considerations

IABC basic provider course
IABC advanced or refresher course
Videotapes
   IAB insertion/removal
   IABC management
   IABC troubleshooting

---

settings have cardiac catheterization laboratories (CCLs) for diagnostic and treatment procedures, as well as cardiac surgery programs. In this setting, IAB catheters can be inserted and managed in the ED, ICU, CCL, or operating room (OR) by cardiologists or cardiac surgeons with assistance of such other healthcare providers as nurses, perfusionists, or technologists. Most community hospitals will have IABC console(s) available, well equipped ICUs, and healthcare providers experienced in IAB catheter insertion and patient management. Transport is usually only necessary for IABC patients requiring cardiac surgery or transplantation.

A significant barrier to successful IABC management is the lack of a clearly defined IABC program, including policies and procedures relevant to IABC. Other barriers include a lack of (1) sufficient number of consoles, (2) defined referral system agreements, and (3) timely transport.

Referral hospital setting

In the referral hospital setting, both medical management and the IABC program need to consider comprehensive medical and surgical support for IABC patients, as well as outreach IABC support programs for community and rural hospitals. The IABC can be inserted in the ED, ICU, CCL, or OR, but the referral hospital also provides transport and management of patients requiring IABC support from rural or community hospitals. Barriers to successful IABC management are the same as those in the community hospital. In addition, a comprehensive healthcare system approach to IABC may be adversely affected by a lack of consistent standards of care and medical management among critical care units.

Once the scope of the IABC program is determined, total quality management is implemented through a collaborative healthcare team approach. The physician and critical care nurse each have an area of expertise and skills that complement each other; together they become a synergistic unit more powerful than either working alone.[8] No one healthcare professional can observe and focus on everything involved in the complex care of the IABC patient, nor can he or she master all knowledge available from each discipline.[8] Therefore a team approach is necessary for total quality management of the IABC program and patient.

INTRAAORTIC BALLOON TEAM

The medical director, nursing director, and IABC first responders comprise the IABC team. They work closely with the direct IABC bedside providers who are responsible for both patient care and IABC management.

An effective IABC program defines roles and responsibilities for both medical and nursing directors of the IABC team, as well as roles, responsibilities, and certification or privileging for physicians, nurses, and other healthcare team members providing IABC management and patient care for IABC patients.

Medical direction

The IABC team medical director provides expert medical direction and support to the IABC program. The medical director should be experienced in the use of IABC in various settings and should also be clinically available for consultation and problem solving related to IABC.

Principal accountabilities of the medical director include the following:

• Developing and implementing IABC policies and procedures

IABC PHYSICIAN CERTIFICATION GUIDELINES

POLICY STATEMENT: Only IABC certified physicians may insert and remove IAB catheters and manage IABC patients. Attending physicians and other staff must complete preceptored clinical training until certification is recommended by the IABC Medical Director and granted by the Hospital Credentialing Committee.

Certification requirements

1. Review of IABC videotapes
   IABC preparation and IAB insertion
   IABC console operation
   IAB removal
2. Timing review session with IABC team medical or nursing director
3. Clinical experience
   One observation of IAB insertion
   Two successful precepted IAB insertions
   One observation of IAB removal
   Two successful precepted IAB removals

From *Certification guidelines for intraaortic balloon placement*, Salt Lake City Veterans' Administration Medical Center, Salt Lake City, Utah, 1992.

- Providing medical education and consultation
- Serving as a physician preceptor for IABC insertion, management, and removal
- Recommending IABC credentialing and privileging of qualified applicants to the hospital credentialing committee
- Monitoring and evaluating physician standards of practice relative to IABC
- Providing education, consultation, and support to the IABC team
- Facilitating problem solving and conflict resolution related to IABC resource management
- Facilitating multidisciplinary care and ethical decision making for the IABC patient

An example of a physician certification program is found in the box above.

Nursing direction

The IABC team nursing director provides expert nursing direction and support to the IABC program. The nursing director should be experienced in use of IABC in various settings such as the ED, ICU, CCL, and OR and must be clinically available for consultation and problem solving related to IABC.

Principal accountabilities of the nursing director include the following:

- Developing and implementing IABC policies and procedures
- Providing nursing education, consultation, and support for IABC bedside providers and IABC team members

- Serving as a nursing preceptor during IAB catheter insertion and removal and for nursing management of the IABC patient
- Providing IABC certification for IABC bedside providers and IABC team members
- Monitoring and evaluating nursing standards of practice and standards of patient care for the IABC patient
- Facilitating problem solving and conflict resolution related to IABC resource management
- Facilitating multidisciplinary care and ethical decision making for the IABC patient
- Providing leadership and quarterly IABC team meetings
- Ensuring maintenance of IABC consoles in conjunction with the vendor maintenance program or hospital bioengineering department
- Maintaining adequate IABC supplies in conjunction with the hospital supply services department

Although any experienced IABC nurse may provide nursing direction for the IABC team, the ICU nurse manager or clinical specialist are often selected because of their availability for clinical consultation and troubleshooting.

IABC team first responders

Frequently, the IABC is inserted on an urgent or emergent basis, which requires rapid mobilization of the IABC console, equipment, supplies, and IABC team first responders with expertise in management of both the IABC and unstable critical care patients. IABC team first responders must be readily available 24 hours a day by pager to ensure rapid IABC implementation, consultation, and troubleshooting. It is essential for IABC first responders to be available within 20 minutes if they are not within the hospital setting 24 hours a day.

Although many hospitals use perfusionists and/or technicians as well as nurses to provide initial management of the IABC console during insertion, critical care nurses are uniquely suited to this role. During cardiac surgery, the primary responsibility of the perfusionist is to manage the cardiopulmonary bypass machine. During cardiac catheterization, the primary responsibility of the cardiac catheterization technologist is to manage the patient and CCL equipment. Therefore use of a dedicated IABC team critical care nurse who is responsible for immediate IAB catheter insertion and/or IABC troubleshooting enhances effectiveness of the team approach in this emergent situation. Advantages of using critical care nurses in the role of IABC team first responder include the following:

- Primary responsibility for IABC rather than dual responsibility during insertion and management of the IABC patient
- Expertise in management of unstable cardiac patients
- Hemodynamic and pharmacological knowledge and skills
- Clinical experience in management of the IABC console

IABC TEAM FIRST RESPONDER CERTIFICATION GUIDELINES

POLICY STATEMENT: Certified IABC team first responders will be available 24 hours a day to assist with insertion, removal, consultation, and troubleshooting for IABC.

Certification requirements

1. Completion of IABC basic provider course
2. Completion of IABC advanced provider course
3. Timing review session with IABC nursing director
4. IABC direct bedside provider clinical experience
      120 hours of independent IABC
5. IABC team first responder preceptored clinical experience until proficient in the following:
      Set-up of the IABC console in the OR, ICU, ED, or CCL
      Management and troubleshooting of IABC console
      Insertion/removal of IAB catheter
6. Availability for independent on-call assignment

Ongoing certification requirements

1. Attendance at three out of four IABC quarterly meetings
2. Review of IABC cases at quarterly meetings
3. Preceptoring IABC first responder candidates
4. Preceptoring IABC direct bedside providers
5. Teaching in IABC basic and advanced provider courses
6. Developing, implementing, evaluating, and revising IABC policies, procedures, teaching materials, and standards of care
7. Availability for on-call assignment

From *Intraaortic balloon pump team*, Salt Lake City Veterans' Administration Medical Center, Salt Lake City, Utah, 1992.

The IABC team first responders include the nursing director and, ideally, sufficient critical care nurses to provide in-hospital availability 24 hours a day. In smaller community and rural hospital settings, this may not be possible. These settings should ensure the availability of an IABC team first responder within 20 minutes by beeper system. An example of certification for IABC team first responders is found in the box above.

IABC direct bedside providers

In some hospitals, the responsibility for providing direct bedside care for IABC patients includes managing all aspects of the IABC, whereas at other hospitals, this responsibility is shared among nursing staff who manage patient care and perfusionists and/or technicians who manage the IABC console.[9] Unless these individuals are available within the ICU for immediate consultation and intervention on a 24 hour a

---

IABC DIRECT BEDSIDE PROVIDER CERTIFICATION GUIDELINES

POLICY STATEMENTS: Certified IABC direct bedside providers will be available 24 hours a day to provide management of the IABC patient and IABC console.

Certification requirements

1. Completion of the IABC basic provider course
   2-day hospital-based course or 1-day manufacturer's course with second-day hospital-based course
2. Completion of the IABC written examination at 84% or better
3. Completion of clinical skills lab and timing review session with IABC nursing director
4. Completion of clinical skills lab test
5. IABC team first responder preceptored experience until proficient in the following:
   Management of the IABC patient
   Troubleshooting and management of IABC console

From *Intraaortic balloon pump team*, Salt Lake City Veterans' Administration Medical Center, Salt Lake City, Utah, 1992.

day basis, management of both the patient and the IABC console is more effectively provided by the critical care nurse.

The critical care nurse is able to continuously and accurately assess the effect of IABC on the patient's hemodynamic status and integrate IABC into the overall medical management of the patient, including manipulation of vasoactive drugs, oxygen transport, ventilatory support, fluid balance, and other therapies.[9]

If a hospital does elect to use perfusionists and/or technicians for IABC console management, the critical care nurse must still be very familiar with counterpulsation principles, IABC console troubleshooting, effects of IABC on the hemodynamic status of the patient, and integration of IABC into the overall patient management.[9]

An example of IABC direct provider certification is found in the box above.

IABC PROGRAM POLICIES AND PROCEDURES

After defining the scope of the IABC program and roles and responsibilities of IABC team members, establishing IABC policies and procedures is essential to provide formal organizational structure and accountability for the IABC program. A useful working definition of **"policy"** is an administrative statement defining who may do what and under what circumstances, which thereby provides direction for decision making in a given situation.[10] Important policies related to IABC are listed in the box on p. 376.

A **"procedure"** may be defined as a delineated series of steps to be followed in a

---

IABC POLICIES

1. IABC program
2. IABC team roles and responsibilities
3. IABC physician certification guidelines
4. IABC team first responder certification guidelines
5. IABC direct bedside provider certification guidelines
6. IABC standby scheduling or activation
7. IABC intraagency borrowing and lending
8. IABC referral and transport

---

regular and orderly fashion to achieve a desired result.[11] Important procedures related to IABC are listed in the box below.

It is helpful to centralize all policies and procedures related to IABC with the manufacturer's reference manuals in an IABC binder for quick reference. These policies and procedures are also included in unit policy and procedure reference manuals.

IABC EQUIPMENT AND SUPPORT SERVICES

Each hospital must ensure an adequate number of available IABC consoles to manage both elective standby requests for cardiac surgery or invasive cardiac procedures and unscheduled emergent or urgent insertion situations. Backup IABC consoles must be immediately available in case of IABC console failure as well. Many hospitals share IABC console resources when the number of IABC consoles required exceeds the number of IABC consoles owned by the hospital. Intrahospital resource sharing agreements should be clearly defined in writing to facilitate this process in

---

IABC PROCEDURES

1. IABC set-up and IAB catheter insertion
2. IABC nursing management and documentation
3. IABC weaning
4. IAB catheter removal
5. Emergency management of IAB—manual inflation
6. Documentation of clinical training time
7. Documentation of IAB catheter insertion and removal

---

an emergency. In large metropolitan areas, IABC consoles can often be leased from medical equipment companies or obtained from IABC manufacturers providing local support to high-volume areas. Proficiency in managing various IABC models that might be obtained from other hospitals or companies is important for both IABC team members and direct bedside providers.

In the event of IABC console failure, hospital biomedical personnel or manufacturer biomedical personnel provide diagnostic troubleshooting and repair support. Telephone numbers for 24-hour availability should be attached to each IABC console for quick reference. Another important support function is the regular maintenance program of IABC consoles by hospital biomedical personnel or through a contract with the manufacturer to minimize IABC console failure. Lastly, IABC team members and direct bedside providers need to be aware of any IABC console software updates installed by the hospital biomedical department or manufacturer to minimize confusion during IABC.

IABC insertion and removal in the ED, ICU, MBU, or CCL is easier if the essential equipment and supplies are readily available in a centrally located mobile IABC cart that can be taken to the patient care area. It is often kept in the ICU to ensure regular monitoring of the IABC cart for completeness and outdated supplies. The availability of some IABC equipment and supplies in the OR and CCL minimizes insertion delays in these high-risk areas. Another time-saving strategy is to regularly apply the IABC electrocardiogram (ECG) leads on all cardiac patients with the potential for IABC support to markedly reduce disruption of the sterile field during insertion and startup of IABC.

Although checking the IABC cart is usually the responsibility of the IABC team, an IABC cart equipment checklist and signature form should be kept with the IABC cart for reference by the ICU nurses responsible for ensuring that emergency equipment and essential supplies are available. The equipment checklist should include the ordering number from the hospital supply department or vendor for quick reference by the IABC team members or individuals responsible for maintaining stock levels. An example of an IABC cart equipment checklist is provided in Table 23-1.

IABC EDUCATION AND CLINICAL TRAINING

In modifying Alspach's definition of critical care nursing education, IABC education can be defined as "education directed at facilitating application of the knowledge, skills, and attitudes required for competent critical care nursing practice related to care and management of the IABC patient and management of the IABC console."[12]

The educational process for a successful IABC program includes completing a needs assessment of both the IABC team members and direct bedside providers, planning a didactic educational curriculum and clinical skills experience, imple-

Table 23-1. IABC cart equipment checklist

Location on cart	Equipment
Top of cart	IAB 40 cc (2)
	IAB 30 cc (1)
Drawer #1	Three-way stopcock (2)
	36-inch arterial pressure tubing (2)
	6-inch arterial pressure tubing (2)
	Accudynamic (2)
	Sheath dilators
	6-inch (4)
	11-inch (2)
	Guidewires
	Arterial line pressure monitoring kit
Drawer #2	Razors (2)
	ECG electrodes (3)
	Scrub brush (1—Hibiclens; 1—Betadine)
	Povidone-iodine solution (3 bottles)
	Towels (sterile) (4 pkg.)
	Restraints (2)
	4×4 (single pkg. ×6)
Drawer #3	10 cc syringes (3)
	3 cc syringes (4)
	Needles (assorted sizes)
	Alcohol sponges
	Lidocaine (1 bottle)
	Scalpels
	Size 10 (2)
	Size 11 (2)
	Size 15 (2)
	Scalpel blades
	Size 10 (2)
	Size 11 (2)
	Size 15 (2)
	Suture removal kit
	Suture set (2)
	Elastoplast tape
	4×4 10 pkg. tub (2)
	Suture (2-4 pkg. of each):
	0 silk with cutting needle
	3-0 silk with cutting needle
	2-0 silk with cutting needle
	2-0 silk with straight needle
Drawer #4	Sterile medium sheets (2)
	Sterile gowns (3)
	Sterile gloves (assorted sizes)
	TPN/CVP tray (2)
Bottom of cart	Caps
	Masks
	Sterile full-length sheets (2)

PRINCIPLES OF THE TEACHING-LEARNING PROCESS

- Learning is a self-activity of the learner.
- Learning is intentional.
- Learning is an active and interactive process.
- Learning is a unitary process of the learner, the teacher, and the learning situation.
- Learning is influenced by learner motivation.
- Learning is influenced by learner readiness.
- Learning is social.
- Learning is influenced by the learning environment.
- Learning is optimized by organization and clear communication.
- Learning is facilitated by positive and immediate feedback.
- Learning retention is facilitated by early review and summary combined with performance feedback.
- Learning is creative.
- Learning is inferred from behavioral changes demonstrated as a result of a learning experience rather than directly observed.
- Learning is influenced by the nature and variability of the learning experience.

From Alspach JG: *The educational process in critical care nursing*, St Louis, 1986, Mosby–Year Book.

menting the educational program, and evaluating the educational program in terms of meeting behavioral objectives.[13] The IABC educational process considers general education and experience of the nurses, teaching and learning principles, and principles of adult education.[14] Principles of the teaching-learning process are presented in the box above, and important distinguishing characteristics of critical care nurses and adult learners are presented in the box on p. 380.

IABC educational needs assessment

A comprehensive IABC program provides basic IABC education to meet the needs of the direct bedside providers, advanced IABC education to meet the needs of experienced bedside providers, refresher education to meet the needs of first responders and direct bedside providers when IABC is infrequently used, and significant case review education to meet continuing educational needs of the IABC team members.

Manufacturers of IABC consoles provide basic IABC education to critical care nursing staff with the purchase of an IABC console or basic and advanced IABC educational offerings on request. Frequently, regular city-wide educational offerings at both basic and advanced levels are available and may be held in conjunction with user networking group meetings. Basic and advanced level IABC educational offerings are also provided at regional and national nursing symposia.

DISTINGUISHING CHARACTERISTICS OF CRITICAL CARE NURSES AND ADULT LEARNERS

Adult learners

- Adults learners are highly differentiated, or heterogenous, as a group.
- Adult learners expect to command the respect that is due them as mature individuals.
- Adult learners have multiple personal and professional responsibilities.
- Adults value and bring a large reservoir of personal and professional experience to the learning situation.
- Adults often learn more slowly than do younger individuals.
- Adults are often less flexible than are younger individuals.
- Adults frequently have negative past learning experiences that produce feelings of inadequacy, fear of failure, and diminished self-confidence.
- Adults are usually voluntary learners who engage in learning activities for a variety of reasons.
- Adults typically engage in learning activities with the intention of immediately applying what they learn to solve problems in their present roles and responsibilities.
- Adults' readiness for learning depends on demands already present or impending in their current situation.
- Adults work best with teachers who interact with them as knowledgeable colleagues, who facilitate learning, and who are subject to the same human shortcomings as they are.
- Adults expect to be given the opportunity to evaluate learning experiences in terms of their own goals and expected outcomes of the experience.

Critical care nurses

- Critical care nurses place a high value on their advanced knowledge and clinical skills; their self-concepts and the respect of peers and colleagues are closely tied to their knowledge and skills.
- Critical care nurses value current and accurate information.
- Critical care nurses may be more amenable to making changes or modifications in their practice based on participation and perceived need.
- Critical care nurses are often direct, vocally assertive individuals who dispense respect for peers somewhat judiciously after it is earned.

From Alspach JG: *The educational process in critical care nursing*, St Louis, 1982, Mosby–Year Book.

If the IABC program is dependent on these educational resources, it is important to have an additional day of hospital-specific education planned to manage organizational-specific content such as policies and procedures or roles and responsibilities, to provide adequate individualized console instruction, and to provide adequate educational review of timing, triggering, and troubleshooting. The IABC team members will require orientation or review of organizational settings such as the OR, ED, and CCL vs. the ICU for insertion and startup. A variety of teaching methods can be employed in all IABC educational courses to increase effectiveness of the educational process, including lectures, small-group task solving, handling of equipment, and discussion of case studies. Content outlines for basic and advanced and/or refresher IABC educational courses are presented in the boxes on pp. 382-383 and 384.

Clinical training and testing

Clinical training is initiated in the skills lab of the basic IABC educational course, but many nurses need additional content review time, which can be facilitated with use of videotapes, IABC clinical simulators, and abbreviated operator's manuals. Videotapes are available from manufacturers on concepts of IAB pumping, insertion and removal procedures, and nursing care of the IABC patient. Journal articles and reference texts can be used to provide additional reading materials. Experience in using the abbreviated operator's manual, in conjunction with the IABC simulator and IABC console to initiate IAB pumping, develops confidence in the basic direct bedside provider when he or she is managing this stressful treatment modality.

When a direct bedside provider has completed the didactic educational content, written assessment testing, clinical skills testing, and preceptored clinical experience provide ideal clinical application and skills evaluation. An example of a clinical skills lab test is presented in the box on p. 385. An individual record of IABC clinical training and pumping, as shown in Fig. 23-1, provides documentation of didactic and clinical experience for hospital documentation requirements and regulatory agencies. IABC team members and direct bedside providers should be responsible for maintaining their own records.

Evaluating the IABC educational program

A written test can be used to assess the didactic information presented during the IABC educational program. Test questions should reflect behavioral objectives of the program didactic component.[9] A competency based clinical skills lab test or check-off tool is useful to evaluate clinical application of IABC theory and psychomotor skills required for IABC console management.[9] Course evaluation tools, written tests, and a clinical skills lab test are useful in considering effectiveness of the IABC education program and total quality management of the IABC education program. Finally, preceptored observation and assessment of each provider's ability to assume primary management of IABC patients and the IABC console should be considered along with the self-assessment of individual readiness by the critical care nurse.

IABC MANAGEMENT ISSUES

IABC management includes medical management issues, nursing management issues, and collaborative management issues. *Text continued on p. 387.*

IABC BASIC PROVIDER COURSE CONTENT OUTLINE

COURSE OBJECTIVES: At the end of the course, the student will be able to do the following:
- State the determinants of cardiac output
- Recognize symptoms of a cardiac failure
- State the indications and contraindications of IABC
- Recognize early and late IAB inflation and deflation using the arterial pressure and helium gas waveforms
- Demonstrate proper startup and alarm troubleshooting of the IABC console
- Develop a nursing plan of care for the IABC patient based on unit standards of care and patient assessment

Day one
I. *General concepts of IABC*
  A. History of IABC
  B. Cardiac anatomy and physiology
    1. Anatomy
    2. Review of the determinants of cardiac output
    3. Compensatory mechanisms
    4. Oxygen supply and demand
    5. Myocardial failure
  C. Principles of counterpulsation
    1. Balloon structure and position
    2. IAB inflation
    3. IAB deflation
    4. Physiological pressure waveform changes
    5. Clinical assessment
II. *IABC*
  A. Indications
  B. Contraindications
  C. Expanding applications
  D. Complications
  E. Escalation of treatment
  F. Ethical problem solving
III. *Medical management*
  A. Insertion
  B. Treatment goals and plan of care
  C. Weaning
  D. Removal
IV. *Nursing management*
  A. Insertion
  B. Nursing management of IABC patient
    1. Nursing diagnoses
    2. Standard of patient care—Patient outcomes
    3. Standard of nursing practice—Nursing interventions
    4. Nursing documentation

IABC BASIC PROVIDER COURSE CONTENT OUTLINE—cont'd

C. Nursing management of IABC console
  1. Set-up and insertion
  2. Timing
  3. Triggering
  4. IABC console operation and troubleshooting
  5. Patient transport
  6. Removal
  7. Emergency management of IAB catheter and console

V. *Clinical skills demonstration and individual experience*
  A. IAB catheters, insertion kits
  B. IAB cart
  C. IABC console(s)
  1. Console features
  2. Console operation
  3. Console alarms
  D. Breakout sessions for individual clinical skills lab

Day two

I. *IABC team*
  A. IABC medical director—Role and responsibilities
  B. IABC nursing director—Role and responsibilities
  C. IABC team first responders—Role and responsibilities
  D. IABC direct bedside providers—Role and responsibilities
  E. Collaborative team approach—Case conferences
  F. Review of policies and procedures

II. *Practice timing exercises*
  A. ECG, arterial, and helium waveform analysis
  B. Early and late inflation
  C. Early and late deflation
  D. Other timing considerations
  E. Documentation of timing

III. *Nursing care of IABC patient*
  A. Case studies
  B. Ethical problem solving and patient/family advocacy

IV. *Documentation and certification*
  A. Documentation of course work
  B. Documentation of clinical experience
  C. Documentation of insertion, management, and removal
  D. Certification as direct bedside provider
  E. Certification as IABC first responder

V. *ICU, CCU, OR, CCL, ED tours*

From Salt Lake City Veteran's Administration Medical Center: *IABC basic provider course*, Salt Lake City, Utah, 1992.

IABC ADVANCED OR REFRESHER COURSE CONTENT OUTLINE

COURSE OBJECTIVES: At the end of the course, the student will be able to do the following:
- Determine appropriate treatment modalities for IABC patients based on hemodynamic subsets
- Recognize early and late inflation and deflation based on the arterial pressure waveform and helium gas waveform
- Troubleshoot causes of abnormal helium gas waveforms
- Perform return demonstration on proper IABC console operation
- Resolve IABC problems with console equipment, alarms, and unit-specific monitoring conditions

I. Introduction and review
    A. Oxygen transport
    B. Medical treatment plan
    C. Hemodynamic subsets
    D. Case studies

II. IABC
    A. Principles of counterpulsation
    B. Review of ECG, arterial, and hemodynamic waveforms
    C. Optimal timing vs. safe timing
    D. Triggering modalities

III. IABC in alternative settings
    A. ICU
    B. CCL
    C. OR
    D. ED
    E. Transport

IV. Clinical skills lab experience
    A. IAB catheters
    B. IAB cart
    C. IABC console(s)
        1. Console features
        2. Console operation
        3. Console alarms
    D. Breakout sessions for individual clinical skills lab

V. Ethical dilemmas and collaborative problem solving
    A. Issues
    B. Collaborative practice
    C. Patient/family rights
    D. Critical care nurse as an advocate
    E. Case studies

From Salt Lake City Veteran's Administration Medical Center: *IABC advanced or refresher provider course content outline*, Salt Lake City, Utah, 1992.

IABC CLINICAL SKILLS LAB TEST

(Initials of IABC team director, in the spaces provided, indicate successful completion of the task)

_____ Demonstrates proper set-up and power-up

_____ Demonstrates changing helium tanks

_____ Demonstrates proper recorder function and paper change

_____ Demonstrates proper use of cables for:

      simulating ECG, arterial, and pulmonary artery
          monitoring on IABC simulator

      initiating indirect patient ECG, arterial, and
          pulmonary artery monitoring used in ICU

_____ Demonstrates proper use of OPERATION MENU to:

      select pumping ratio

      select appropriate trigger mode (pattern, peak, atrial
          fibrillation, ventricular pacing, atrial pacing,
          arterial pressure, or internal) based on various
          IABC and patient conditions

      initiate ESIS function

      increase and decrease IAB inflation volume

_____ Demonstrates proper use of CALIBRATION MENU to:

      calibrate hemodynamic monitoring lines

      select appropriate hemodynamic monitoring displays

_____ Demonstrates proper use of ALARM MENU to:

      turn alarms on and off

      review alarm conditions

      select alarm auditory levels

_____ Demonstrates proper use of RECORDER MENU to:

      change recorder speed

      select waveforms for channel 1 and channel 2 recording

      change time

      use update function

_____ Demonstrates battery operation and termination:

      appropriate battery use

      battery alarm conditions

_____ Empties water drain

_____ Demonstrates circuit breaker reset on patient headwall

_____ States proper method to activate IABC first responder

_____ Demonstrates manual IAB inflation technique

From Salt Lake City Veteran's Administration Medical Center: _IABC clinical skills lab test_, Salt Lake City, Utah, 1992.

Name _____ Unit _____

IABC Basic Provider Course Day I _____ Day II _____

    Basic Provider Course Written Examination Score _____

    Clinical Skills Experience and Lab Testing Score _____

IABC Preceptored Clinical Experience:

Date/Shift	Unit	IABC Patient	Preceptor	Other

IABC Competency Certification by IABC Nursing Director _____

IABC Review and Refresher Experience:

IABC Advanced or Refresher Course   Date _____

    Clinical Skills Experience and Lab Score   _____

IABC Videotape Review:

    IABC Preparation and IAB Insertion   _____

    IABC Console Operation   _____

    IABC Nursing Management   _____

    IAB Removal   _____

IABC Simulator Practice   Cumulative Hours _____

IABC Clinical Experience:

Date/Shift	Unit	IABC Patient	Preceptor/Comments

First Responder Certification by IABC Nursing Director   _____

Fig. 23-1. IABC clinical training record. (From *Record of clinical training for IABC*, Veterans' Administration Medical Center, Salt Lake City, Utah, 1992.)

Medical management

Medical management issues are usually related to patient selection, medical treatment, and complications of IABC therapy. Patient selection considerations include routine medical and surgical indications, contraindications, and expanding applications for IABC. Patient selection criteria are influenced by the national standards of medical practice, individual physician experience, and hospital policies. Patient selection criteria is discussed in Chapter 8.

Comprehensive medical treatment and support therapies for the IABC patient focus on maintaining adequate oxygenation, perfusion, acid-base balance, fluid balance, and support to all body systems while minimizing complications related to IABC therapy or the underlying cause of cardiac failure. Monitoring, evaluation, and successful resolution of medical management issues is the responsibility of the IABC team medical director.

Nursing management

Nursing management issues are usually related to staffing considerations, nursing education, IABC nursing experience, nursing management of the IABC patient, and nursing documentation. Staffing of IABC patients is usually 1:1, unless the patient is extremely unstable and requires two nurses to safely provide care or the patient is extremely stable and may be paired with a patient requiring minimal observation and nursing interventions. Staffing considerations when making assignments for care of the IABC patient are listed in the box below.

STAFFING CONSIDERATIONS WHEN MAKING IABC PATIENT ASSIGNMENT

IABC patients will be assigned to nursing staff based on the following considerations:
- The complexity of the patient's condition and required nursing care
- The dynamics of the patient's status, including the frequency with which the need for specific nursing care activities changes
- The complexity of the assessment required by the patient, including the knowledge and skills required of the nurse to effectively complete the required assessment
- The type of technology employed in providing medical and nursing care, with consideration given to the knowledge and skill required to effectively use the technology
- The degree of supervision required by the nurse based on previously assessed level of competence and current competence in relation to the nursing care needs of the patient
- The availability of supervision appropriate to the assessed and current competence of the nurse being assigned responsibility for providing the care to the IABC patient
- Relevant infection control and safety issues

From The standards for nursing care and scoring guidelines. In *Accreditation manual for hospitals*, Oakbrook Terrace, Ill, 1992, Joint Commission on Accreditation of Healthcare Organizations.

IABC education programs described in the boxes on pp. 382-383 and 384 are designed to ensure clinical competency of the critical care nurse in IABC patient and console management in addition to quality patient and family care. Inadequate educational support will severely limit effectiveness of any IABC program, and therefore administrative financial support for nursing education must be considered in program planning.

IABC preceptored clinical experience is often jeopardized by scarce nursing resources, but the IABC team nursing director must ensure adequate didactic education and clinical experience before certifying direct bedside providers and IABC team members. Fig. 23-1 illustrates a record that can be kept to record each IABC team member's clinical training and education. Adequate administrative financial support for preceptored clinical experience should be part of the planning and included in the IABC program support budget.

Comprehensive nursing management and interventions for the IABC patient are discussed in Chapter 20. Key nursing diagnoses are listed in the box below. Inclusion of appropriate nursing standards of care related to these nursing diagnoses for

---

NURSING DIAGNOSES FOR THE CARE OF THE IABC PATIENT

Alterations in cardiac output related to:

• Left ventricular failure requiring IABC therapy

Potential alteration in cardiac output related to:

• Impaired myocardial contractility
• Incorrectly timed IABC
• Dysrhythmias

Potential mechanical problems of IABC secondary to:

• Loss of trigger
• Balloon leak or catheter disconnect
• Kink in IAB catheter system
• Loss of augmentation
• Failure in pneumatics
• Low helium tank
• System failure
• Autofill failure

Potential for vascular complications secondary to:

• Traumatic insertion or removal of IAB catheter resulting in excessive bleeding at insertion site
• Peripheral embolism during IAB catheter insertion, pumping, or removal
• Peripheral ischemia
• Bleeding from anticoagulation therapy or coagulopathies
• Thrombocytopenia

NURSING DIAGNOSES FOR THE CARE OF THE IABC PATIENT—cont'd

Potential alteration in tissue perfusion secondary to:

- Arterial obstruction of the subclavian, carotid, renal, or femoral artery
- Transient arterial spasm
- Inadequate limb perfusion related to invasive lines or IAB catheter
- Embolus dislodged during IAB catheter insertion, pumping, or removal
- Emboli formation related to IAB catheter immobility
- Rupture of undiagnosed thoracic or abdominal aneurysm

Potential for decrease in renal function related to:

- Occlusion of renal arteries by IAB catheter
- Hypotension or cardiogenic shock
- Electrolyte imbalance

Potential for impaired gas exchange related to:

- Inadequate pulmonary status
- Bedrest
- Extended intubation

Potential alteration in bowel elimination secondary to:

- Immobility
- Decreased gastrointestinal motility
- Tube feedings

Potential for alteration in nutritional intake secondary to:

- Prolonged intubation
- Decreased activity and appetite
- Stress of illness
- Possible occlusion of mesenteric artery
- Strict fluid restriction

Potential alteration in skin or muscle integrity secondary to:

- Immobilization and inadequate tissue perfusion
- Poor nutrition
- Invasive procedures and lines
- Use of thrombolytics

Potential alteration in immunological defense system secondary to:

- Wound, systemic, or nosocomial infection
- Invasive procedures and lines
- Debilitated condition

Potential alteration in level of consciousness related to:

- Carotid artery obstruction from incorrect IAB catheter placement or IAB catheter migration
- Cerebral embolization
- Psychosis
- Oversedation
- Decreased cerebral perfusion secondary to decreased cardiac output

Continued.

NURSING DIAGNOSES FOR THE CARE OF THE IABC PATIENT — cont'd

Potential alteration in thought process related to:
- Potential ICU psychosis
- Frequent administration of narcotics or drugs
- Unfamiliar surroundings

Alteration in comfort related to:
- Angina or postoperative pain
- Immobility
- IAB catheter insertion, manipulation, or removal
- Environmental stress from noise, cold, heat, overstimulation or understimulation, and light

Potential anxiety related to:
- Fear of the unknown, including IABC
- ICU environment
- Loss of independence
- Fear of dying

High risk for alteration in family process related to:
- Lack of knowledge about medical treatment plan or IABC therapy
- Fear of the unknown, including ICU
- Alterations in life-style
- Loss of control
- Fear of death or dying by loved one
- Inability to interact with loved one
- Feelings of helplessness or hopelessness
- Burden of making decisions related to care

From Nespeca JG: *Plan of care for the patient/family requiring intra-aortic balloon pump therapy in a nursing diagnosis framework*, Paramus, NJ, 1987, Datascope.

each hospital will assist in maintaining the total quality management of IABC care by all IABC team members and direct bedside providers.

Important aspects of IABC documentation include the record of IAB insertion and removal by IABC team members (Figs. 23-2 and 23-3), flowsheet charting by direct bedside providers (Fig. 23-4), progress note charting related to the medical treatment plan by physicians, and progress note charting related to patient outcomes or goals for the nursing diagnoses listed in the box above.

Monitoring, evaluation, and successful resolution of nursing management issues are the responsibility of the IABC team nursing director, clinical specialist, and nurse manager.

Text continued on p. 395.

Patient Name _____ ID No. _____

Age _____ Sex _____ Height _____ Weight _____

Diagnosis _____ Date _____ Time _____

Location of Insertion: OR   Cath Lab   MICU   SICU

Physician(s) Inserting IAB _____

IAB First Responder _____

IAB Bedside Provider _____

IAB Brand _____ Catheter Size _____ Volume _____

Lot Number _____ Serial Number_____ Exp Date_____

Insertion Site _____

Indication(s) for Insertion _____

Complications During Insertion _____

Timing / Augmentation Verification Strip:

Verification of Position by x-ray _____

Removal Date _____ Time _____

Physician(s) Removing IAB _____

Complications During Removal _____

Comments _____

Fig. 23-2. Record of intraaortic balloon insertion. The record is maintained in the IABC team log book for documentation, education, and research purposes. It is filled out by the IABC team first responder and reviewed by the IABC team during quarterly meetings. (From *Record of intraaortic balloon insertion,* Veterans' Administration Medical Center, Salt Lake City, Utah, 1992.)

Patient Name _____ ID No. _____

Age _____ Sex _____ Height _____ Weight _____

Diagnosis _____ Date _____ Time _____

Location of Insertion: OR   Cath Lab   MICU   SICU

Physician(s) Inserting IAB _____

_____

IAB First Responder _____

IAB Brand _____ Catheter Size _____ Volume _____

Lot Number _____ Serial Number_____ Exp Date_____

Indication(s) for Insertion _____

Patient Peripheral Vascular Assessment:

Pedal Pulses Before Procedure _____ After _____

Ankle Arm Index _____ Capillary Refill _____

Insertion Technique:

  Transthoracic with Open Chest Femoral Cutdown

  Percutaneous Sheath/Guidewire   Percutaneous Sheathless/Guidewire

Verification of Position by X-ray _____

Complications During Insertion _____

Timing/Augmentation Verification Strip:

Comments _____

_____

Signature of First Responder _____

Fig. 23-3. IABC patient procedure summary. The summary is an adhesive sticker placed in the progress notes of the patient chart for documentation. It is filled out by the IABC first responder after balloon insertion. (From *Virginia Mason Medical Center intraaortic balloon pump insertion record.*)

ASSISTED ARTERIAL WAVEFORM (1:2)

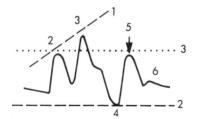

1) PAEDP: Patient Aortic End Diastolic Pressure
2) PSP: Peak Systolic Pressure
3) PDP: Peak Diastolic Augmented Pressure
4) BAEDP: Balloon Aortic End Diastolic Pressure
5) APSP: Assisted Systolic Pressure (Systole after IAB Deflation)
6) DN: Dicrotic Notch

TIME											
IABP Type *(circle)*	KAAT/K2000 Document Q4° or with △'s										
Trigger											
Ratio											
Balloon Fill Volume											
Helium Level Check											
Site/Check											
StripMount Q4°											
PAEDP											
PSP											
PDP											
BAEDP											
APSP											
Mean Pressure											
Heart Rhythm											
Radial Pulses	R / L										
Pedal Pulses	R / L										
Ankle Arm Index	R / L										

A

TRIGGER CODE		PULSE SCALE	SITE CODE
PE—Peak	AP—Atrial Pace	3+—Bounding	F—Femoral
P—Pattern	VP—Vent Pace	2+—Normal	T—Thoracic
AF—Afib		1+—Weak	S—Subclavian
		D—Doppled	

Fig. 23-4. A, Front of IABC flowsheet charting form. (From *ICU 24-hour flowsheet*, Veterans' Administration Medical Center, Salt Lake City, Utah, 1992.)

Continued.

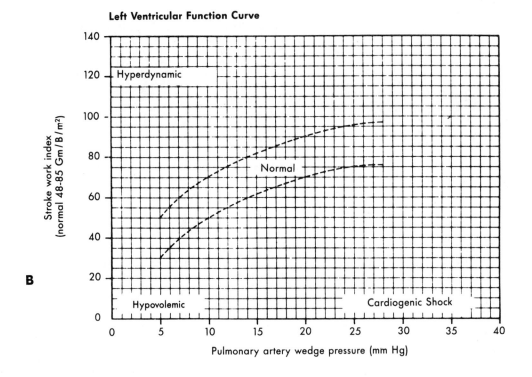

Fig. 23-4, cont'd. B, Back of IABC flowsheet charting form.

Collaborative management issues

Significant collaborative management issues include IABC-dependent patients, escalation of treatment therapies, and patient and family decision making. Because of the increased risk of morbidity and mortality in IABC patients and the complexity of multidisciplinary care required, multidisciplinary care conferences should be used to address these collaborative management issues. The following are issues related to clarity of patient goals and communication among the healthcare providers, patient, and family members that should trigger a multidisciplinary care conference[15]:

- Unclear perception of treatment goals by any member of the multidisciplinary team
- Unpredictable ICU transfer date resulting from poor patient progress
- Inadequately documented medical or nursing care plan
- Lack of consensus among members of the multidisciplinary team related to treatment goals or care plan
- Patient or family concerns
- Patients with major unresolved complications and prolonged stays

It has been said that "the finest gift a man can give to his age and time is the gift of constructive and creative life."[16] But the multidisciplinary team is often called upon to "give of ourselves when we give the gifts of the spirit: prayer, vision, beauty, aspiration, peace, and faith" at the end of life and when the dying IABC patient will not benefit from further treatment.[15] At this time, the patient, family, and entire multidisciplinary team benefit from the support provided by collaborative care conferences.

Monitoring, evaluation, and successful resolution of collaborative management issues is the responsibility of all members of the multidisciplinary team; however, direction and guidance frequently come from the IABC nursing and medical director or nurse manager.

THE NURSE MANAGER AS A FACILITATOR

The nurse manager is accountable for implementation, monitoring, and evaluation of adherence to the American Association of Critical Care Nurses Standards for Nursing Care of the Critically Ill.[17] To this end, the nurse manager is ultimately accountable for total quality management of the IABC program and IABC patient. The nurse manager can facilitate total quality management in IABC patient care by establishing an effective hospital-based IABC program, ensuring multidisciplinary monitoring and evaluation of medical and nursing care of the IABC patient, providing nursing education, and nurturing a collaborative healthcare environment. "With the unique combination of clinical, fiscal, and management expertise, the critical care nurse manager is in a key position to promote effective and cost efficient care of patients in the critical care environment."[18]

CONCLUSION

Today's healthcare system is complex and rapidly changing as social and economic forces challenge quality patient care in a financially constrained environment.[19] Total quality management is the process of managing quality despite these forces and constraints. As IABC technology and medical interventions evolve, critical care nurses will be increasingly challenged to master new concepts and techniques in the science of nursing. The art of nursing will continue to nurture "the deep sensitivity in the critical care nurse by which we may suffer and know tragedy, and die a little, but through which we will also experience the grandeur of human life."[20]

REFERENCES

1. Moulopoulos SD, Topaz S, Kolff WJ: Diastolic balloon pumping (with carbon dioxide) in the aorta—a mechanical assistance to the failing circulation, *Am Heart J* 63:669, 1962.
2. Kantrowitz A, Tjonneland S, Freed PS et al: Initial clinical experience with intraaortic balloon pumping in cardiogenic shock, *JAMA* 203:135, 1968.
3. Buckley MJ, Leinbach RC, Kastor JA et al: Hemodynamic evaluation of intra-aortic balloon pumping in man, *Circulation* 46(suppl II):130, 1970.
4. Bregman D, Goetz RH: Clinical experience with a new cardiac assist device: the dual-chambered intraaortic balloon assist, *J Thorac Cardiovasc Surg* 62:577, 1971.
5. McEnany MT, Kay HR, Buckley MJ et al: Clinical experience with intraaortic balloon pump support in 728 patients, *Cardiovasc Surg* 58(suppl I):123, 1978.
6. Alcan KE, Stertzer SH, Wallsh E et al: The expanding role of intra-aortic balloon counterpulsation in critical care cardiology in a community-based hospital, *Cardiovasc Reviews Reports* 3:61, 1982.
7. American Association of Critical Care Nurses: *Scope of critical care nursing practice*, Newport Beach, Calif, 1986, The Association.
8. Clemmer TP, Orme JF: An integrated approach to the patient with acute respiratory failure. In Clemmer TP, Orme JF, eds: *Critical care medicine*, Salt Lake City, 1981, LDS Hospital.
9. Goran SF: Establishing a nursing education program on intra-aortic balloon pumping: experience at the Maine Medical Center, *Cardiac Assist Educator Update* 1:1, 1992.
10. Joint Commission on Accreditation of Healthcare Organizations: Glossary. In *AMH accreditation manual for hospitals*, Oakbrook Terrace, Ill, 1992, Joint Commission on Accreditation of Healthcare Organizations.
11. American Nursing Association: Definitions adopted for standards, guidelines, *Am Nurse*, March 1991.
12. Alspach JG: *Issues in critical care education*, Keynote address presented at the American Association of Critical Care Nurses Leadership Institute, Chicago, 1983.
13. Alspach JG, Bell J, Canobbio MM et al: *AACN education standards for critical care nursing*, ed 1, St Louis, 1986, Mosby–Year Book.
14. Alspach JG: *The educational process in critical care nursing*, ed 1, St Louis, 1986, Mosby–Year Book.
15. Osguthorpe SG: Collaborative practice. In Birdsall C, ed: *Management issues in critical care*, St Louis, 1991, Mosby–Year Book.
16. Peterson WA: The art of giving. In Peterson WA, ed: *The art of living*, New York, 1961, Simon & Schuster.
17. Sanford SJ, Disch JM: *AACN standards for nursing care of the critically ill*, ed 2, Norwalk, Conn, 1989, Appleton & Lange.
18. American Association of Critical Care Nurses: *Role expectations for the critical care manager*, Newport Beach, Calif, 1986, The Association.

19. Arthur Andersen & Co, American College of Healthcare Executives: *The future of healthcare: changes and choices*, Chicago, 1987, Arthur Andersen & Co.
20. Peterson WA: The art of awareness. In Peterson WA, ed: *The art of living*, New York, 1961, Simon & Schuster.

CHAPTER 24

Weaning from the intraaortic balloon pump

Adrian Kantrowitz, **Raul R. Cardona**, and **Paul S. Freed**

The intraaortic balloon pump (IABP) is now the most commonly used left ventricular assist device (LVAD). With the experience accumulated worldwide since the clinical introduction of balloon pumping in 1967,[9] its adjunctive management, outcomes, and side effects have been defined with some precision. In turn, considerable insight into risk-benefit ratios has been obtained and a substantial consensus on indications and contraindications achieved. Yet the question of when and how to wean the patient from balloon pumping is still being elucidated.

Weaning from the IABP may be defined as the process of bringing about a physiological transition to the condition in which cardiac action is no longer supported by mechanical circulatory assistance. From the outset of clinical intraaortic balloon pumping, nursing has had a critically important role in carrying out the procedure and refining aspects of patient management, including weaning.[15] On most contemporary IABP teams, the nurse's role includes substantial responsibility for clinical and hemodynamic monitoring and assessment of the patient. It follows that the evolving topic of weaning from IABP is one that will continue to be strongly relevant to critical care nursing.

In this chapter we discuss criteria and methods for initiating, continuing, and ending the weaning process; we also comment on the selection of weaning method. Urgent situations that necessitate immediate interruption of IABP do not afford time for weaning and are not within the scope of this chapter. Such urgent indications include, for example, severe ischemia of the leg through which the balloon was inserted or a leak in the balloon. In such situations IABP can often be resumed using the other extremity for insertion of a new IABP catheter.

HISTORICAL NOTE

In its first few years, the implications of weaning from the IABP were not uniformly appreciated in the then-small community of clinical investigators studying the technique. Reporting a multicenter trial (initiated by us) of the IABP in patients with postinfarction cardiogenic shock, Scheidt et al.[18] noted inconsistent weaning techniques among the nine participating centers:

During the initial period of the study attempts were generally made to wean patients . . . as soon as they were hemodynamically stable. . . . In some cases, balloon counterpulsation was stopped altogether after an arbitrary period of circulatory assistance . . . and was not restarted unless shock recurred. In other patients, intermittent assistance (e.g., 15 minutes on, 15 minutes off) was given before use of the device was discontinued.

These practices differ from those suggested earlier by Krakauer et al.[12] of our laboratory:

It has not been possible to establish positive criteria for the termination of intraaortic balloon pumping, which therefore has been attempted on a trial basis. Once clinical shock had been reversed and all metabolic defects corrected, pumping was continued for several hours. If no change in the patient's status appeared, circulatory assistance was interrupted. If there were no immediate untoward changes, the patient was closely observed for half an hour without intraaortic balloon pumping. Mechanical circulatory assistance was then resumed for 30 minutes. If resumption of pumping did not bring about improvement in the patient's status, the procedure was terminated. . . . [I]f resumption of pumping after a 30 minute trial interruption led to improvement in the patient's condition, then assistance was continued for several hours longer.

Since then, progress in the design and manufacture of IABP consoles enabled two other techniques of weaning to be implemented, discussed on pp. 401 and 403.

CRITERIA OF READINESS FOR WEANING

In the patient undergoing balloon pumping because of acute left ventricular dysfunction, weaning is undertaken when the circulation is stable. In particular, clinical and hemodynamic parameters should be as follows in a patient no longer receiving vasoactive drugs:

Clinical parameters:
1. Blood gas values, fluid volume, temperature, cardiac rhythm, and hemoglobin, hematocrit, and electrolyte levels must all have been corrected.
2. Urinary output must be greater than 0.5 cc/kg/hr (in the adult).

Hemodynamic parameters:
1. Systolic arterial pressure must be greater than 90 mm Hg.
2. Mean arterial pressure must be greater than 70 mm Hg.
3. Cardiac index must be greater than 2.1 L/min/m^2.
4. Systemic vascular resistance must be less than 2100 dynes/sec/cm^{-5}.
5. Pulmonary capillary wedge pressure must be greater than 18 mm Hg.

There should be good recovery of left ventricular function and clinical evidence of adequate perfusion of the brain. Useful parameters include the left ventricular ejection fraction and left ventricular function, as assessed on the basis of wall motion analysis. Both of these parameters can be obtained by means of transesophageal echocardiography, as discussed below.

It bears emphasis that satisfying these criteria is not sufficient to ensure that weaning will be successful. This is confirmed by the many instances in which patients who are hemodynamically stable during assistance suffer relapses during or directly after weaning. Furthermore, not much is known about the additional factors on which successful weaning depends. Restoration of myocardial substrate depleted in the course of left ventricular dysfunction and its antecedents may be important. Satisfactory clinical indicators of substrate restoration, however, are lacking. In light of present knowledge, a quantitative assessment of whether a patient is ready for weaning is not possible. The practical consequence is that weaning is still performed essentially on a trial-and-error basis.

In our experience with patients undergoing balloon pumping because of acute left ventricular dysfunction, weaning was typically attempted in patients with a cardiac index of 2.2 L/min/m^2 or more, a pulmonary capillary wedge pressure below 18 mm Hg, and normal arterial pressure.[4] This improvement generally persisted for several hours before weaning was initiated.

As a matter of interest, we note that recently transesophageal echocardiography (TEE) has been used to provide important information for patient management and to help in determining the optimal time to wean the patient. Kyo et al.[14] reported on the use of biplane TEE to follow the cardiac status of patients receiving mechanical circulatory assistance after heart surgery. Of the patients they studied, 28 were supported with the IABP. In 16, the IABP had been inserted preoperatively for cardiogenic shock and the procedure was continued after surgery. In 12, balloon pumping was initiated to allow weaning from cardiopulmonary bypass. In the initial postoperative period, TEE examination was performed to assess the need for further surgery, to measure the size of the ventricle, and to obtain data for LV wall motion analysis. In the 89% (25 patients) who were weaned from IABP, good recovery of LV function was demonstrated by TEE (wall motion analysis), as well as by hemodynamic data. In 11% (3 patients), IABP support could not be discontinued because of failure to recover adequate left ventricular function. Kyo et al. concluded that biplane TEE is practical in the ICU setting, by its usually providing an adequate echo window and allowing measurement of coronary flow and sequential wall motion of the ventricles.

TECHNIQUES OF WEANING

Two methods of weaning are currently recommended, namely, frequency ratio and volume weaning. Before describing them, we must remind the reader that in planning to undertake weaning, allowance must be made for the need to stop heparin administration 4 hours before removal of the IABP from the patient.

Frequency ratio weaning

Frequency ratio weaning, described—among many others—by Hagemeijer et al.,[6] requires the IABP console operator to reduce the ratio of assisted to the total number of heart beats. When balloon pumping is initiated, the patient is assisted on each heart beat; the ratio of assisted to total heart beats is therefore 1:1 (Fig. 24-1). In the frequency ratio approach, the frequency of assistance is reduced until the patient is being assisted on every second or fourth beat (Figs. 24-2 and 24-3). It is evident that this procedure exposes the patient's heart muscle to large variations in afterload from one moment to the next; necessarily, the patient is also exposed to large changes in the amount of external work the myocardium is expected to perform. Although no relevant experimental studies have been reported, a related issue was addressed by Fuchs et al.[5] In their study of the effect of IABP on regional myocardial blood flow in patients with unstable angina, they measured great cardiac vein flow as

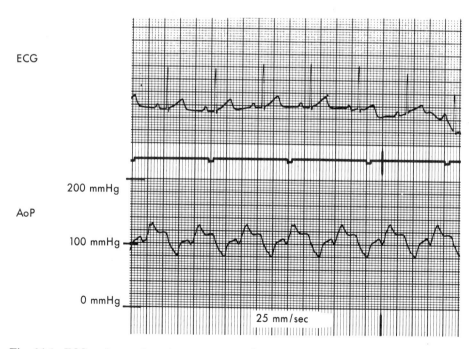

Fig. 24-1. ECG and central aortic pressure waveform during IABP at 1:1 assist ratio. *ECG*, electrocardiogram; *AoP*, central aortic pressure.

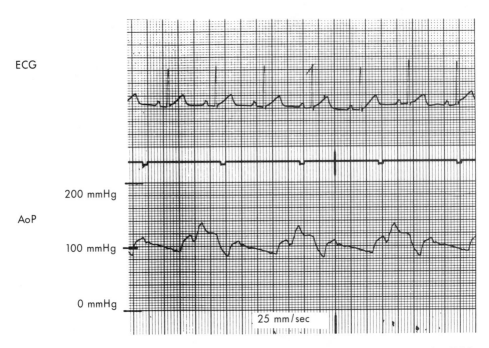

Fig. 24-2. ECG and central aortic pressure waveform during IABP at 1:2 assist ratio. *ECG,* electrocardiogram; *AoP,* central aortic pressure.

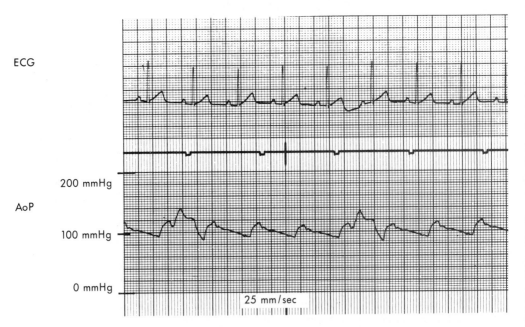

Fig. 24-3. ECG and central aortic pressure waveform during IABP at 1:4 assist ratio. *ECG,* electrocardiogram; *AoP,* central aortic pressure.

an indicator of the ability of balloon pumping to augment diastolic perfusion of beds fed by poststenotic portions of the left anterior descending coronary artery. They found that at 1:1 assist ratios, full-volume and intermediate-volume IABP did increase great cardiac vein flow. However, assist ratios of less than 1:1 led to no increase in great cardiac vein flow. These observations suggest the possibility that reduced assist ratios may not represent an intermediate level of balloon assistance but, to the contrary, may be hemodynamically equivalent to turning the balloon off. Bavin[1] gave a comparable analysis.

Volume weaning

The more physiological approach, in our view, is provided by volume weaning. Here, the volume of gas with which the balloon is inflated is gradually reduced to effect weaning. At first, we reduce the balloon volume by 20%. Assistance is continued for 15 to 30 minutes while the patient's hemodynamic parameters are observed closely. If they remain essentially at the same level as immediately before the first decrement in balloon volume, the volume is further reduced by approximately 20%. If the patient's response is favorable, balloon volume is further reduced in 20% decrements every 15 to 30 minutes. However, the volume is not reduced below approximately 20%.

On the other hand, if a more variable hemodynamic response to the first reduction in volume is observed, assistance at this volume is continued for a longer period. If the patient seems to be slipping back into hemodynamic decompensation, full-volume IABP is resumed for some hours.

Volume weaning, in our estimation, allows the clinician to make gradual adjustments in the magnitude of assistance according to the patient's needs. It entails no sudden significant increments in the load on the heart, as frequency ratio weaning necessitates. Volume weaning, however, is not recommended by some manufacturers of balloon pumps and balloon consoles, out of concern for the risk of clot formation on the balloon surface. It is true that the movement of the balloon surface lessens when its volume is reduced, which theoretically could increase the chances of clotting. Nevertheless, this risk is highly unlikely if a small volume of gas (for example, 20% of the full balloon stroke volume) is cycled through the balloon catheter continually. This procedure, in our experience, makes clotting on the balloon surface highly unlikely.

CRITERIA OF SUCCESSFUL WEANING

Weaning may be considered successful (1) if the patient's hemodynamic parameters remain in the normal range with clinical evidence of adequate perfusion and (2) if the patient's clinical condition is satisfactory, given the initial status, for several hours after the IABP is turned off.

MANAGEMENT OF RELAPSES

If the patient suffers a return to circulatory decompensation during or directly after weaning, full-volume balloon pumping is resumed. Another attempt to wean the patient from the IABP may be made 6 to 12 hours later. Hagemeijer et al.[6] reported that when a patient deteriorated during weaning, they resumed 1:1 assistance and continued it "for at least another week." In our view a briefer period of support may suffice for many such patients. There is no satisfactory evidence that the duration of weaning should be a function of the duration of preceding IABC, as Bolooki recommends.[2]

A patient who cannot be weaned is balloon-dependent. In all likelihood, the patient in whom balloon pumping is the primary treatment will already have been evaluated and found unsuitable for surgical treatment. The reported rate of patient who become balloon dependent is wide: 5% to 37%.[7,16,19] Sturm et al.,[19] in a study of 35 patients who experienced left ventricular dysfunction after myocardial infarction severe enough to require IABP, found that those who became balloon-dependent were relatively young (aged 40 to 55 years). These patients survived the first 50 hours of IABP support but neither improved nor worsened during the second 50 hours of balloon pumping; they remained in class B (CI >1.2 L/min/m^2 but <2.1 L/min/m^2 and SVR <2100 dynes/sec/cm^{-5}) for 7 to 10 days and did not experience life-threatening ventricular arrhythmias.[19]

For a balloon-dependent patient in whom a definitive surgical treatment has been excluded, the remaining possibilities include cardiac transplantation and a permanently implanted LVAD. Of several types of LVAD now being developed, one—a permanent form of the intraaortic balloon pump (Fig. 24-4)—is designed to replace a portion of the wall of the thoracic aorta in the same operating location as the IABP. The current device (in-series LVAD) incorporates a newly developed reliable long-term percutaneous access for power transfer. If successful, this permanent IABP will offer balloon-dependent patients the advantages of nonobligatory operation and documented efficacy in chronic CHF.[8]

SUMMARY

Since our initial implementation of balloon pumping in patients in cardiogenic shock in 1967,[9] the IABP drive unit has evolved substantially. First-generation drive units did not afford control of weaning variables such as balloon volume and assist frequency. Second-generation consoles allow the frequency ratio and volume-weaning techniques addressed in this chapter.

As the discussion of weaning has indicated, the weaning procedure is quite complex, requiring frequent correlation of hemodynamic and clinical observations, adjustments of console parameters, and close monitoring of the patient response. "Au-

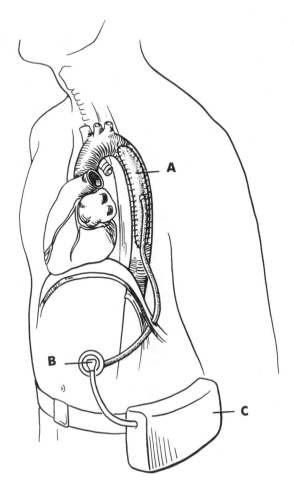

Fig. 24-4. The permanent intraaortic balloon pump has two implantable components. The blood pump (**A**), which can be used intermittently, and the percutaneous access device (**B**). The patient can detach the connector to the external drive unit (**C**) when the blood pump is passive.

tomated weaning," in which the IABC console would gradually implement reduced support over a period determined by the physician, is not yet commercially available, but recent progress is encouraging.

A computerized system that could adjust IABC parameters beat by beat in response to changes in the hemodynamic status of the patient, and particularly in response to arrhythmias, had long been sought.[13,17,20] With the Aisin Seiki Company of Japan and academic collaborators, we are now developing such a third-generation IABP system (Fig. 24-5). The reconfigured balloon pump incorporates an aortic

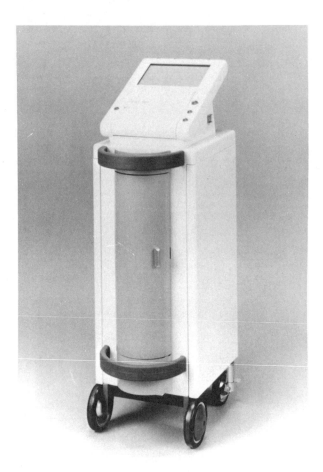

Fig. 24-5. AISIN/LVAD prototype of third generation closed-loop, totally automatic intraaortic balloon pump drive unit. (Courtesy Aisin Human Systems Co, Ltd. Kariya City, Japan.)

pressure sensor and ECG electrodes to detect physiological signals, affording continuous optimization of diastolic augmentation without operator intervention. An initial trial in 10 patients confirmed the feasibility of using the computer-based system in the clinical setting.[3,10,11] Safety and efficacy of the system are being further investigated in a multicenter trial.

The advent of this third-generation IABP controller is now making automated weaning feasible. Of course, clinical assessment of the patient response remains essential, but such assessments clearly would benefit from the advantages conferred by computer-based control of the IABP.

REFERENCES

1. Bavin TK: Weaning from intra-aortic balloon pump support, *Am J Nurs* 91(10):54, Oct 1991.
2. Bolooki H: Weaning from balloon pump assist. In Bolooki H, ed: *Clinical application of intra-aortic balloon pump*, Mt Kisco, NY, 1984, Futura Publishing.
3. Cardona RR et al: Experimental model for studies of a closed-loop, fully automatic intraaortic balloon pump. In *Proceedings of the AAMI Cardiovascular Science and Technology Conference*, Bethesda, Md, December 2-4, 1991.
4. Freed PS et al: Intraaortic balloon pumping for prolonged circulatory support, *Am J Cardiol* 61:554, 1988.
5. Fuchs RM et al: Augmentation of regional coronary blood flow by intra-aortic balloon counterpulsation in patients with unstable angina, *Circulation* 68:117, 1983.
6. Hagemeijer F et al: Report on therapy: effectiveness of intraaortic balloon pumping without cardiac surgery for patients with severe heart failure secondary to a recent myocardial infarction, *Am J Cardiol* 40:951, 1977.
7. Kantrowitz A: The physiologic bases of in-series cardiac assistance and the clinical application of intra-aortic devices. In Davila JC, ed: *Second Henry Ford Hospital International Symposium on Cardiac Surgery*, New York, 1977, Appleton-Century-Crofts.
8. Kantrowitz A: In-series temporary and permanent cardiac assistance. In Kantrowitz A, ed: *ASAIO primers in artificial organs, no 3, Ventricular assist devices*, Philadelphia, 1988, JB Lippincott.
9. Kantrowitz A et al: Initial clinical experience with intraaortic balloon pumping in cardiogenic shock, *JAMA* 203:135, 1968.
10. Kantrowitz A et al: Initial clinical trial of a closed-loop, fully automatic intraaortic balloon pump, *ASAIO Trans* 21:46, 1992 (abstract).
11. Kantrowitz A et al: Initial clinical experience of a closed-loop, totally automatic intraaortic balloon pump, *ASAIO Trans* 38:3, Sept 1992.
12. Krakauer JS et al: Clinical management ancillary to phase-shift balloon pumping in cardiogenic shock, *Am J Cardiol* 27:123, 1971.
13. Kuklinski WS: *Closed loop control of intraaortic balloon pumping: studies using a computer simulation and animal experiments*, Kingston, 1979, University of Rhode Island (dissertation).
14. Kyo S et al: Transesophageal Doppler echo monitoring of cardiac function during assist circulation. In Erbel R et al, eds: *Transesophageal echocardiography*, Berlin, 1989, Springer-Verlag.
15. Lane C: Intra-aortic phase-shift balloon pumping in cardiogenic shock, *Am J Nurs* 69:1654, 1969.
16. Lorente P et al: Multivariate statistical evaluation of intraaortic counterpulsation in pump failure complicating acute myocardial infarction, *Am J Cardiol* 46:124, 1980.
17. Moskowitz MS et al: A system for evaluation of computer control of intraaortic balloon pumping. In Proceedings of the 28th Annual Conference on Engineering in Medicine and Biology, New Orleans, 1975.
18. Scheidt S et al: Intra-aortic balloon counterpulsation in cardiogenic shock: report of a cooperative clinical trial, *N Engl J Med* 288:979, 1973.
19. Sturm JT et al: Quantitative indices of intraaortic balloon pump (IABP) dependence during postinfarction cardiogenic shock, *Artificial Organs* 4:8, 1980.
20. Zelano JA et al: A closed-loop control scheme for intraaortic balloon pumping, *IEEE Trans Biomed Eng* 37:182, 1990.

PART FIVE

IABC INSTRUMENTATION

CHAPTER **25** _____

The historical account

As derived by **Susan J. Quaal**

This chronicle is derived, in part, from two recent historical papers written by Adrian Kantrowitz, a giant in the field of intraaortic balloon pumping. These articles appeared in the *ASAIO Transactions* series: "A Moment in History and in the Annals of Thoracic Surgery," as one of the "Classics in Thoracic Surgery" Series.*

THE CONCEPT OF DIASTOLIC AUGMENTATION

Intraaortic balloon pumping (IABP) is the product of an endeavor begun more than 3 decades ago to explore first the concept and then the uses of diastolic augmentation. The foundation for this research was a precise understanding of cardiac cycle events, particularly the arterial pressure pulse. These events were explored in the laboratories of great cardiac physiology pioneers over scores of years.

Among these pioneer physiologists was Carl Wiggers, who headed the Cardiovascular Physiology Laboratory at Case Western Reserve University. Adrian Kantrowitz served as a U.S. Public Health Service Trainee in Wiggers' Laboratory from 1951 to 1952. Other faculty members included Robert Alexander, Ewald Selkurt, Gerhart Brecher, Matthew Levy, and Robert Berne, who continued to illuminate cardiovascular physiology throughout their careers.

Although its optical manometers would today seem primitive, the Wiggers laboratory was a superb environment in which Kantrowitz performed experiments to test his theory that it was possible to alter timing of pressure events during a heartbeat and whether there were any advantages to doing so. Adrian Kantrowitz and his brother, Arthur Kantrowitz (then on the Cornell physics faculty and later at the AVCO Corporation), performed a series of experiments that demonstrated that coronary pressure and flows could be manipulated during the cardiac cycle.[1] Their re-

*Reproduced in part from Kantrowitz A: Introduction of left ventricular assistance, *ASAIO Trans* 10:(1):39, 1987, and Kantrowitz A: Origins of intraaortic balloon pumping, *Ann Thorac Surg* 50:672, 1990, with permission of Adrian Kantrowitz, MD and the publishers of *ASAIO Transactions* and *Annals of Thoracic Surgery*.

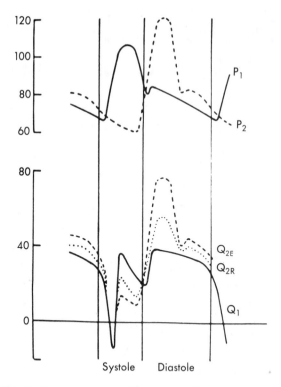

Fig. 25-1. Heavy lines indicate normal aortic pressure (P_1) and phasic coronary flow (Q_1). Dashed and dotted lines indicate predicted flows when the anterior descending coronary artery is perfused with pulse pressure out of phase with myocardial systole. P_2 represents proposed delayed coronary pressure; Q_{2R}, calculated flow in presumed rigid coronary system; Q_{2E}, calculated flow in presumed elastic coronary system. (From Kantrowitz A:*ASAIO* 10:(1) 39, 1987.)

sults demonstrated that it was possible to change blood flow patterns in the left coronary artery (Fig. 25-1).

This work eventually led to a cooperative effort between Kantrowitz's research group at Maimonides Hospital in Brooklyn and the AVCO-Everett Research Laboratory in Boston. Their goal was to develop a permanent mechanical assist device that would provide diastolic augmentation for the relief of chronic left ventricular failure. They concluded that it might be feasible to devise a surgical procedure, based on the principle of diastolic augmentation. This was realized by Kantrowitz and associates, as well as other researchers, in a succession of small steps via a journey still far from its end.

FIRST APPLICATION: A BIOLOGICAL AUXILIARY VENTRICLE

Before 1953, there was no lack of imaginative workers searching for surgical methods of increasing the blood supply to an ischemic myocardium. Certainly there already were major accomplishments in the development of pump oxygenators to allow intracardiac surgery. However, the possibility of using mechanical means to increase the functioning myocardium for patients with chronic left ventricular failure had not been reported.

Kantrowitz's first thought for translating the concept of diastolic augmentation into a surgical procedure was to use the diaphragm's motor power to share the myocardium's workload. In initial experiments, the diaphragm was wrapped around the heart and the left phrenic nerve was stimulated synchronously with each systole. This procedure did not raise arterial pressure significantly. The diaphragm sheath acted like a restrictive pericarditis; the heart lost some of its compliance and was unable to dilate sufficiently during diastole to accept diastolic filling.

In a second group of animals, the left leaf of the diaphragm was peripherally mobilized, so as to preserve its blood supply and innervation. This time, the hemidiaphragm was wrapped around the distal portion of the thoracic aorta and stimulated during each diastole, which increased diastolic pressure significantly as compared with control studies (Fig. 25-2).[2] This work was presented at the 1960 meeting of the American Society for Artificial Internal Organs.[3] Stanley Sarnoff was in the audience and at once scolded, lauded, and lectured on his seminal tension-time index.[4]

Dr. Kantrowitz, I think you're underestimating the advantages you really have. If I understand your basic orientation correctly, it's a desire to propel blood through the body while diminishing the energy requirements of the presumably defective myocardium. . . . I would guess that you're not entirely aware of the fact that the oxygen requirement of the heart is in no way, shape, or form related to the work done by the heart. The oxygen requirement of the heart, to the best of my knowledge, is a function of the amount of tension the myocardium develops, not the amount of work, which is the pressure times stroke volume delivered by the heart.

Your position, therefore, is actually stronger than that which you've stated, namely that you are promoting a higher aortic pressure and therefore a larger circulating volume per minute without requiring the heart to develop the peak tension that it would do without your auxiliary heart.

To extend these experiments to a chronic preparation, the phrenic nerve had to withstand long-term stimulation. Kantrowitz and associates began to study this problem and soon found themselves with a number of spinoff projects involving neuromuscular stimulation—the development of an implantable cardiac pacemaker, neurogenic bladder control, paralytic ileus, and paralyzed limbs.[5-7]

Advantages of a biological power source for cardiac assistance were clear. All the

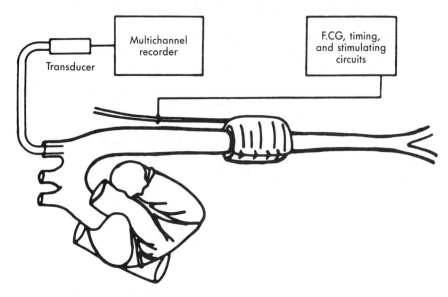

Fig. 25-2. Schematic of hemidiaphragm wrapped around the distal thoracic aorta to produce diastolic augmentation. (From Kantrowitz A:*ASAIO* 10:(1) 39, 1987.)

patient would have to do is eat a good breakfast. They also envisioned that perfecting the prerequisite long-term phrenic nerve stimulation was a daunting undertaking. As an alternative to use of autologous muscle, they began to investigate a mechanical prosthesis as a mechanical ventricle in a series of studies. These experiments enabled Yukihiko Nosé, a research associate newly arrived at Maimonides Hospital Laboratory from Hokkaido, Japan, to establish an important principle. After examining the relationship between anatomic location of an auxiliary ventricle and its hemodynamic effects, Nose', in 1963, demonstrated that the closer the pump is to the heart, the more effective the circulatory assistance[8] (Fig. 25-3).

MECHANISM AND APPLICATION FOR TEMPORARY CARDIAC ASSIST

The concept of counterpulsation was also investigated by a number of other researchers. Two groups working in Boston—Dwight Harken, Armand Lefemine, and associates[9] and Ralph Deterling, William Birtwell, and Harry Soroff[10]—used a femoral access to remove blood during systole and rapidly replace it during diastole, in an effort to increase coronary perfusion.

There were, however, difficulties with this system, chiefly related to the fact that one had to exert very high pressures and high vacuum through the femoral artery to remove any significant quantity of blood and replace it as rapidly as necessary to

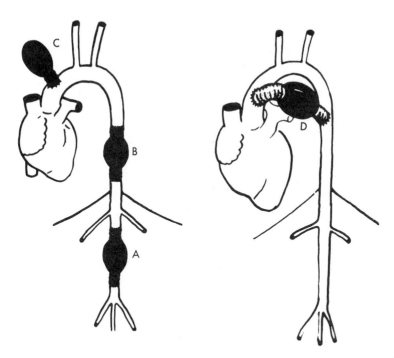

Fig. 25-3. Prostheses were implanted (**A**) in abdominal aorta; (**B**) in thoracic aorta; (**C**) end-to-side, making blind anastomosis with ascending aorta; and (**D**) end-to-side in ascending and descending aorta, bypassing the aortic arch. (From Kantrowitz A:*ASAIO* 10:(1) 39, 1987.)

influence arterial pressure in the desired ways. This led to considerable hemolysis. Further, the amount of blood that could be moved in the short time available was only 5 to 10 ml. The combination of this limitation and the fact that blood was being withdrawn and infused at the femoral arteries, far away from the aortic valve, appeared to foreclose the possibility of achieving significant benefit.

Clauss et al.[11] described an invention to improve coronary collateral circulation surrounding an area of acute myocardial infarction. A pump actuator was used to withdraw a fixed volume of blood from bilateral femoral arterial catheters during systole, which reduced pressures in the aortic root. This volume was reinfused during diastole. Each exchange was "timed" to the electrocardiogram. In the normotensive patient, left ventricular work decreased and coronary perfusion was increased; myocardial oxygen supply and demand were improved. This concept was initially enthusiastically received. However, the extracorporeal handling of blood proved to be clinically difficult.

Conception, design, assembly, and testing of an IABP also took place in Dr. Willem Kolff's laboratory at the Cleveland Clinic in 1961.[12] Stephen R. Topaz, a mechanical engineer, and Spyridon Moulopoulos, a cardiologist from Athens, tested

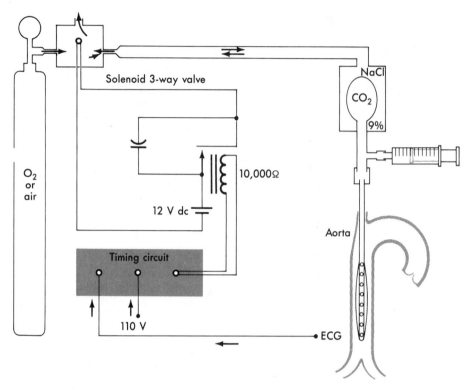

Fig. 25-4. Diagram of the balloon pump designed by Moulopoulos and Topaz. NaCl indicates the sterile 0.9% solution of sodium chloride around the outside balloon to decrease the dead space in the system. The amount of carbon dioxide can be regulated with the syringe. (From Moulopoulos SD, Topaz S, Kolff WJ: *Am Heart J* 63(3):669, 1962.)

their balloon pump on a mock circulatory loop. They placed a distensible balloon condom over a catheter and introduced it into the aorta. A latex tubing (0.95 cm in diameter and 20 cm in length) was tied around the end of a polyethylene catheter (external diameter, 3.25 mm; internal diameter, 2.16 mm; length, 60 cm) with multiple side holes. The distal end of the polyethylene catheter was occluded so that the tubing could be inflated and deflated through the side holes in the catheter (Fig. 25-4).

Use of a latex balloon ensured that the device would be occlusive in the aorta. When inflated with carbon dioxide, this balloon displaced a volume of blood in the aorta, corresponding to that removed by the actuator in the earlier Clauss design. Over a 6-month period the balloon pump was modified, and tested in animal models and a cadaver.[12]

Other researchers began publishing various new ideas for assisting the failing heart. A diastolic leg compression method of reproducing effects of arterioarterial pumping without entering the arterial tree was studied by Dennis et al.,[13] Osborn et al.,[14] and Birtwell et al.[15] The legs were compressed suddenly during diastole and released suddenly during systole. The tracheal airway was also used to produce synchronous intrathoracic pressure variations.[16] Goldfarb et al.[17] developed a blind-end pump triggered by a peripheral arterial pulse and tried it in one comatose patient. Working in Denver, Colorado, Watkins, Duschesne, and Callaghan developed and clinically used the "SIMAS" myocardial augmentation system.[18a,18b]

In a second family of approaches, Salisbury[19] demonstrated the value of left ventricular bypass, demonstrating its theoretical applications in experimental heart failure. Dennis reported a technique for acute left heart failure, using a large-bore cannula for transjugular/transseptal drainage of the left atrium, which made left ventricular bypass possible without thoracotomy. By 1964 they had used the procedure in 12 patients.[20]

CLINICAL USE OF A PERMANENT LEFT VENTRICULAR ASSIST DEVICE

By the mid-1960s, after further experimental work by Nosé, Russell, Gradel et al.[21] with a valveless, pneumatic, ellipsoidal left ventricular device, Kantrowitz's group shifted to a new geometry, a U-shape, which bridged the aortic arch[22] (Fig. 25-5). Some of the U-shaped devices were made in Adrian Kantrowitz's laboratory and some in the AVCO-Everett Research Laboratory directed by Arthur Kantrowitz.

This left ventricular assist device (LVAD) was extremely powerful, because the pump inlet was placed within centimeters of the aortic valve and it had a stroke vol-

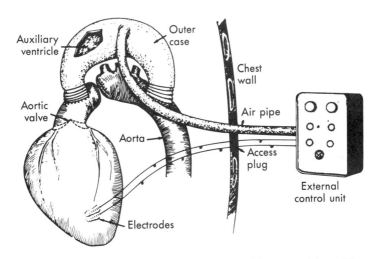

Fig. 25-5. The U-shaped, first-generation mechanical auxiliary ventricle and its power supply. (From Kantrowitz A: *ASAIO* 10:(1) 39, 1987.)

ume that far exceeded that of the left ventricle. The device consistently effected major improvement of hemodynamic parameters in dogs with induced heart failure.[23] The avalvular design permitted intermittent pumping. Animals appeared to tolerate the LVAD well, and there was no evidence of hemolysis or clotting.

When the system had demonstrated long-term reliability and effectiveness in the laboratory and when the cumulative experience indicated that side reactions were likely to be minimal, they concluded that the time was ripe for trial in patients with progressive left ventricular failure who had passed beyond the compass of any known standard therapy.

In February 1966 the first patient, a 33-year-old man, died of an uncontrollable tachycardia less than 24 hours after operation. The second implantation, in a 63-year-old woman, took place in May 1966. The patient's thoracic anatomy deviated markedly from that expected and necessitated fitting the LVAD with a long efferent limb. Despite these variances from the protocol established in animals, intermittent pumping with the LVAD was highly effective during the first several postoperative days. At one point, after a 2-hour deactivation period, Kantrowitz came to examine the patient and found her in frank congestive failure. Ventricular support was resumed. Within minutes, the patient's lungs began to clear, and she became alert and oriented. It was a dramatic confirmation of the assist device's hemodynamic effectiveness in alleviating fulminant left ventricular failure. In spite of the marked clinical improvement brought about by diastolic augmentation, the patient experienced a stroke 12 days after implantation and she died soon afterward. Autopsy disclosed a thrombus in the long efferent limb of the auxiliary left ventricle.[24]

INTRAAORTIC BALLOON PUMPING: A CLINICAL MODALITY

Another modality of left ventricular support showed promise in Kantrowitz's laboratory. After the patient experience with the U-shaped LVAD—in which it was possible to quickly return central venous, left ventricular, end-diastolic pressure, and cardiac output to normal ranges—it was felt that it would be relatively easy to achieve a cardiac assist device that was intended for temporary use. Kantrowitz et al.[25] were then convinced that there were many patients in acute heart failure who could benefit from short-term support. They decided to try to design an IABP that would be useful in treating patients with medically refractory acute heart failure. It was at this time that Adrian and Arthur Kantrowitz decided to work independently. Adrian continued to work with his group of engineers and surgical research associates at Maimonides Hospital in Brooklyn, and Arthur collaborated with the research group at Massachusetts General Hospital.

During 1966, Adrian Kantrowitz and associates designed and fabricated animal balloon pumps. They quickly learned the advantage of using helium as the driving gas. This gas, which has 1/20th the density of carbon dioxide, could be shuttled much more quickly and therefore achieve more precise diastolic augmentation. They also realized the negative effect of a completely occlusive IAB and explored alternative balloon configurations. Following up on Nosé's work on optimal assist device location, they even designed a balloon that traversed the aortic arch, so that the tip lay within 1 cm of the aortic valve. It, however, proved too cumbersome. Their efforts were therefore concentrated on producing a simple, effective balloon that would be placed in the lumen of the thoracic aorta.

They secured human subjects' approval at Maimonides Hospital for use of their prototype balloon system in a limited number of patients in cardiogenic shock. On June 29, 1967, they were called to examine a patient whose condition the cardiologists considered hopeless. The patient was a 45-year-old female, who had sustained a posterior wall myocardial infarction and was in deep cardiogenic shock, comatose, and anuric. She was receiving a continuous infusion of high-dose levophed (18 mg in 500 cc). Over a 7-hour period, balloon pumping restored normal circulatory dynamics. The most impressive moment occurred when the urine collection bag began to fill with urine. This patient recovered and was discharged.

When word of success with IABP reached the medical community, a small army of visitors arrived at Adrian Kantrowitz's laboratory, requesting permission to use IABP in their own patients. The equipment that they had developed to date consisted of a polyurethane balloon (Fig. 25-6) and control unit (Fig. 25-7). At that time it was concluded that if IABP were to have broad application, other physicians would need the opportunity to evaluate it independently with their own patients. One way to accomplish this was through a cooperative study.

Adrian Kantrowitz decided to explore this possibility and invited physicians representing nine medical centers to meet with him at Maimonides Hospital. Thomas Killip of Cornell Medical Center brought a delegation, including Stephen Scheidt, Diana Argyros, Robert Ascheim, and V. A. Subramanian. Edmund Sonnenblick and Jacob Matloff of the Peter Bent Brigham Hospital were delayed by weather. Others attending included Edward Diethrich from Baylor University; Stephen Ayres, Foster Conklin, and Stanley Giannelli, Jr., from St. Vincent's Hospital, New York; Fred Kittle and Leon Resnekov from the University of Chicago; Alfred Goldman from the Cedars-Sinai Medical Center; Clarence Dennis and Philip Sawyer from the State University of New York, Downstate Medical Center; Robert Cline from Duke University; and Gerald Wolff and John Collins from Barnes Hospital in St. Louis. All wanted to participate in this study; therefore sources of funding were investigated. Others who later took part in the study were listed in a subsequent publication.[26]

The John A. Hartford Foundation was approached for funding. Their trustees were enthusiastic about the study and awarded a grant to fund the equipment, data coordination, travel, and other costs. Adrian Kantrowitz's personal funds were used to duplicate his laboratory's balloon-fabrication equipment in a location near the

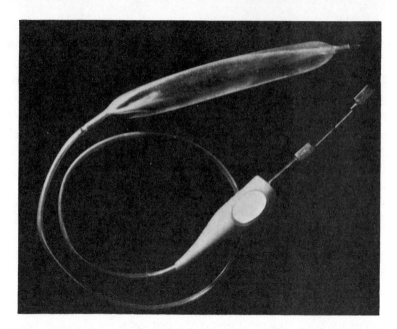

Fig. 25-6. Intraaortic balloon pump used in initial patients. It was fabricated of polyurethane and exposed to transmembrane pressure of 50 mm Hg during operation but could withstand 300 mm Hg without undergoing elastic deformation. Markedly higher pressure were required to burst the balloon. In accelerated life tests, balloons were operated for 15,000,000 cycles at 200 mm Hg pressure without failure. (From Kantrowitz A: *ASAIO* 10:(1) 39, 1987.)

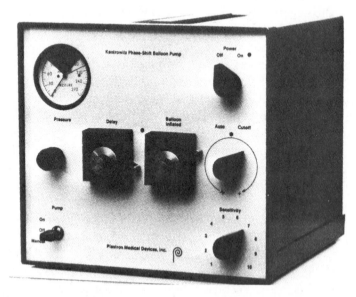

Fig. 25-7. Early control unit for intraaortic balloon pumping used in initial patients. In addition to operation in automatic mode, inflation and deflation could be manually controlled as adjunct to resuscitation after cardiac arrest. (From Kantrowitz A: *ASAIO* 10:(1) 39, 1987.)

hospital. Their objectives were to meet the equipment needs of the cooperating groups and to have an established healthcare company take over manufacturing and marketing of the balloon pump. Both objectives were realized. Multiple balloon pump systems were given to each group.

By 1970 the Kantrowitz team had treated 30 patients with IABP. Other groups also began reporting on their clinical experiences. At the April 1970 meeting of the American Society for Artificial Internal Organs, Bregman, Kripke, and Goetz described their use of a IABP in the treatment of four patients with cardiogenic shock. Within 30 minutes of assist, all were alert and one patient was alive and well at 5 months.[27] In May 1970, Buckley et al., working with Arthur Kantrowitz, reported the results of treating their first eight patients in cardiogenic shock, also with a sole survivor, at the Massachusetts General Hospital.[28]

In June 1970, Kantrowitz moved his laboratory, staff of 25, and research equipment to Sinai Hospital in Detroit. He continued to pursue further patient IABP studies with the cooperative study group. Scheidt and co-workers reported on 87 IABP patients from this cooperative study group in 1973.[26] Thus IABP had been convincingly demonstrated and promised to be useful in acute low-output left ventricular failure.

FURTHER ADVANCES

Feola[29] advanced the technique of balloon pumping by studying counterpulsation under fluoroscopy. He produced data that indicated that timing of inflation and deflation was of critical importance. Hemodynamic benefits were arduously researched by Buckley,[30] initially in animal models and later in humans. Buckley confirmed that balloon inflation in diastole augmented perfusion, but equally important, he also confirmed how balloon deflation just before systole markedly reduced resistance to left ventricular ejection and thereby reduced cardiac work and myocardial oxygen consumption.

Mundth and associates[31] extended the application of IABP to patients who required cardiac surgery after myocardial infarction. By 1976 more than 5000 patients with circulatory failure after cardiotomy had received IABP. An equal number of patients underwent IABP in other countries.[32]

In 1972, Bregman and Goetz[33] developed a dual-chambered balloon that was designed with a large proximal balloon and smaller distal balloon. The rationale behind this design was to produce a unidirectional blood flow proximally to the brain and coronary arteries by initial inflation of the distal, smaller balloon. This resulted in a blocking of the distal blood flow and an augmenting of proximal or forward flow.

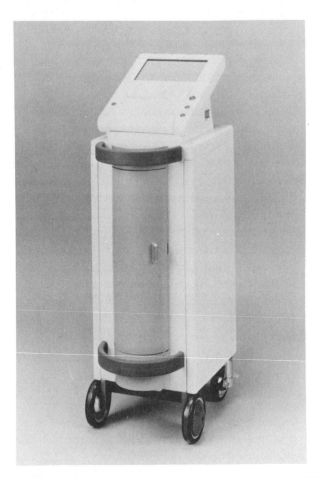

Fig. 25-8. Prototype of a new generation closed-loop, fully automatic IABP drive unit. (Courtesy of Aisin Human Systems Co. Ltd.)

A new generation closed loop fully automated IABP

Kantrowitz and associates[34] recently published clinical studies of a new generation, closed loop fully automated IABP (CL-IABP) that continuously optimizes diastolic augmentation, beat by beat, without operator intervention (Fig. 25-8). With current equipment it is extremely difficult, or even impossible, to maintain precise synchronization during an arrhythmia. The problem of optimizing the ability of a balloon console to operate in accord with physiological, clinical, and engineering criteria has long been recognized.[35,36] Ten patients were studied who met standard indications for IABP. These patients were pumped by the fully automatic IABP system for an average of 20 hours. As soon as the system was activated, it provided consistently beneficial diastolic augmentation without any further operator intervention. This study suggested that a fully automated IABP is feasible in the clinical setting and may have advantages relative to current generation IABP systems.

SUMMATION OF 3 DECADES OF IABP HISTORY

The history of IABP extends over 3 decades. Despite what must have appeared to be seemingly insurmountable obstacles, these dedicated researchers persistently pieced together the mosaic that evolved into the era of IABP as we know it today. Kantrowitz[37] beautifully summarized how IABP reached its genesis as follows:

Any new idea, if it is to succeed, requires the courage and depth of understanding of its inventor to pursue the thought to its conclusion. The least challenges in the development of IABP were solving the many technical problems. More formidable were the intrainstitutional political agendas and their obstructive consequences. That IABP was not aborted in its infancy is a witness to the remarkable support to us from the National Institutes of Health, from the John A. Hartford Foundation, from many residency and research staff members and from independent-minded colleagues and investigators in the cooperative study, all of whom participated in this exciting adventure.

In a recent publication,[38] Kantrowitz concluded:

Despite its secure position in contemporary cardiac care, the concept is by no means static, and a number of intriguing possibilities are being pursued:

Since 1980, serious efforts are being made to develop IABP for pediatric patients. Most applications thus far are in children with refractory low cardiac output syndrome after cardiac surgery. Reported results indicate an immediate survival of 50% to 67% and a long-term survival of 25% to 33%—outcomes comparable to those in adults.[39] Technical issues are being pursued vigorously.

The first clinical case in which pulmonary artery balloon counterpulsation was implemented was reported by Miller in 1980.[40] Adequate pulmonary artery diastolic augmentation was achieved, enabling discontinuation of cardiopulmonary bypass in a patient who probably would not have survived. The goals of recent efforts are to construct a dedicated intrapulmonary artery balloon and to improve the efficiency of pulmonary artery counterpulsation using valveless pulsatile assist devices with stroke volume of up to 100 ml.

Permanent in-series left ventricular assist by means of a balloon pumping-like pumping chamber implanted in the wall of the thoracic aorta has been advanced to the stage where clinical trial is imminent for selected congestive heart failure patients. The intravascular surface of this system possesses documented hemocompatibility.[41] The system is valveless and minimally alters the topography of the aorta, allowing deactivation for extended periods of time without jeopardizing the patient.

If the balloon pump is to assist each heart beat, including those generated during arrhythmias, a totally automated closed-loop system is essential.[42] Working with the Aisin Seiki Company of Japan and university colleagues, our laboratory has developed a new-generation intraaortic balloon pump that automatically makes and implements timing decisions for balloon inflation and deflation on a beat-by-beat basis. Studies in a large series of dogs in sinus rhythm and experimentally induced arrhythmias have provided data indicating that this system correctly responds to tachyarrhythmias (205 beats/min) and rapid atrial fibrillation, as well as other arrhythmias. A trial in 10 patients documented the feasibility of clinical implementation of this technique.[43]

A SECOND PERMANENT LVAD

At Sinai Hospital, Kantrowitz and associates resumed experimental work on the permanent aortic-wall LVAD. Their findings corroborated their earlier evidence of the hemodynamic capability of this type of left ventricular assistance (Fig. 25-9). Because the device operated on the same principle as the balloon pump and was in the same intraaortic location, they felt that a trial of balloon pumping would enable them to predict just how the permanent LVAD would work. When this device satisfied criteria for use in human subjects and with institutional review committee approval, they performed the first implant in September 1971.

The patient was a 65-year-old man who survived 96 days.[44] It turned out that this patient's preoperative trial of balloon pumping indeed predicted the benefits provided by permanent LVAD. These benefits were substantial. As in the balloon used preoperatively, the LVAD returned left ventricular end-diastolic pressure, pulmonary capillary wedge pressure, and cardiac output to normal values. The patient improved from having been bedridden to the point where he could walk several hundred yards in the hospital. The patient was discharged from the hospital with his implanted pump deactivated and untethered to any external apparatus. While at home on an intermittent pumping regimen he was able to take walks in the neighborhood for the first time in 2 years. This was an incredible accomplishment, considering that it has taken almost 20 years before another patient with an implantable VAD has even been able to leave the hospital temporarily on pass during the day.

MECHANICAL ASSISTANCE ON THE HORIZON

Conceptual approaches to mechanical assistance for the failing heart were delineated in the 1950s and 1960s. Since then, of the many techniques studied, only one method for temporary left ventricular assistance—intraaortic balloon pumping—has gained wide clinical acceptance. Worldwide, at least 75,000 patients undergo IABP annually.[38] Although this technique is still used to treat patients in cardiogenic shock, the main indications for its use are inability to discontinue cardiopulmonary bypass after open-heart surgery and unstable angina.

The need for a permanent LVAD for irreversible failure is therefore obvious. The number of candidates for mechanical assistance who are in terminal failure is estimated to be 17,000 to 35,000 new patients a year. If one considers patients in

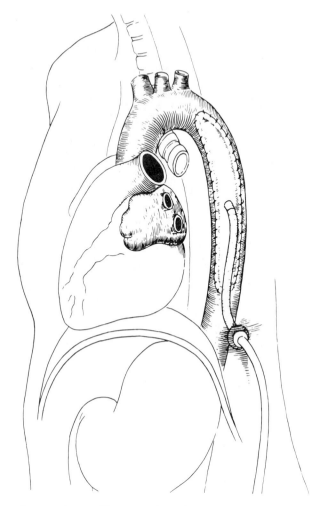

Fig. 25-9. Second-generation auxiliary ventricle (the dynamic aortic patch) showing implantation site in the descending thoracic aorta. (From Kantrowitz A: *ASAIO* 10:(1) 39, 1987.)

whom the first diagnosis of irreversible failure has been made, the number is much larger, perhaps as many as 100,000 per year. Such patients' chances of living more than 1 year are 50%. After 2 decades of support by the National Heart, Lung and Blood Institute Devices Branch, a cluster of totally implantable left ventricular assist systems in now undergoing clinical trials. The groups involved in this program are Novacor, collaborating with Stanford; Thermo Cardiosystems with Children's Hospital of Boston and Texas Heart Institute; Nimbus with Johnson & Johnson Interventional Systems and multiple clinical trial centers; Abiomed with the Massachu-

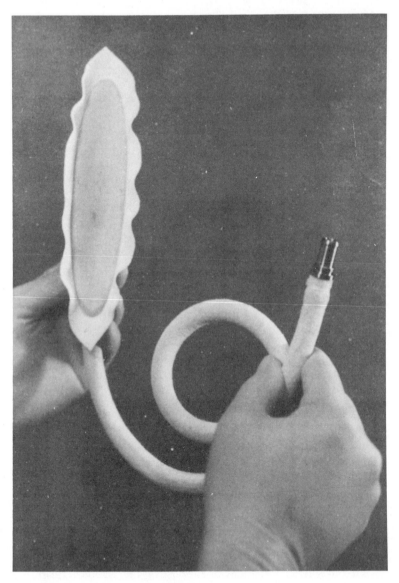

Fig. 25-10. Third-generation auxiliary ventricle, a simple pumping bladder of unilayer construction with no valves. (From Kantrowitz A: *ASAIO* 10:(1) 39, 1987.)

setts General Hospital; and Pierce's group at Hershey, Pennsylvania, working with Thoratec and Sarns 3M.

Kantrowitz's second-generation LVAD was plagued with infection at the skin access site for external pneumatic power, which led his group to voluntarily suspend this trial. Currently, after some 12 years of studying a device with a surface of autologous cells, he believes he has developed a successful skin access device (implants in swine for more than 3 years with no clinical evidence of infection) and is readying a third-generation LVAD system for clinical trial (Fig. 25-10).

These LVAD systems on the horizon differ from one another in more than one respect. First, there is the difference between the parallel and in-series systems—that is, bypassing the left ventricle to take over most, if not all, of its work—vs. augmenting a partially functioning left ventricle. Second, there is the difference between implanting all the components (pump, energy converter, compliance chamber, back-up battery, transcutaneous energy transmission receiver) and restricting the implanted components to the minimum (pump and skin access device), leaving the power source outside the patient's body for ease of repair or replacement. Finally, there is the difference between the obligatory continuous operation of the parallel systems and discretionary operation (intermittent or continuous), depending on the patient's needs, a capability of the in-series systems. In future years, benefits and risks of each approach will be matched to the particular patient requirements.

Kantrowitz, truly a giant in the history of mechanical assistance, began his legacy by demonstrating the principle of diastolic augmentation, which laid the foundation for successful clinical implementation of IABP. Incisive and original, he has led the ardous effort to expand mechanical assist device development beyond IABP to the achievement of a totally implantable LVAD. He summarized the future of LVADs beyond balloon pumping as follows[45]: "We stand on the threshold of an era of great excitement in which permanently implanted LVADs of various types will play an important role in restoring a reasonable lifestyle, for a reasonable length of time, to the multitude of patients who have intractable heart failure."

The reader is directed to a companion resource to this book for further information on the various types of LVADs and associated patient management.[46]

REFERENCES

1. Kantrowitz A, Kantrowitz A: Experimental augmentation of coronary flow by retardation of the arterial pressure pulse, *Surgery* 34:678, 1953.
2. Kantrowitz A, McKinnon WMP: The experimental use of the diaphragm as an auxiliary myocardium, *Surg Forum* 9:266, 1959.
3. Kantrowitz A, McKinnon G: Functioning autogenous muscle used experimentally as an auxiliary ventricle, *Trans Am Soc Artif Intern Organs* 6:305, 1960.
4. Sarnoff SJ, Braunwald E, Welch CH Jr et al: Hemodynamic determinants of oxygen consumption of the heart with special references to the tension-time index, *Am J Physiol* 192:148, 1958.
5. Kantrowitz A: Electronic physiologic aids. In *Proceedings of the Third IBM Medical Symposium*, Armonk, NY, IBM Corp. (Initially presented at the Surgical Forum, American College of Surgeons, San Francisco, November 1960.)

 6. Schamaun M, Kantrowitz A: Management of neurogenic urinary bladder in paraplegic dogs by direct electric stimulation of the detrusor, *Surgery* 54:640, 1963.
 7. deVilliers DR, Saltiel I, Nonoyama A, et al: Control of postoperative adynamic bowel in dogs by electric stimulation, *Trans Am Soc Artif Intern Organs* 9:351, 1963.
 8. Nosé Y, Schamaun M, Kantrowitz A: Experimental use of an electronically controlled prosthesis as an auxiliary left ventricle, *Trans Am Soc Artif Intern Organs* 9:351, 1963.
 9. Maccioli GA, Lucas DDS, Norfleet EA: The intra-aortic balloon pump: a review, *J Cardiothorac Anesth* 2:365, 373, 1988.
10. Birtwell WC, Soroff HS, Well M et al: Assisted circulation. I. An improved method for counterpulsation, *Trans Am Soc Artif Intern Organs* 8:35, 1962.
11. Clauss RH, Birtwell WC, Albertal G et al: Assisted circulation. I. The arterial counterpulsator. *J Cardiovasc Surg* 41:447, 1961.
12. Moulopoulos SD, Topaz S, Kolff WJ: Diastolic balloon pumping (with carbon dioxide) in the aorta—a mechanical assistance to the failing heart, *Am Heart J* 63:669, 1962.
13. Dennis C, Moreno JR, Hall DP et al: Studies on external counterpulsation as a potential measure for acute left heart failure, *Trans Am Soc Artif Intern Organs* 9:186, 1963.
14. Osborn JJ, Russi M, Salel A et al: Circulatory assistance by external pulsed pressures, *Am J Med Electronics* 3:87, 1964.
15. Birtwell W, Giron F, Soroff H et al: Support of the systemic circulation and left ventricular assist by synchronous pulsation of extramural pressure, *Trans Am Soc Artif Intern Organs* 11:43, 1965.
16. Osborn JJ, Main FB, Gerbode FL: Circulatory support by leg or airway pulses in experimental mitral insufficiency, *Circulation* 28:781, 1963.
17. Goldfarb D, McGinnis GE, Balinger WF II: Am improved system for diastolic augmentation, *Trans Am Soc Artif Intern Organs* 11:31, 1965.
18a. Watkins DH, Duchesne ER: Postsystolic myocardial augmentation, *Arch Surg* 82:839, 1961.
18b. Watkins DH, Callaghan PB: Postsystolic myocardial augmentation, *Arch Surg* 90:544, 1965.
19. Salisbury PF, Cross CE, Rieben PA et al: Physiological mechanisms which explain the effects of veno-arterial pumping and of left ventricular bypass in experimental heart failure, *Trans Am Soc Artif Intern Organs* 6:176, 1960.
20. Dennis C, Hall DP, Moreno JR et al: Left atrial cannulation without thoracotomy for total left heart bypass, *Acta Chir Scand* 123:267, 1962.
21. Nosé Y, Russell F, Gradel F et al: A long-term operation of an electronically controlled, plastic, auxiliary ventricle in conscious dogs, *Trans Am Soc Artif Inter Organs* 10:140, 1964.
22. Kantrowitz A, Gradel FO, Akutsu T: The auxiliary ventricle, IEEE International Convention Record, part 12:20, 1965.
23. Chaptal PA, Skutsu T, Kantrowitz A: Hemodynamic effects of a mechanical auxiliary ventricle following induced heart failure in dogs, *J Thorac Cardiovasc Surg* 52:3786, 1966.
24. Kantrowitz A, Akutsu T, Chaptal PA et al: A clinical experience with an implanted mechanical auxiliary ventricle, *JAMA* 197:525, 1966.
25. Kantrowitz A, Krakauer JS, Rosenbaum A et al: Phase-shift balloon pumping in medically refractory cardiogenic shock: results in 27 patients, *Arch Surg* 99:739, 1969.
26. Scheidt S, Wilner G, Mueller H et al: Intraaortic balloon counterpulsation in cardiogenic shock. Report of a co-operative clinical trial, *N Engl J Med* 288:979, 1973.
27. Bregman D, Kripke DC, Goetz RH: The effect of synchronous unidirectional intraaortic balloon pumping on hemodynamics and coronary blood flow in cardiogenic shock, *Trans Am Soc Artif Intern Organs* 16:439, 1970.
28. Buckley MJ, Lenbach RC, Kastor JA et al: Hemodynamic evaluation of intraoartic balloon pumping in man, *Circulation* 46(suppl II):130, 1970.
29. Feola M, Adachi M, Akers WW et al: Intraaortic balloon pumping in the experimental animal. Effects and problems, *Am J Cardiol* 27:129, 1971.
30. Buckley MJ: Hemodynamic evaluation of intraaortic balloon pumping in man, *Circulation* 41(suppl II):130, 1970.

31. Mundth ED, Yurchak PM, Buckley MJ et al: Circulatory assistance and emergency direct artery surgery for shock complicating acute infarction, *N Engl J Med* 283:1382, 1970.

32. Normal JD: Mechanical circulatory assistance and replacement: an evolving perspective, *Bull Texas Heart Institute* 4:445, 1980.

33. Bregman D, Goetz RH: A new concept in circulatory assistance—the dual-chambered intraaortic balloon, *Mt Sinai J Med* 39:123, 1972.

34. Kantrowitz A, Freed PS, Cardona PR et al: Initial clinical trial of a closed loop, fully automated intra-aortic balloon pump, *ASAIO Trans* 38:M617, 1992.

35. Zelano JA, Li JKJ, Welkowitz A: A closed loop control scheme for intraaortic balloon pumping, *IEEE Trans Biomed Eng* 37:182, 1990.

36. Philipe E, Clark JW, Lande A et al: Microprocessor control of intra-aortic balloon pumping, *Ann Biomed Eng* 8:209, 1980.

37. Kantrowitz A: Origins of intraaortic balloon pumping, *Ann Thorac Surg* 50:672, 1990.

38. Kantrowitz A, Cardona RR, Freed PS: Percutaneous intraaortic balloon counterpulsation, *Crit Care Clin* 8:819, 1992.

39. Pollock JC, Charlton MC, Williams WG et al: Intraaortic balloon pumping in children, *Ann Thorac Surg* 29:522, 1980.

40. Miller DC, Moreno-Cabral RF, Stinson EB et al: Pulmonary artery balloon counterpulsation for acute right ventricular failure, *J Thorac Cardiovasc Surg* 80:760, 1980.

41. Kantrowitz A: In-series temporary and permanent cardiac assistance. In Kantrowitz A, ed: *ASAIO primers in artificial organs, no 3, Ventricular assist devices*, Philadelphia, 1988, JB Lippincott.

42. Cardona RR, Rios C, Freed PS et al: Experimental models for studies of a closed loop, fully automatic intraaortic balloon pump. In *Programs and Abstracts of the AAMI Cardiovascular Science and Technology Conference*, Bethesda, MD, 1991.

43. Kantrowitz A, Cardona RR, Au J et al: Intraaortic balloon pumping in congestive heart failure. In Hosenpud JD, Greenberg BH, eds: *Congestive heart failure: pathophysiology, differential diagnosis, and comprehensive approach to therapy*, New York, Springer-Verlag (in press).

44. Kantrowitz A, Krakauer J, Rubenfire M et al: Initial clinical experience with a new permanent mechanical auxiliary ventricle: the dynamic aortic patch, *Trans Am Soc Artif Intern Organs* 18:159, 1972.

45. Kantrowitz A: Introduction of left ventricular assistance, *ASAIO Trans* 10:39, 1987.

46. Quaal SJ, ed: *Cardiac mechanical assistance beyond balloon pumping*, St Louis, 1993, Mosby–Year Book.

CHAPTER 26

St. Jude Medical, Inc., Cardiac Assist Division Model 700 IABP Control System

Pamela Kasold

SYSTEM COMPONENTS

The St. Jude Medical, Inc., Cardiac Assist Division Model 700 IABP Control System[1,2] (Fig. 26-1) can be divided into two sections—the top panel and the side panel. The top panel contains the message center, two-channel monitor with recorder, monitor controls, and the pump drive controls. The right side panel contains the volume limiter disk (VLD), helium tank and gauge, and the I/O panel for ECG and transducer cables.

Top panel

The top panel consists of the message center, monitor, recorder, and lead selection (Fig. 26-2).

Message center. The message center displays VLD volume (size) of 30, 40, or 50 cc; and heart rate and alarm/status messages.

Monitor. On the monitor, channel 1 displays patient ECG. Channel 2 displays either the arterial pressure, balloon pressure, or assist marker waveform.

Recorder. The operator has the choice to record upper trace (ECG) or lower trace (arterial pressure, balloon pressure, or assist marker).

Lead selection. The operator when using the ECG (skin lead) cable may select Lead I, II, or III.

Monitor controls

Channel 2—Three-position switch. Operator may select to view arterial pressure, balloon pressure, or assist marker waveform.

Pressure Range—Three-position switch. Operator may choose scale of 0 to 60, 0 to 150, or 0 to 300 mm Hg.

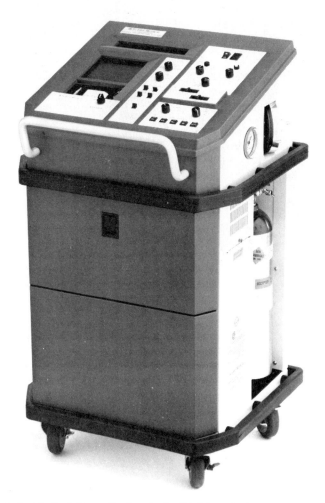

Fig. 26-1. St. Jude Medical, Inc., Cardiac Assist Division Model 700 IABP Control System.

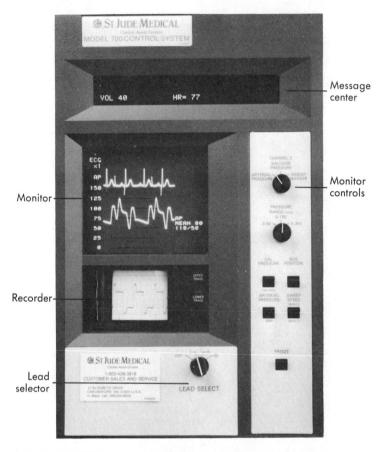

Fig. 26-2. Model 700 IABP Control System: top panel shows the message center, monitor, monitor controls, recorder, and lead selector.

Arterial pressure

Zero. When direct transducer is used, after opening to the atmosphere, the operator must depress and hold the zero switch for 2 seconds.

Calibration. Depressing the switch establishes 100 mm Hg square wave calibration signal.

ECG position

Two-position switch allows operator to change position of ECG on monitor screen.

Sweep speed

Two-position switch with the choice of 25 or 50 mm/sec sweep.

Freeze

Two-position switch to freeze/unfreeze monitor screen.

Pump controls

Pump controls are illustrated in Fig. 26-3.

Power control and indicators—Rocker switch establishes power. Indicator lamps communicate the following with the operator: *green,* console connected to AC power (wall outlet); *yellow,* power is ON (AC); *blue,* power is ON (battery).

Alarm indicator—Red light flashes indicate status/alarm message.

Trigger indicator—White light flashes once with each trigger event.

ECG input–Rotary switch—Operator may select signal from skin leads or external monitor.

ECG gain–Rotary switch—Clockwise rotation increases amplification of ECG signal.

Trigger mode–rotary step switch—Operator may select one of the following: R sense, QRS sense, Pacer reject, AV Sequential Pacer Arterial pressure, or Internal 80 BPM (see Table 26-1).

Inflate/deflate controls–slide pots—These controls allow operator to adjust timing earlier or later in the cardiac cycle. Numerical references of 0 to 5 are included, with midpoints (2.5/2.5) noted in red.

Wean control–rotary step switch—Operator may select assist ratio of 1:1, 1:2, 1:4, or 1:8.

% Volume–rotary step switch—Full clockwise rotation delivers 100% volume displacement of VLD.

Pump drive controls–push buttons—Once depressed, button is illuminated and activates functions as follows:

OFF	Stops pumping, vents line of helium
STN	Standby—Stops pumping, operator may initiate manual fill by depressing button for 4 seconds
FILL	Initiates auto-purge
ON	Initiates pumping
AUTO	Initiates activation of gas surveillance and leak alarms

Side panel

The side panel is illustrated in Fig. 26-4.

The VLD is inserted into the housing and is locked in place by putting lever in DOWN position. The helium gauge (0 to 3000 psi) indicates helium remaining in tank. The I/O panel contains connector fittings for ECG cable or phono jack connec-

Text continued on p. 438.

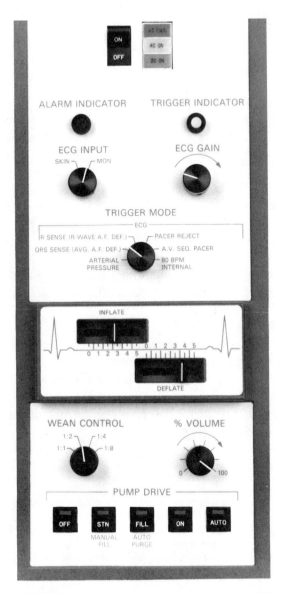

Fig. 26-3. Model 700 IABP Control System: pump controls. Power ON, alarm/trigger indicator lights, ECG input, ECG gain, trigger selector, inflate/deflate controls, wean control, % volume, and pump drive controls.

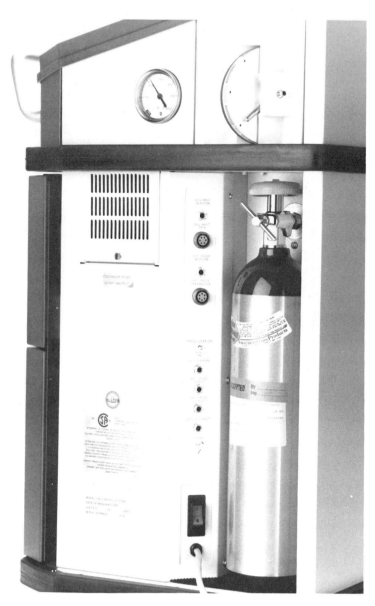

Fig. 26-4. Model 700 IABP Control System: side panel. VLD, helium tank and gauge, and I/O panel.

Table 26-1. Model 700 trigger modes

Trigger	Signal detected		Use for	Not recommended for
QRS Sense (Avg AF DEF)	QRS complex Deflection and reversal of polarity over 135 msec window (pacer spikes rejected) Irregular rhythm: averages 8 R-R intervals for inflate and deflate	135 msec	Normal QRS Most wide QRS Paced rhythms	Ventricular block Extremely variable QRS width Paced rhythms with loss of capture
R-Sense (R wave AF DEF)	R wave/pacer spike Deflection over 25 msec window Irregular rhythm: deflates only on R wave, deflate control inoperative	25 msec	Normal QRS Wide QRS V-paced rhythms	A-paced rhythms A-V paced rhythms
Pacer Reject	R wave Pacer spike rejected Deflection over 25 msec window	Reject 25 msec	A-paced rhythms A-V paced rhythms	Paced rhythms with loss of capture

Continued.

Table 26-1. Model 700 trigger modes—cont'd

Trigger	Signal detected	Use for	Not recommended for
A-V Sequential Pacer	Interval pattern V-A interval (long) A-V interval (short) then trigger	100% *fixed* A-V paced rhythms	Demand paced rhythms
Arterial Pressure	≥20 mm Hg difference between systole and diastole	"Back-up trigger" ECG trigger/signal is unobtainable Cardiac arrest, use with CPR	Arterial lines with interference due to manipulation (frequent, zero, flushing, or blood drawing) Irregular rhythms due to change in systolic upstroke
Internal	Asynchronous mode 80 = (1:1), 40 = (1:2), 20 = (1:4), 10 = (1:8)	Cardiac arrest Cardiopulmonary bypass	Patient with existing rhythm, pulse, and blood pressure

tions, arterial pressure transducer or phono jack, calibration pot for transducer, output connections, and alarm volume.

Air intake filter is a plastic foam filter that maintains electronic components dust free. The circuit breaker–rocker switch should be ON at all times.

THEORY OF OPERATION

The St. Jude Medical, Inc., Cardiac Assist Division Model 700 IABP is designed to shuttle a predetermined amount of helium to and from the IAB catheter. This is accomplished by a VLD (Fig. 26-5).

The VLD is available in 30, 40, or 50 cc sizes. The disk size should match that of the IAB. The VLD is made of aluminum and contains a diaphragm to isolate the helium to the patient side of the disk. When the operator presses and holds the standby STN switch for 4 seconds, a Manual Fill is initiated. The fill valve will open, and the patient side of the VLD will fill with helium. Pressure and vacuum are applied alternately to the instrument side of the diaphragm, causing it to move, shuttling the helium in and out of the balloon. This is demonstrated in the schematic drawing of the VLD in Fig. 26-6.

Each VLD is color coded and marked with the volume it displaces. A light bar-coding device in the console analyzes the bar code on the disk. The size is then displayed on the message center. To ensure proper operation, the VLD should be re-

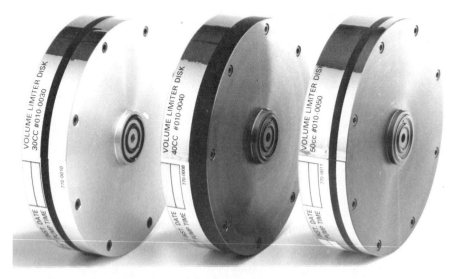

Fig. 26-5. VLD: 30, 40, and 50 cc sizes.

placed after every 1000 hours or 6 months of use. For a summary of set-up instructions, see the box on p. 441.

TIMING

The Model 700 uses a physiologically based *triggering* signal in conjunction with operator synchronized *timing* to regulate balloon inflation and deflation relative to the diastolic phase of the cardiac cycle.

Relative or "rough" timing may be established before initiating counterpulsation. Inflation and deflation controls may be seen on the ECG (inflate marker as a positive deflection, deflate marker as a negative deflection) to assist the clinician. By placing the inflate and deflate controls on 2.5 and 2.5, respectively, the inflate and deflate markers should appear on the ECG as seen in Fig. 26-7. NOTE: If R wave deflation is occurring, the deflate marker will be within the QRS complex.

The operator may also use the Assist Marker for assessment of relative timing. By placing the Channel 2 selector on Assist Marker, the ECG inflate and deflate markers are removed and an analog square wave will be seen on Channel 2. This square wave represents the inflate/deflate cycle.

Once pumping is initiated, assess the arterial waveform for optimal inflation and deflation. The Model 700 will adjust automatically for changes in heart rate on a beat-to-beat basis; however, the operator may intervene and adjust the timing as necessary.

SYSTEM ALARMS INTERPRETATIONS AND RESPONSES

For a summary of alarm interpretations and responses, see Table 26-2.

TROUBLESHOOTING GUIDELINES

Use the following four Priority Checkpoints with the balloon pressure waveform to assist in troubleshooting:

√ Patient   √ Condensation
√ Blood   √ Loose connections or kinks in airway tubing

Cardiac arrest/defibrillation

In the event of cardiac arrest, the Model 700 may be placed on either Arterial Pressure or Internal 80 BPM trigger modes. The system is protected up to 500 joules should defibrillation be necessary.

Text continued on p. 444.

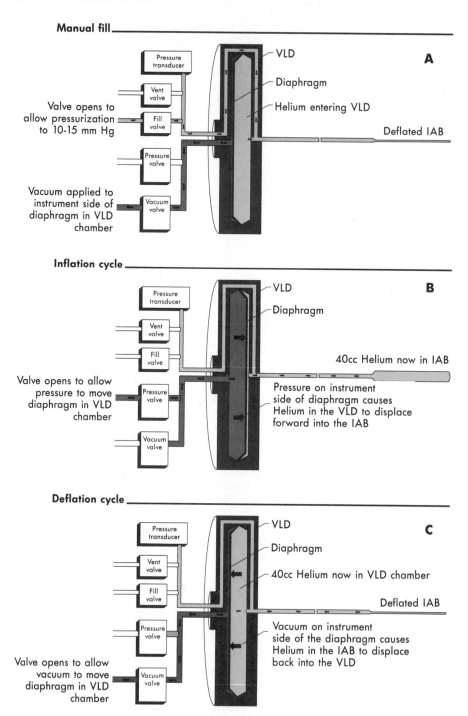

Fig. 26-6. A, Manual fill (operator initiated by pressing and holding the standby (STN) button for 4 seconds). **B,** Inflation cycle. **C,** Deflation cycle.

SET-UP INSTRUCTIONS FOR MODEL 700 IABP CONTROL SYSTEM

The three quick steps for start-up

Step 1—Power up
Verify AC circuit breaker (red switch) is ON.
Plug console into AC outlet.
Turn console power ON.

Step 2—Remember the "HEART" acronym

H	Helium	Is the tank open?
		≥200 psi on gauge?
E	ECG	Attach ECG skin leads or phono cable.
		Select ECG Input—skin or monitor.
		Select best lead and adjust ECG
		gain as needed.
A	Arterial line	Attach transducer or phono cable.
		Zero transducer.
R	Relative timing	Place inflate/deflate controls on 2.5/2.5 (*red* markers).
		Assess timing markers.
T	Trigger	Choose *most* appropriate one for patient's rhythm.
		Verify trigger light flashing appropriately.

(NOTE: Check message center before proceeding to Step 3.)

Step 3—Attach IAB catheter and initiate pump drive

OFF	Stops pumping.
	Vents line of helium.
STN	Stops pumping. Helium remains in system.
	To initiate Manual Fill—Hold for 4 sec. Check balloon pressure waveform (BPW) for fill baseline of 10 to 15 mm Hg.
FILL	Initiates Autopurge. Auto is necessary *only* for initial start-up and when airway tubing has been opened to atmosphere.
	On completion, system will alarm and display "Purge Complete."
ON	Initiates pumping.
	"Manual" mode GAS ALARMS OFF.
	NOTE: Gas surveillance *off*. Operator *must* autopurge every 1 to 2 hours to compensate for normal helium diffusion.
AUTO	Initiates leak detection (alarms).
	Initiates gas surveillance.

Once pumping is initiated, assess timing and fine tune as necessary to achieve optimal results.

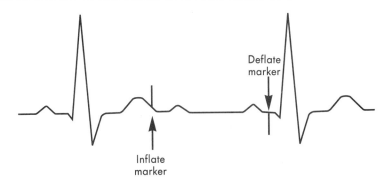

Inflate
marker

Deflate
marker

Fig. 26-7. ECG timing markers are adjusted using the inflation and deflation slide controls. Proper placement is achieved by positioning the inflate marker just after the T wave and the deflate marker between the P wave and the QRS complex.

Table 26-2. System alarms interpretations and responses

Alarm/message	Possible cause	Solution
High gas leakage (auto mode only)	IAB leak/abrasion	Check for blood in tubing. Stop pumping. Contact physician to remove IAB as soon as possible.
	Condensation in extension tubing or VLD	Remove condensation from tubing *and* VLD. Refill, autopurge, and resume pumping.
	Kink in IAB catheter or tubing	Check catheter and tubing for kinks or loose connections. Refill and resume pumping.
	Tachycardia: Insufficient fill pressure baseline due to rapid shuttle of helium	Change wean control to 1:2 or operate in ON (manual) mode. NOTE: *Gas alarms off in ON mode. Autopurge IAB every 1-2 hours and monitor BPW closely.*
	Malfunctioning or loose VLD	Replace or tighten VLD. Refill, autopurge, and resume pumping.
Balloon line block (auto mode only)	System leak	Contact St. Jude Medical Field Service.
	Kink in IAB catheter or tubing	Check catheter and tubing for kinks. Refill and resume pumping.
	IAB did not unfurl	Contact physician to manually inflate IAB, reposition sheath or IAB catheter.
	Sheath positioned too high, or IAB positioned too high Condensation in tubing and/or VLD	Remove condensation from tubing *and* VLD. Refill, autopurge, and resume pumping.
	Balloon too large for aorta	Decrease % volume control by one notch.
	Malfunctioning/incorrect size VLD	Replace VLD, refill, autopurge, and resume pumping.
No ECG trigger	Inadequate signal	Adjust ECG gain, change lead/trigger mode.
	Lead disconnected	Replace lead.
	Improper ECG Input (skin/monitor) selected	Adjust ECG input to appropriate mode (skin or monitor).
No AP trigger	Arterial line dampened	Flush line.
	Arterial line open to atmosphere	Check connections on arterial pressure line. Attempt to pump in ECG.
Trigger mode change	Trigger mode changed while pumping	Resume pumping.
Irregular rhythm	Patient in irregular rhythm (atrial fibrillation, ectopics, and so on)	Change to R sense or QRS sense (if necessary) to accommodate irregular rhythm.

Erratic AV pacing	Demand paced rhythm while in AV Sequential Pacer trigger	Change to Pacer Reject trigger or QRS sense.
Noisy ECG signal	Check leads	Replace leads/check ECG cable.
	Electrocautery in use	Switch to Arterial Pressure trigger.
Internal trigger	Trigger mode set on Internal 80 BPM	Select alternative trigger if patient has heart beat or rhythm. NOTE: *Internal trigger should be used only during cardiopulmonary bypass or cardiac arrest.*
Autopurge ON	Autopurge initiated	Initiate pumping when message "Purge Complete" is displayed.
Purge complete	Autopurge cycle completed	Initiate pumping.
Purge incomplete	Operator depressed OFF during autopurge, interrupting purge cycle	Initiate autopurge again or initiate pumping.
High fill pressure	Malfunctioning VLD	Replace VLD, refill, autopurge, and resume pumping.
	Occluded vent line or valve	Attempt to resume pumping. If unsuccessful, contact St. Jude Medical Field Service.
No drive pressure	Possible compressor or system malfunction	Contact St. Jude Medical Field Service.
No vacuum	Loose VLD; catheter disconnected	Verify placement of VLD; check connections.
	Malfunctioning VLD	Replace VLD.
	System malfunction	Contact St. Jude Medical Field Service.
	No VLD	Insert VLD, lock securely in place.
No balloon drive	Tubing disconnected	Reconnect tubing, refill, autopurge, and resume pumping.
Check timing	Inflate and deflate controls improperly set	Place inflate/deflate controls at midpoints. Reassess timing, adjust as necessary.
Low % volume	% Volume control not on 100%	Assess reason for decreased volume, reset if necessary.
Helium low	Helium tank turned off	Open helium tank.
	Helium tank has less than 15 psi	Change helium tank.
Low battery	Less than 20 minutes battery time remaining	Plug into AC outlet. Check circuit breaker to assure proper setting.
Gas alarms OFF	Circuit breaker (red switch) OFF	Press Auto to initiate Gas Surveillance/Leak Alarms.
	System in Manual (ON) mode	If unable, monitor balloon pressure waveform closely and autopurge system every 1-2 hours.
	Gas surveillance/leak alarms off	
Pumping stopped	Pumping interrupted by operator/system in standby	Resume pumping.

Battery operation

To place the IABP on battery, do the following:
1. Verify AC circuit breaker is on.
2. Unplug console from wall outlet.
3. Verify DC Main light is on.
4. Battery has 1.5 hours time limit.
5. "LO BATT" message will be displayed and console will beep once every 20 seconds when less than 20 minutes battery time remains.
6. Plug into wall outlet to recharge. Charge time is 12 hours.

NOTE: To maintain a fully charged battery, keep console plugged in at all times.

Condensation removal

Condensation may develop in the airway extension tubing and VLD with prolonged use. This moisture should be removed periodically to ensure optimum functioning of the system.

To remove condensation, do the following:
1. Place pump drive to STN.
2. Disconnect IAB airway tubing from VLD.
3. Place pump to ON to remove moisture from VLD. Allow system to pump for 15 to 20 seconds.
4. Disconnect IAB tubing at white connector junction and do one of the following:
   a. Gently shake tubing to dispel moisture.
   b. Connect tubing to O_2 outlet or suction source to remove moisture.
5. Place pump drive to STN or OFF.
6. Reconnect IAB tubing to patient *and* IABP console.
7. Press STN for four seconds to initiate Manual Fill.
8. Press FILL to initiate Auto Purge.
9. When purge complete, press ON and AUTO to resume pumping.

USE OF THE BALLOON PUMP CONSOLE IN AIR TRANSPORT

The Model 700 IABP can also act as a full-function IABP for use during ground or air transport situations. No special equipment is required for transport outside the hospital setting other than 115 V AC power supply if intending to use the IABP for longer than the battery capacity.

SYSTEM SPECIFICATIONS
General

Size	18 × 20 × 36 inches (45.72 × 50.80 × 91.44 cm)
Weight	180 lb (81.8 kg) including helium tank and batteries

ECG section

Common Mode Rejection	>100 lb with respect to chassis ground (at 60 Hz)
Input	Protected against damage from 500 J defibrillator and electrosurgery voltages
Patient Isolation	Fully isolated
Lead Selection	I, II, III
ECG Position	Channel 1, fully adjustable
Input Connector	MS Type 6 pin
Patient Cable	3-Lead, low noise, filtered
System Output	×1000 gain ±5% single ended
High Level Input	Standard ¼″ Phono Cable

Pressure section

Ranges (display only)	Front panel selective:
	0-60 mm Hg
	0-150 mm Hg
	0-300 mm Hg
Transducer	Part #070-0016 or equivalent for Physio Control VSM-1 Monitor
Input Connector (Transducer)	MS Type 6 pin
Input Connector (High Level)	¼″ Phono Cable 100 mm Hg/V

Triggering section

ECG Mode	R Sense
	QRS Sense
	Pacer Reject
Pressure Mode	Arterial Pressure
Internal	Internal, 80 BPM

Analog display section

Sweep Speeds	25 and 50 mm/sec free running (switch selectable)
Display Type	Dual trace
Channel 1	ECG
Channel 2 (Selectable)	Arterial pressure, balloon pressure or assist marker
Freeze Capability	Freezes both traces simultaneously
Alphanumeric Display	Status and alarm messages
	Heart rate
	VLD volume (size)
	Pressures:
	Peak Systolic
	End-Diastolic
	Mean

Recorder section

Dual Channel Recorder	Single trace; selectable to channel 1 or channel 2. Thermal dot matrix Standard 4 cm strip chart paper 2 speeds; 25 or 50 mm/sec

Alarm section

Audible Alarm	Volume Control (min-max)

Pneumatics section

Pumping volume	Controlled by operation selection and insertion of a calibrated volume limiter disk (VLD) 30, 40, or 50 cc size
Shuttle Gas	Medical grade helium D size cylinder

Power section

AC Power Input	Factory Set 105-125 V AC or 210-250 AC (50 Hz) and 90-110 V (50/60 Hz) <4 A peak at 115 V 5 A surge current
Battery Capacity	1.5 hours full system operation, fully charged
Battery Recharge Time	12 hours

RESOURCES

St. Jude Medical, Inc.
Cardiac Assist Division
12 Elizabeth Drive
Chelmsford, Mass 01824
508-250-8020 (Mass only)
1-800-438-3818 (outside Mass)
508-250-1722 (Fax)

St. Jude Medical Europe, Inc., Belgian Branch
Excelsiorlaan 79
1930 Zaventem
Brussels, Belgium
011-32-27-196-811 (Telephone)
011-32-27-255-162 (Fax)

REFERENCES

1. St. Jude Medical, Inc., Cardiac Assist Division: *Operator's Manual for the Model 700 IABP*, Chelmsford, Mass.
2. St. Jude Medical, Inc., Cardiac Assist Division: *Redi-Guide for the Model 700 IABP*, Chelmsford, Mass.

CHAPTER 27

Datascope Systems 95 and 90T

Debra L. Joseph and **Kathleen Beaver**

The Datascope Systems 95 (Fig. 27-1) and 90T (Fig. 27-2) IABPs share similar theories of operation and troubleshooting guidelines. The System 95 is a console unit used primarily at the patient's hospital bedside. The System 90T is a transport IABP designed for air or ground transport, as well as in the hospital. The specifications for Systems 95 and 90T are listed in Tables 27-1 and 27-2. In this chapter, the theory of operation, set-up, triggers, alarm systems, and troubleshooting guidelines are discussed.

THEORY OF OPERATION

Datascope IABP Systems are designed to operate under three key guidelines: (1) maximal patient safety, (2) simplicity of operation, and (3) wide-ranging capability.

Patient safety

All Datascope IABP Systems use a closed gas system featuring total patient isolation. A fixed volume of gas is shuttled between the System 90T safety chamber or the System 95 safety disk and the patient balloon. This fixed volume is continually monitored to alert operators to potential gas losses or increases in gas pressure that may indicate a restricted catheter. The closed system is automatically purged and refilled every 2 hours to ensure that the volume and purity of the gas system is maintained for maximal pumping efficiency and accurate alarm operation. A unique diastolic augmentation alarm alerts operators to changes in patient conditions that cause the augmented diastolic pressure to fall below operator-selected limits. The System 95 automatically sets the augmentation alarm on initial set-up.

Simplicity of operation

Whenever possible, the Datascope IABP is designed to free operators from tedious timing and other operational adjustments, allowing the operator to focus on patient care. On initial set-up, both Systems 95 and 90T automatically default to the

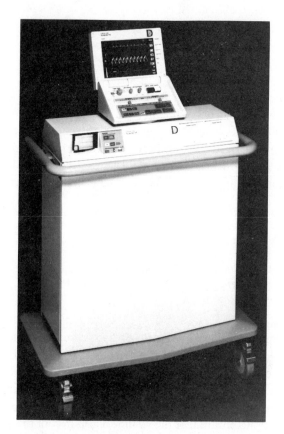

Fig. 27-1. The Datascope System 95 IABP.

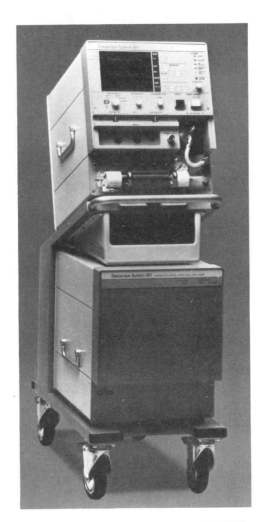

Fig. 27-2. The Datascope System 90T IABP.

Table 27-1. Key technical specifications of the Datascope System 95 IABP*

Feature	System 95
Trigger selections	ECG
	Arterial pressure
	Pacer A
	Pacer V/A-V
	Internal—variable 40 to 120 beats/minute
Heart rate range	0 to 198 beats/minute
Electrosurgical interference suppression	Automatic when internal ECG amplifier is used
Pacer rejection	Automatic
Weaning selections and frequency	1:1, 1:2, 1:3
Volume weaning	Yes
Portable operation	1.5 hours minimum
ECG trigger threshold	120 μV ± 20 μV (ECG gain = NORM)
ECG gain	NORM position × 1000
	Variable ×150 to ×3000
Pressure trigger threshold	15 mm Hg
Alarm categories	System surveillance
	Trigger
	IAB catheter
	Pneumatic drive
Alerts	Messages are displayed in the ADVISORY section
Status/Prompts	Messages are displayed in the ADVISORY section
ECG leads	I, II, III, AVR, AVL, AVF, V
Voltage interface requirements	
ECG	1 V/1 mV nominal
Pressure	1 V/100 mm Hg
Size	48"H × 33"W × 19"D
Weight	80 kg
Recorder	Dual channel chart recorder
Trend	8-hour trend

* More detailed specifications are available from the manufacturer.

most commonly used monitoring parameters. Set-up steps for Systems 95 and 90T are listed in the boxes of pp. 452-454. The automatic timing system instantaneously adjusts to changes in patient rate and rhythm, once the operator sets the initial timing appropriately. Electrosurgical interference suppression and pacemaker rejection are fully automatic in ECG trigger. Optimal fill volume is maintained through periodic automatic purging and refilling of the systems once every 2 hours. The alarm system is designed to alert operators to changing patient and pump conditions but interrupts pumping only when conditions require immediate operator intervention. Concise messages direct operators to the cause of an alarm condition. The System 95 provides user-selected HELP screens for assistance in troubleshooting alarm and alert conditions.

Table 27-2.   Key technical specifications of the Datascope System 90T IABP*

Feature	System 90T
Trigger selections	ECG
	Arterial pressure
	Pacer V
	Pacer AV
	Internal
Heart rate range	0 to 198 beats/minute
Electrosurgical interference suppression	Automatic when internal ECG amplifier is used
Pacer rejection	Automatic
Weaning selections and frequency	1:2, 1:3
Volume weaning	Yes
Portable operation	2 hours typical
ECG trigger threshold	120 μV ± 20 μV
Pressure trigger threshold	15 mm Hg
Alarms	Trigger
	Gas loss
	IAB catheter
	Pneumatic drive
	System failure
Alerts	Diastolic augmentation
	Low helium
	Low battery
ECG leads	I, II, III, aVR, aVL, aVF, V
Voltage interface requirements	
Arterial pressure	1 V/100 mm Hg
ECG	1 V/1mV
Size	Monitor and pump modules: 16"H × 14"W × 18"D
Weight	50.4 kg
Other	Disconnect mode
	Stretcher configuration
	Aircraft mounting brackets

* More detailed specifications are available from the manufacturer.

Wide-ranging capability

While simplicity of operation is a key design goal, Datascope also recognizes that certain patient conditions may warrant intervention and IABP capability beyond normal operation. Therefore the Systems 95 and 90T feature optional manual timing and fill capability to allow the operator to optimize the timing and fill for those circumstances when fully automatic operation is not optimal. Manual timing allows the operator to adjust inflation and deflation over the complete range of the cardiac cycle without overriding the safety of the R-wave deflation. Manual fill allows the operator to use pediatric catheters effectively, as well as provides a backup system in the event of a fill system failure.

SET-UP OF DATASCOPE SYSTEM 95 IABP

Step 1: Establish power.

A. Plug power cord into AC outlet.
B. Main power switch—ON.
C. Pull and turn TRIGGER SELECT switch—ECG.

NOTE: The system will automatically perform a system check. When the check is completed, "SYSTEM TEST OK" will appear on the monitor screen. This test takes approximately 10 seconds.

Step 2: Establish gas pressure.

A. Open helium tank.

Step 3: Establish ECG and pressure.

A. Plug ECG cable into ECG six-pin connector.
B. Attach arterial line to Datascope-compatible transducer and plug into PRESSURE TRANSDUCER. "NO ZERO" will appear on the monitor screen next to SYSTOLIC.

Step 4: Zero the transducer.

A. Open the transducer to air.
B. Depress the ZERO key for 3 seconds. Two audible clicks and a spike on the pressure trace will appear.
C. Close the transducer. Systolic, diastolic, and mean pressure values will be displayed.

Step 5: Confirm initial pump settings.

A. Front panel controls
   Trigger select—ECG
   IAB frequency—1:1
   IAB augmentation—OFF
   IAB inflation—Midpoint
   IAB deflation—Midpoint
B. Override controls
   Timing—Auto
   IAB fill—Auto
   Slow gas loss alarm—ON
C. Auxiliary controls
   ECG gain—Norm
   Internal trigger—Fixed 80 beats/minute

Step 6: Set the initial timing.

A. Adjust the IAB INFLATION and DEFLATION controls to position the intensified portion of the arterial waveform to begin at the dicrotic notch and end before the upstroke of the systolic pressure.

Step 7: Fill the IAB catheter.

A. Attach the IAB catheter and the appropriate extender to the safety disk.
B. Depress and hold the IAB FILL switch until the "AUTO FILLING" message appears in the upper left corner of the display. When the message clears, proceed.

SET-UP OF DATASCOPE SYSTEM 95 IABP—cont'd

Step 8: Initiate pumping.

A. Depress the ASSIST/STANDBY switch.

B. Rotate the IAB AUGMENTATION dial to MAX. Observe proper diastolic augmentation on the screen.

C. Fine-tune the timing for optimal augmentation and hemodynamic unloading by adjusting the IAB INFLATION and DEFLATION controls if needed.

Step 9: Verify AUG ALARM.

A. Verify that the AUG ALARM setting is approximately 10 mm Hg less than the patient's diastolic augmentation pressure.

B. Adjust, if needed, by depressing AUG ALARM and using the arrow keys to change the value displayed on the screen.

SET-UP OF DATASCOPE SYSTEM 90T IABP

Step 1: Establish power.

A. Plug power cord into AC outlet.

B. Mains power switch—ON.

C. Pull and turn TRIGGER SELECT switch—ECG.

NOTE: The system will automatically perform a system check. Alarm lights will illuminate, and then each will illuminate for 2 seconds. When the check is completed, "SYSTEM TEST OK" will appear on the monitor screen.

Step 2: Establish gas pressure.

A. Open helium tank.

Step 3: Initial control settings.

A. Front panel controls
   IAB frequency—1:1
   IAB augmentation—Min
   IAB inflation—At the midpoint
   IAB deflation—At the midpoint
   Timing—Auto
   IAB fill—Auto
   Slow gas loss alarm—ON

Step 4: Establish ECG and pressure.

A. Plug ECG cable into ECG six-pin connector.

B. Attach arterial line to Datascope-compatible transducer and plug into PRESSURE TRANSDUCER of System 90T. Flashing "XXX" will appear on the monitor screen next to SYS.

Continued.

SET-UP OF DATASCOPE SYSTEM 90T IABP—cont'd

C. Zero the transducer by opening the transducer to air and pushing the ZERO button for 3 seconds. Two audible clicks and a spike on the pressure trace will appear. "MEAN PRESSURE ONLY" will be displayed on the monitor screen.

Step 5: Initial timing.

A. Adjust IAB INFLATION and IAB DEFLATION controls to position the intensified portion of the arterial waveform to correspond to diastole.

Step 6: Preload the IAB.

A. Attach the IAB catheter with the appropriate extender to the safety chamber.
B. Press IAB FILL for 1 second. The AUTO FILLING message will appear on the monitor screen. When the message clears, proceed.

Step 7: Initiating IABC.

A. Depress the ASSIST/STANDBY switch.
B. Rotate the IAB AUGMENTATION dial clockwise until optimal diastolic augmentation is observed during diastole. Optimize augmentation by marking the peak of diastolic augmentation with the reference line. Slowly turn the augmentation dial counterclockwise until diastolic augmentation falls just below the reference line.
C. Fine-tune INFLATION and DEFLATION points for optimal augmentation and hemodynamic unloading.
D. Depress the DISPLAY KEY. Systolic, diastolic mean, and diastolic augmentation pressure valves will now appear on the screen.
E. Depress the AUG ALARM SET. Adjust the ALARM VALUE, if necessary.

TRIGGERS AND TIMING
Trigger

The Systems 95 and 90T feature five trigger modes. The trigger modes available on the System 95 include ECG, Pressure, Pacer A, Pacer V/A-V, and Internal. The trigger modes on the System 90T include ECG, Pressure, Pacer V, Pacer A/V, and Internal. The following reviews the trigger modes for the Systems 95 and 90T.

ECG trigger (Systems 95 and 90T)

The most commonly used and most reliable trigger mode is ECG. In this trigger, the onset of the cardiac cycle is signaled by the arrival of the patient R wave on the ECG. The R wave may be positive or negative, but the system requires that the R-wave amplitude be equal to or greater than 120 uV. The trigger circuit dynamically adjusts the R-wave amplitude to ensure that triggering on tall T waves does not occur. Electrosurgical interference suppression and pacemaker rejection are automatically active in ECG trigger.

The System 95 provides the operator with an adjustable ECG gain. When an extremely low or high level ECG signal is encountered, the signal strength can be altered by adjusting the ECG gain located in the auxiliary controls.

Pressure trigger (Systems 95 and 90T)

The Pressure trigger mode of the Systems 95 and 90T uses the systolic upstroke of the arterial pressure waveform to signal the onset of the cardiac cycle. A zeroed transducer and a 15 mm Hg pressure rise are required for adequate trigger recognition. Because of the mechanical delays associated with use of Pressure trigger, this systolic upstroke comes too late in the cardiac cycle to be used as a deflation command, and use of pressure trigger will require that deflation be set before the onset of systole. A status message, "DEFLATE EARLIER," will be displayed to alert the operator if timing is inappropriately set. Note that the Pressure trigger should not be used in the presence of irregular rhythms.

Pacer V (System 90T)

The Pacer V trigger mode uses the ventricular pacer spike to indicate the onset of the cardiac cycle. Pacer V trigger is designed to be used only when the patient R wave is of insufficient amplitude for adequate trigger. Use of Pacer V requires that the patient be 100% paced.

Pacer A/V (System 90T)

Pacer A/V trigger also uses the ventricular pacer spike to signal the onset of the cardiac cycle and, similar to Pacer V, requires that the patient be 100% paced. Because the system must distinguish between the atrial and ventricular pacer spikes, the use of Pacer A/V also requires that the paced rate be less than 110 beats/minute and the A/V interval must be no less than 50 msec and no greater than 250 msec.

Pacer V/A-V (System 95)

In this trigger mode the System 95 has the ability to automatically identify and display the appropriate V or A-V pacer type. The system triggers on the ventricular pulse for either type of pacer, provided there is a 100% paced rhythm. The system recognizes the presence of a ventricular pacer, provided the ventricular pacing interval is fixed and the rate is less than 185 beats/minute. The system recognizes the presence of an atrial-ventricular sequential pacer, provided the A-V interval is between 80 to 225 msec and the rate is less than 125 beats/minute.

Pacer A (System 95)

In Pacer A trigger, the System 95 triggers on the R wave without interference from atrial pacer artifact. This trigger selection is recommended only if atrial pacer tails interfere with R-wave detection when using ECG trigger. Fixed or demand atrial pacing can be used in this trigger mode.

Internal (Systems 95 and 90T)

Internal trigger is designed to be used only when the patient has no cardiac cycle, such as during cardiopulmonary bypass or during ventricular standstill when chest compressions are unable to generate a trigger.

Should the patient begin to generate a valid ECG during use of this trigger, the system will alert the operator with a tone and the message "ECG DETECTED" will be displayed. To ensure patient safety under this condition, both of the systems will automatically deflate whenever a valid R wave is detected.

During Internal trigger, the IAB is inflated and deflated asynchronously at a preset rate. On the System 90T the preset rate is determined by the setting of the IAB frequency switch.

1:1— 120 beats/minute
1:2— 60 beats/minute
1:3— 40 beats/minute

On the System 95 the Internal trigger rate can be adjusted from 40 to 120 beats/minute using the variable Internal trigger switch located in the Auxiliary Controls. In the fixed position the Internal trigger rate is 80 beats/minute.

Timing

The Systems 95 and 90T provide the operator with both AUTO and MANUAL timing.

Auto timing. Auto timing is based on a proprietary algorithm that uses basic physiological principles that have been documented in the literature. In auto timing, the IABP will automatically adjust both inflation and deflation with changes in patient rate and rhythm. During the initial set-up of the IABP, the operator uses the inflation and deflation slide controls to position the intensified waveform on the arterial trace to correspond with diastole. Inflation is positioned to begin at the dicrotic notch, the beginning of diastole. Deflation is positioned to occur just before the upstroke of the next systole. Optimal timing of the IABP results in maximal diastolic augmentation and systolic unloading, as evidenced by alterations in the arterial pressure waveform and positive changes in patient hemodynamics. Changes in heart rate and rhythm result in an instantaneous change in inflation, with deflation changing as a result of an average of the previous four deflation points. The R wave always results in deflation of the patient IAB, if it has not already deflated.

Manual timing. Manual timing is used in those patients that fall outside the range of the auto timing algorithm and in the pediatric IABC patient. Inflation and deflation points are determined using the intensified portion of the arterial waveform as in auto timing. The difference now is that the operator must manually move inflation and deflation points with changes in patient heart rate of $\pm$ 12 beats/minute. In manual timing, each increment on the inflation and deflation slide controls represent 125 msec. The R wave will cause deflation of the patient IAB, if it has not already deflated.

ALARMS, ALERTS, AND STATUS/PROMPTS—SYSTEM 95

In the presence of an alarm, alert, and/or status/prompt condition, messages are displayed in the upper left-hand corner of the monitor screen. Table 27-3 lists the messages and causes for the messages.

Table 27-3. Alarm, alert, and status/prompt messages and causes—System 95

Message	Cause
Trigger	
No trigger	Valid trigger does not exist
No pressure trigger	Valid trigger does not exist while in PRESSURE trigger
No pressure trigger/ zero transducer	Pressure trigger is selected, and transducer has not been zeroed
Trigger interference	Electrosurgical noise while in pacer trigger
Check pacer timing	Pacer trigger requirements have not been met
ECG detected	Electrical activity exists while in internal trigger
Pneumatic alarms	
Autofill failure	IAB could not be automatically filled
Autofill failure/ no helium	IAB could not be adequately filled due to inadequate supply of helium
Autofill required	There has been a switch from manual fill to autofill mode, and an autofill is required
IAB disconnected	IAB or extension tubing disconnected
Rapid gas loss	Large leak in IAB
Leak in IAB circuit	Small gas loss or slow leak in IAB
Check IAB catheter	IAB not fully unwrapped, or a clinically significant kink exists
Blood detected	Blood has migrated into the autofill tubing due to a leak in the IAB
High drive pressure	Component failure in pneumatics
Low vacuum	Insufficient compressor vacuum
System surveillance	
Electrical test fails code	Electrical failure during power-up diagnostics
System failure	Microprocessor or other electronic failure
Safety disk test fails	Leak in safety disk or fittings

Continued.

Table 27-3.   Alarm, alert, and status/prompt messages and causes—System 95—cont'd

Message	Cause
Alerts	
Augmentation below limit set	Diastolic augmentation has dropped below limit set
No patient status available	Software communications failure
Heart rate low	Heart rate <40 beats/minute
Low helium	Helium supply is below 24 fill reserve
Low battery	Battery operation time is 30 minutes or less
Deflation set too late	Pressure trigger with deflation set too late or in the presence of irregular rhythms
Status/Prompts	
Unplug disk outlet	Instructions given during safety disk test
Plug disk outlet	
Leak testing safety disk	
IAB not filled	IAB has not been filled
Manual fill IAB	Notifies the operator when to manually fill the IAB catheter
Autofilling	Notifies the operator the system is refilling the IAB circuit
Slow gas loss override on	Notifies the operator that the alarm disable has been selected
Gas loss and catheter alarms disabled	Operator has selected the manual fill mode
System test OK	Power-up diagnostics test passes
System trainer	Indicates Series 90 trainer in use
Help available for manual fill	Displayed on bottom of screen when user selects manual fill

The System 95 provides the operator with comprehensive HELP SCREENS for all alarms and alerts. In the presence of an alarm or alert message, the operator can use the HELP screens by depressing the HELP key on the control panel. The operator will be provided with step-by-step troubleshooting instructions.

ALARM conditions cause pumping to stop, and a steady tone is sounded.

ALERT conditions do not stop pumping but signal the operator that immediate corrective action is required. A double beep tone will sound.

STATUS/PROMPTS do not sound any tones and are advisory in nature.

The alarm/alert tone can be muted for 30-second intervals by depressing alarm mute.

TROUBLESHOOTING

When troubleshooting the IABP, the operator must be prepared to manage critical patient conditions. The following section highlights specific patient conditions.

Atrial fibrillation

In atrial fibrillation use auto timing and ECG trigger. Adjust the IAB INFLA-TION/DEFLATION controls to position the intensified portion of the arterial waveform to correspond to the period of diastole. IAB DEFLATION may be moved to the extreme right, allowing deflation of the balloon on the R wave.

Ectopy

The Systems 95 and 90T will automatically deflate when an ectopic R wave is sensed, resulting in deflation of the patient balloon. No adjustment of the IABP is required. Treat the ectopy as appropriate.

Ventricular fibrillation

The Systems 95 and 90T are completely isolated from the patient. No danger of harm to the unit or the patient exists during defibrillation. When the signal for "all clear" is given, keep in mind that this now includes all clear of the IABP console.

Cardiac arrest

Use ECG or arterial pressure trigger during CPR. The IABP trigger will synchronize to the chest compressions. Note that the IAB should not be immobile for greater than 30 minutes, due to the potential for thrombus formation around the IAB. When using the System 90T, if chest compressions do not provide adequate trigger to allow balloon movement, turn the TRIGGER SELECT to INTERNAL, IAB FREQUENCY to 1:2, and IAB AUGMENTATION to a level where movement of the safety chamber balloon is observed. When using the System 95, turn the TRIGGER SELECT to INTERNAL, and reduce IAB AUGMENTATION to a level where the IAB STATUS INDICATOR is observed at the halfway point on the monitor screen. If the patient begins generating an ECG during the resuscitation, a message will alert the operator to return to ECG trigger. Reevaluate and readjust timing, once the ECG is reestablished.

Water condensation

During the course of IABC therapy, a fine mist or small droplets of water may be observed in the external pneumatic system. The presence of condensation is normal; however, if excessive condensation is allowed to accumulate, it may affect the pneumatic performance of the IABP. To remove the condensation, follow these steps:

1. Set IAB FILL to MANUAL.
2. Set ASSIST/STANDBY to STANDBY.
3. Disconnect the balloon catheter extender from the patient IAB.
4. Point the tip of the extender downward.

5. Set ASSIST/STANDBY to ASSIST.
6. Pump for approximately 20 to 30 seconds, allowing the water to be expelled from the catheter extender.
7. Set ASSIST/STANDBY to STANDBY.
8. Reconnect the catheter extender to the patient IAB.
9. Set IAB FILL to AUTO.
10. Preload patient balloon by pushing IAB FILL.
11. Resume pumping by pushing ASSIST/STANDBY.

Portable operation

To go from AC power to battery operation, simply unplug the power cord from the AC outlet. The Systems 95 and 90T will automatically switch to portable operation. An amber LED will illuminate to indicate battery operation. When the available battery power falls below 30 minutes, an audible tone will sound. On the System 95 the message LOW BATTERY will be displayed until AC power is resumed. To return to AC power, plug the AC power cord into an AC outlet. The Systems 95 and 90T will automatically switch to AC operation. A green LED will flash, indicating that the battery is charging. Note the main power must be on for the battery to charge.

In the event of a power failure, the Systems 95 and 90T will automatically switch to battery without any operator intervention.

CONSIDERATIONS FOR AIR TRANSPORT

As IABC therapy continues to expand to community-based institutions, the need to move patients expeditiously to tertiary care facilities has also grown. It is therefore important that certain factors unique to air transport of these patients be considered. Currently, the FAA treats the IABP unit itself as cargo and, as such, requires that it meet the following requirements:
• The pump must be secured in such a way to ensure that it will withstand gravitational forces likely to be encountered in turbulent or crash conditions without breaking loose from its mounting.
• Operation of the pump must not interfere with electronic navigational or radio equipment.

FAA requirements

The System 90T has been specifically designed for air transport, and the unit's mounting brackets have been certified to withstand the forces required (as indicated by a certificate of structural substantiation, 8110-C). This certification indicates that the Datascope-supplied mounting brackets will secure the unit appropriately. Interface between the brackets and the aircraft are the responsibility of the aircraft operator.

The System 90T has been tested to D0160-b to ensure that interference with navigational and other electronic equipment does not occur.

Power considerations

The System 90T is designed to operate on batteries, an inverter, or directly from 24-volt DC aircraft power. The internal batteries of the system will generally provide 2 hours of operation when fully charged and spare battery packs are available. Operators should consider both ground and air time when determining power requirements.

Disconnect mode

When transferring the patient to the aircraft, the System 90T features an IABP disconnect mode that enables the operator to disconnect the patient from the equipment for loading into the aircraft and to return easily to pumping without the need to repeat set-up procedures. All IABP settings are maintained for 15 minutes on initiation of this mode.

Patient considerations for air transport

Management of the IABC patient during air transport can be a challenging undertaking, due mainly to the space limitations inherent in most air ambulances. Care of the critically ill patient should follow established air transport standards of care. There is little that is unique to the IABP transport situation.

Of singular importance in managing the patient in the air is ensuring that changes in altitude do not compromise the operation of the patient balloon. It is recommended that the IABP system be purged and refilled every 2000 feet of ascent and descent to ensure that the maximum IABP efficacy and effective alarm limits are maintained. This procedure should be implemented in both pressurized and nonpressurized cabins. Once cruising altitude is maintained, further IABP intervention is generally not required until descent has begun.

RESOURCE

For further information about operation and troubleshooting of the Datascope Systems 95 and 90T, please contact Datascope Corp., 14 Philips Parkway, Montvale, New Jersey 07645; telephone: 1-800-288-2121.

ACKNOWLEDGMENT

The authors would like to thank Annette Fasnacht for her contributions to the section on the System 90T.

CHAPTER 28

Kontron KAAT II and Model 7000

Debra W. Hartigan

The latest generation of intraaortic balloon pump (IABP) systems manufactured by Kontron Instruments, Inc., is the Model 7000 (console) and the Kontron air ambulance transport (KAAT II).

The Model 7000 and KAAT II are advanced microprocessor-based IABP systems. Each pump is designed for patient safety, simplicity, and flexibility to meet the challenge of balloon counterpulsation in today's critical care settings. Each screen displays three-channel, four-color waveforms with alphanumeric physiological data and operating information. Preset operating parameters and dedicated single function control keys simplify operations, allowing more time for patient management. A continually engaged alarm system with a continuously displayed balloon pressure waveform monitors helium exchange, catheter, and pump performance.

In an alarm condition, automatic display of alarm messages and instructions assist the clinician with troubleshooting, thereby maximizing patient safety.

Automatic rhythm tracking and timing, along with multiple trigger mode options, optimize the ability to pump reliably in varying clinical situations.

Both systems are lightweight. The Model 7000 is equipped with a universal IV pole mount and 90-minute battery life for easier intrahospital transport. The KAAT II has a unique liquid crystal display (LCD) control module that is detachable from the pneumatic drive unit. The control module reduces overall weight, offers mounting flexibility, and reduces power consumption, which increases battery life to 180 minutes and provides flexibility of operation, ease, and safety in transport situations.

TECHNICAL SPECIFICATIONS

Specifications are for both the Model 7000 and the KAAT II unless noted.

General description

Model 7000 (Fig. 28-1). Self-contained, microprocessor-based system using 68000 dual central processor controls; software programmed

463

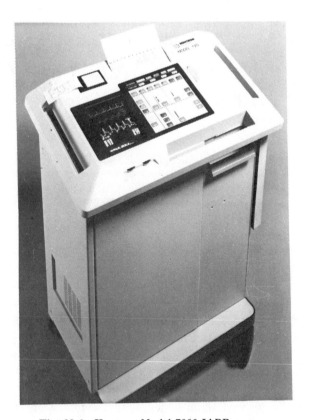

Fig. 28-1. Kontron Model 7000 IABP system.

KAAT II (Fig. 28-2)

Modular, microprocessor-based system using 68000 dual central processor controls; software programmed

Two-part system consisting of monitor/controller and pneumatic drive unit connected by an 8-foot communication cable

Power requirements

90 to 132 or 180 to 264 VAC at 47 to 63 Hz (115/230 nominal). Average power consumption is 225 W. Maximal power consumption is 450 (surge) W.

Fuses

6.25 amp slow-blow and 30 amp (110 V)

3.2 amp slow-blow and 30 amp (220 V)

Battery run time

Model 7000. Approximately 90 minutes

KAAT II. Approximately 3 hours

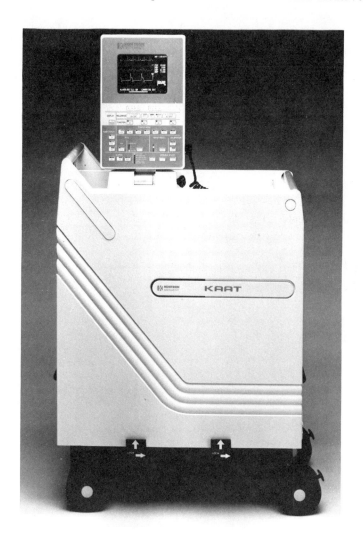

Fig. 28-2. Kontron KAAT II IABP system.

Dimensions

Model 7000. 42.75″ high × 28.5″ wide × 17″ deep (94 cm × 63 cm × 37 cm)

KAAT II *Monitor/controller module:* 13.7″ H × 8.8″ W × 2.4″ D (34.8 cm × 22.4 cm × 6.1 cm)

Pneumatic drive module: 28.2″ H × 12″ W × 25″ D (71.1 cm × 30.5 cm × 63.5 cm)

Wheel cart: 7″ H × 12.5″ W × 22.5″ D (17.8 cm × 31.8 cm × 57 cm)

Weight

Model 7000. 170 lb (77.27 kg) with helium tank installed

KAAT II *Monitor/controller module:* 6 lb (2.7 kg)

Pneumatic drive module: 102 lb (46 kg)

Wheel cart: 10 lb (4.5 kg)

Gas

Helium (recycled); volume and pressure maintained by a closed-loop pressure transducer

Helium tank

Model 7000. Refillable 2000 PSI "D"-size cylinder

KAAT II. Disposable, steel canister with capacity of 500 PSI

Pumping volume

0 to 50 cc in 0.5 cc increments

Pumping rate

40 to 200 beats/minute

Drive

Stepper motor-driven bellows, powered by A/C or internal battery

Water vapor removal

Solenoid, actuated; thermoelectric baffle system (otherwise known as a "cold trap") cools helium and removes moisture from pneumatic lines; collection bottle can be emptied without interrupting operation.

Assist ratios

1:1, 1:2, 1:4, and 1:8

Lead selection

ECG patient cable input (color coded): Lead I, II, or III. *From remote monitor:* Phono to Nicolay (color coded) or phono to phono.

Triggering modes

ECG pattern, ECG peak and *A-Fib* modes use microprocessor-based waveform comparison algorithms. In the A-Fib mode, R-wave detection triggers balloon deflation. *A-Pace* and *V-Pace* modes use pacer recognition system for pacer spikes.

Pulse widths from 0.1 to 0.5 msec require a pulse amplitude of $\pm$ 5 mV or greater, whereas pulse widths greater than or equal to 0.5 msec require a pulse amplitude of $\pm$ 2 mV or greater.

Atrioventricular pacing requires a maximum A-V interval of 250 msec.

Arterial pressure mode requires a microprocessor-based waveform recognition algorithm.

Internal mode is a constant-rate trigger, adjustable from 40 to 120 beats/minute.

Inflation/deflation timing

Automatic timing adjustment for rate changes and arrhythmias using beat-to-beat analysis of the R-R interval

Timing ranges
ECG trigger

Inflation: 20% to 80% R-R interval
Deflation: 30% to 120% R-R interval
Arterial pressure
Inflation: 0% to 35%
Deflation: 35% to 75%
A-Fib
Inflation: 80 to 430 msec after previous R-wave deflation
Deflation: On the R wave

Display

Model 7000. Four-color, three-channel, high-resolution, memory-mapped waveform monitor

KAAT II. Multicolor, three-channel, high-resolution LCD

ECG

Green trace with contrasting color on assisted portions

Arterial pressure

Red trace; calibrated in mm Hg for direct reading

Balloon pressure

Blue trace; sensed through internal strain gauge transducer; calibrated in mm Hg for direct reading

Timing reference display

Bar graph display of inflate/deflate positions relative to the R-R interval

Physiological data

Heart rate (HR)	End diastolic pressure (EDP)
Peak systolic pressure (PSP)	Mean arterial pressure (MAP)
Peak diastolic pressure (PDP)	Sao_2 (KAAT II only)

Heart rate

Derived from ECG or arterial pressure triggering signals
Value averaged over four beats and updated every beat

Arterial pressure data

Each beat sampled and pressure automatically updated every beat
Peak diastolic pressure updated at each assist beat (zero value given when no assist
   seen)

Operating information (continually displayed)

Inflation volume (Model 7000 only)
Balloon volume (Model 7000 only)
Battery voltage (Model 7000 only)
Helium tank pressure
Alarm/battery charging status

Diagnostic alarm messages

   Preprogrammed messages provide procedural steps for troubleshooting specific
patient states, operating conditions, and potential pump malfunctions.

Control function keypad

   The control keys allow for selection of all operating functions. Each key is labeled individually with its corresponding function.

Strip chart recorder

Dual-channel thermal array dot matrix recorder

Records ECG, arterial pressure, and balloon pressure, as well as date, time, physiological parameters, annotation of alarm condition, and trigger mode
Assist interval indicated on top margin of strip when purging and pumping
40 mm grid with 5 mm divisions printed
Records automatically in helium alarm conditions or may be preprogrammed for
   strips at 2, 15, 30, or 60 minutes and 2- or 4-hour intervals
Speed of 25 or 50 mm/sec

Freeze key

   Freezes approximately 5 seconds of patient waveforms

ECG low level filtering

   Diathermy and 50/60 Hz notch; 25 Hz low pass ESIS ON

Applicable standards

Designed to IEC 601-1 and UL 544

Polarity

Automatic processing of positive or negative triggering signals (arterial pressure must be positive)

ECG low level bandwidth

0.5 to 25 Hz with ESIS

Leakage current

Less than 10 mA

Line isolation

120 dB at 60 Hz to ground

Defibrillator protection

Input protected up to 400 J, 5 kV peak defibrillator discharges at 20-second intervals

Pacer rejection

Input amplifier rejects pacer spikes:
At 0.1 to 0.5 msec pulse widths, pulse amplitude of ± 5 mV or greater
At greater than 0.5 msec pulse widths, pulse amplitude of ± 2 mV or greater rejected

ECG (patient cable input)

For input of three-lead patient cable or phono-to-Nicolay cable
Maximal input 10 mV differential

Arterial pressure (transducer cable input)

Compatible with any pressure transducer with output equivalent to Spectramed transducer (50 mV/V/cm Hg)

Balloon connector

Electronic pins sense resistor value of IAB connector for input of IAB size

Data communications—channel 1

DB-25 connector (RS232) for serial transmission of hemodynamic values, current alarms, time, and date

Data communications—channel 2 (KAAT II)

DB-25 connector (RS232) for serial transmission from portable SaO_2 monitors with compatible output

THEORY OF OPERATION
Display

A screen displays ECG trace (green with superimposed assist markers), arterial pressure waveform (red), and balloon pressure waveform (blue); the patient's physiological data are displayed, including HR (with flashing heart icon indicating trigger acceptance), PSP, PDP, EDP, and MAP; operating information is also displayed, including helium supply, alarm/refill status, battery charging status, tutorial prompts, and alarm messages; and a blue horizontal scale at the bottom of the screen shows the inflation/deflation range. The expanding green bar indicates the inflation and deflation set points.

Input/output connections

The Model 7000 and KAAT II interface with most bedside monitors and can also receive inputs directly from patient cables

Input connections

ECG. Nicolay (green) connector for direct three-lead ECG patient cable or phono-to-Nicolay connector from remote monitor.

Arterial pressure transducer cable connection. Nicolay (orange) connector for an arterial pressure transducer; use only transducers with electrical equivalents of 50 mV/V/cm/Hg.

ECG mon input jack. Phono jack for accepting ECG signals (± 6 V DC maximum from remote monitor).

Art press input jack. Phono jack accepts signals (up to ± 6 V DC, 100 mm Hg/V) from a remote arterial pressure monitor; output of the remote monitor must be calibrated at 100 mm Hg/V.

Output connections

ECG. Phono jack provides signal for displaying or recording the ECG trace on an external monitor (maximal output: ± 6 V DC).

Arterial pressure. Phono jack provides signal for displaying or recording arterial pressure trace on an external monitor; output is calibrated at 66 mm Hg/V.

Balloon pressure. Phono jack provides signal for displaying or recording balloon pressure trace on an external monitor; output is calibrated at 58 mm Hg/V.

Assist int. Phono jack provides a signal for use with an interactive simulator (used for training or testing purposes).

Balloon connector

Connection for the IAB catheter to the pump. The pump accepts Kontron's electronically coded balloon connectors, which automatically set pumping volume to match the balloon's maximal volume capacity.

Power switch

The power switch is located directly above the input/output connectors. When the power is turned on, all of the system's preset operating functions are automatically selected for easy set-up. The preset selections are the following:

Recorder: OFF
Trigger mode: PATTERN
Pump status: OFF
ECG lead: II
Assist ratio: 1:2
Calibration: AUTO
Display range (AP): 150 mm Hg
Alarms: ON
Variable adjust: ECG GAIN

Function control keypad (Figs. 28-3 and 28-4)

Inflation control. Adjusts the inflation point; inflation occurs later when control is turned (Model 7000) or pressed (KAAT II) to the right, earlier when moved to the left; allows operator to optimize timing by monitoring the hemodynamic changes produced in the AP waveform.

Deflation control. Adjusts the deflation point; deflation occurs later when control is turned (Model 7000) or pressed (KAAT II) to the right; earlier when moved to the left.

Recorder control keys

ON/OFF: Turns the recorder ON or OFF
ECG: The ECG waveform is recorded on one half of the strip chart
AP: The AP waveform is recorded on one half of the strip chart
BPW: The balloon pressure waveform is recorded on one half of the strip chart
25 mm/sec: Sets strip chart speed to 25 mm/sec
50 mm/sec: Sets strip chart speed to 50 mm/sec

Function control keys

F1: Key that allows the operator to set the year, month, day, hour, and minute on the strip chart recorder
F2: Key that allows the operator to preprogram the recorder to automatically print at 2, 5, 15, or 30 minutes or 2- or 4-hour intervals

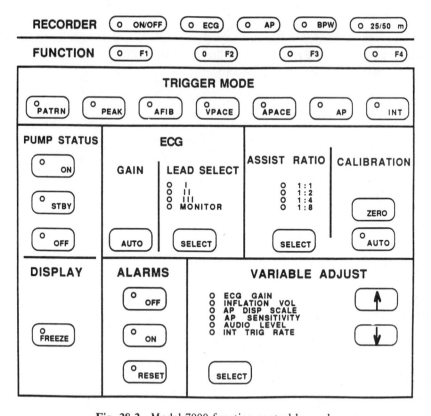

Fig. 28-3. Model 7000 function control keypad.

F3: Used in conjunction with the F1 key to increase selected time parameter

F3 (KAAT II): Used independently, displays elapsed hours of LCD backlit time, battery voltage, and helium tank pressure (in psi)

F4: Used in conjunction with the F1 key to decrease selected time parameter

Trigger control keys

It is necessary to establish an adequate trigger signal before balloon counterpulsation can begin. The computer in the pump requires a physiological signal from the patient to cycle the pneumatic system, which inflates and deflates the balloon. In most cases it is preferable to use the R wave of the ECG as the trigger signal. However, the Model 7000 and KAAT II also give you the option of using pacing spikes or the arterial pressure waveform as the trigger signal.

Pattern. The computer analyzes the slope, height, and width of a positive or negative deflected R wave. The QRS complex must meet a width criteria of 25 to 135 msec. Wider QRS complexes may not be recognized. Automatic pacer rejection

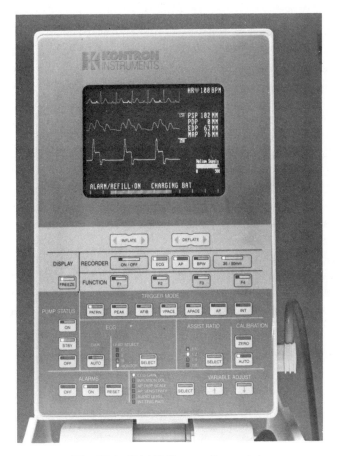

Fig. 28-4. KAAT II controller module.

allows this trigger mode to be used with demand pacing. This is the most commonly used trigger mode.

Peak. The computer analyzes the height and slope of a positive or negative deflected R wave. This may be the trigger mode of choice for rhythms with a widened QRS (e.g., bundle branch blocks, paced rhythms). Automatic pacer rejection allows this trigger mode to be used with demand pacing.

A-Fib. The computer analyzes the R wave as in the PEAK mode (height and slope) for inflation. The R wave is sensed for automatic R wave deflation. This may be the trigger of choice for any rhythm with a varying R-R interval.

V-Pace. The computer uses a ventricular pacing spike as the trigger signal; it may only be used for patients with 100% ventricular or atrioventricular paced rhythms (A/V delay must be 250 msec or less).

A-Pace. The computer uses an atrial pacing spike as the trigger signal; it may only be used for patients with 100% atrial pacing.

AP. The computer uses the rising slope of the arterial pressure waveform as the trigger signal. This mode is available as an option for clinical situations in which an ECG is unavailable or distorted.

Internal. The balloon inflates and deflates at a rate set by the operator and external signals are ignored; the rate is adjustable from 40 to 180 beats/minute. This mode is used only when there is no myocardial activity or ventricular ejection. NOTE: To engage the internal trigger, the key must be selected and pressed a second time.

Pump status

On: Fills the pneumatic system with helium to 2.5 mm Hg and starts pumping; if pressed before PUMP STDBY, pumping starts after two purge cycles.

Standby: If pump is off, it completes a four-beat purge cycle and pressurizes the pneumatic system to 2.5 mm Hg; if pump is on, it immediately stops pumping but does not vent the pneumatic system; class II alarms cause the pump to go into the standby (STBY) mode.

Off: Immediately stops pumping, deflates the balloon and vents the pneumatic system; class I alarms automatically stop the pump.

ECG gain/lead select

Auto: Automatically adjusts the amplitude of the ECG for trigger recognition.

Lead selection: I, II, or III when using a three-lead ECG patient cable; lead II is the only available signal when using a phono-to-Nicolay ECG cable.

Monitor: Model 7000/KAAT II receives signal from ECG monitor; used with phono-to-phono ECG input connection.

Assist ratio keys

These control keys are used to select the percentage of IABP assist the patient will receive. The pump is preset at 1:2 at power-up to allow for timing adjustments. The SELECT key advances the operator through each selection. The illuminated LED indicates assist ratio selected.

Calibration

Zero: Zeroes the pressure source when the transducer is open to atmosphere

Auto: Automatic calibration to 100 mm Hg/V for disposable transducers; NOTE: strain gauge or reusable transducers are zeroed using the ZERO function key and calibrated with variable adjust AP sensitivity and SELECT keys

Freeze key

The freeze key freezes the waveform display; the moving display returns when the freeze key is pressed a second time.

Alarm control keys

Off: Disables pneumatic alarms up to a period of 60 minutes; automatic refill of helium is suspended
On: Restores normal alarm functions if alarms have been disabled
Reset: Silences the audible alarm tone

Variable adjust

Using the SELECT key allows you to change the following selections:
ECG gain: Using the UP and DOWN arrow keys will adjust the amplitude of the ECG waveform
Inflation volume: Using the DOWN arrow keys decreases the balloon volume by 0.5-cc increments; using the UP arrow key increases balloon volume by 2-cc increments; pump must be in the "OFF" mode.
AP display scale: Using the UP and DOWN arrow keys changes the AP-wave display range from 0 to 100 mm Hg, 0 to 150 mm Hg, or 0 to 200 mm Hg.
AP sensitivity: Used for calibration procedure for strain gauge or reusable transducers
Audio level: Using the UP and DOWN arrow keys changes the alarm tone from a range of 10% to 100%
Internal trigger rate: Using the UP and DOWN arrows adjusts the internal trigger rate by 5 beats/minute; preset rate is 80 beats/minute; range is 40 to 120 beats/minute.

SUMMARY OF STEPS TO OPERATION
Power

Plug in power cord.
Turn on console by pressing green switch located in the recessed area of the patient interface panel.

Helium

Model 7000: Turn on tank located in front lower compartment.
KAAT II: Insert disposable tank in receptacle.
Verify helium supply.

ECG

Connect an ECG source using one of the following:
A three-lead ECG patient cable to the green ECG connector
A bedside monitor using a phono-to-Nicolay connector to the green ECG connector
A bedside monitor using a phono-to-phono connector to the phono jack ECG input connector

Select the ECG lead that provides the clearest QRS complex.
Adjust ECG gain if necessary (AUTO GAIN may be used).
Verify trigger recognition indicated by the following:
  Presence of overlay bands on the ECG trace
  Flashing red heart icon next to HR on display screen
  Flashing green LED on selected trigger mode

Arterial pressure

  Connect an AP source to the console by using one of the following:
A bedside monitor using a phono-to-phono connector to the phono jack ART
  PRESS input connector
A compatible pressure transducer connected to the orange ARTERIAL PRESSURE
  input connector.

Purge

Connect the balloon plug securely to the balloon connector; Kontron IAB connectors are electronically coded to automatically deliver a preset volume.
Press PUMP STDBY for automatic purge cycle.

Pump

Press PUMP ON.
Verify correct arterial pressure timing.
Set assist ratio to 1:1 for maximal assist.

TIMING

  Timing is the process of operator-controlled synchronization of the balloon pulse
with the patient's hemodynamics.

  After turning the main power on and initiating counterpulsation, inflation and
deflation will occur at safe preset points. Once timing has been assessed by observing key landmarks on the arterial pressure waveform, the operator may use the in-
flate/deflate control keys (KAAT II) or thumbwheels (Model 7000) to optimize timing. Obtaining a strip chart recording will help to verify and document proper timing. Both the KAAT II and Model 7000 will automatically adjust timing for most
variations in heart rate and arrhythmias.

  The blue horizontal scale at the bottom of the display shows the interval between
trigger points, and the green bar indicates the inflation and deflation set points. The
pump allows adjustment of the inflation and deflation points within certain limits,
defined as a percentage of the interval between trigger points. A safety mechanism
exists to prevent overlap of inflate/deflate settings. There is also an audible alarm

that will sound if there is a gross timing error or if deflation is set beyond 100% of the R-R interval.

ALARMS

The Model 7000 and KAAT II diagnostic alarm systems continuously monitor operating conditions. When an alarm condition occurs, an audible tone is sounded and an alarm message is displayed with troubleshooting steps to corrective actions.

Class I alarms

The following class I (automatic response) alarms alert the operator to potentially serious conditions that require immediate attention:

System error: The computer circuitry has malfunctioned. Press the ALARM RESET key. Correcting this alarm may require turning the power OFF and ON to reset the microprocessor.

Possible helium leak: The system cannot autofill the pneumatic system to +2.5 mm Hg within eight beats, the system attempts a second autofill within 1 minute, or the baseline falls below −10 mm Hg while pumping.

Large helium leak detected: The balloon pressure waveform plateau falls below 5 mm Hg immediately before the onset of deflation, the balloon pressure peak decreases by 50% within five beats, or the balloon-inflated equilibrium pressure drops below 12% of inflation peak pressure within five beats.

Purge failure: The system cannot complete a pneumatic purge sequence because the purge valve on the balloon tubing is open, helium tank is empty, the helium tank is not installed correctly, or no trigger is detected.

High balloon pressure: The balloon pressure baseline exceeds 25 mm Hg.

These alarms cause the system to do the following:

Stop pumping (PUMP OFF key illuminates)

Deflate the balloon

Open the vent valve

Initiate an audible alarm

Display an alarm message

Freeze the waveform

Print approximately the last 5 seconds of the balloon and AP waveforms on the strip chart recorder

Class II alarms

The following class II (automatic response) alarms also require immediate attention:

ECG trigger loss: Eight seconds elapsed without a recognizable trigger point in the ECG waveform (occurs only in Pattern, Peak, A-Fib, V-Pace, and A-Pace trigger modes).

Pressure trigger loss: Eight seconds elapsed without a recognizable trigger point in the AP waveform (occurs only in Art Press trigger mode).

ECG lead fault detected: The system detects high electrical impedance in the ECG leads (usually caused by loose or broken patient leads).

These alarms cause the system to do the following:

Stop pumping (PUMP STDBY key illuminated, system not vented)

Deflate the balloon

Initiate an audio alarm

Display an alarm message

Class III alarms

The class III (information only) alarms alert the operator to less serious conditions. These alarms initiate an audio alarm and a visual message to be displayed:

Deflation >100%: Deflation is set to occur beyond 100% of the R-R interval.

Drain failure: The system was unable to complete a full drain cycle; cold trap requires emptying, or tubing is kinked.

Battery life less than 20, 10, and 5 minutes: Separate alarms indicating remaining battery time before system battery operation shuts down.

System running on battery: AC power was intentionally or accidentally disconnected, and the system has automatically switched to battery power.

Timing error: Inflation and deflation points need to be adjusted (insufficient time to deflate the balloon before the next inflation cycle).

Battery inoperative: The system will not run in battery mode due to a faulty DC power supply fuse.

Class IV alarms

The following class IV (informational alarms) initiate a visual alarm message:

Low helium supply: The helium tank's pressure is less than 100 psi (also occurs if the helium tank is not inserted correctly).

Dead clock battery: Internal clock battery needs replacement (place service call).

Low battery for static RAM: Internal battery needs to be replaced (place service call).

TROUBLESHOOTING

The balloon pressure waveform displayed on the third channel of the display screen represents the helium pressure during inflation and deflation of the balloon. This transduced waveform can tell us much about the interaction of the balloon within the patient's aorta. Understanding normal and abnormal balloon pressure waveforms is an additional troubleshooting tool for the clinician, along with monitoring of the patient's hemodynamic status. The balloon pressure waveform will as-

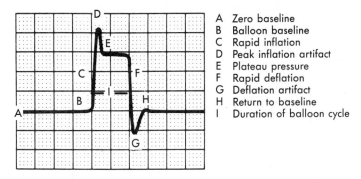

A   Zero baseline
B   Balloon baseline
C   Rapid inflation
D   Peak inflation artifact
E   Plateau pressure
F   Rapid deflation
G   Deflation artifact
H   Return to baseline
I   Duration of balloon cycle

Fig. 28-5. Normal balloon pressure waveform.

sist the clinician in making an educated decision in troubleshooting potential problems and ensuring better patient management and safety. A normal balloon pressure waveform is illustrated in Fig. 28-5.

Class I automatic response alarms

The following are examples of class I "automatic response alarms" with appropriate strip chart recording of the balloon pressure and arterial pressure waveforms:

Alarm: possible helium leak (Fig. 28-6). Possible causes:

Leak in tubing or connections
Kinked catheter
Blood in catheter tubing
Ectopic beats
    Corrective actions:
Check all connection points including catheter tubing and balloon connector.
Find kink and straighten out catheter; be sure that the IAB membrane has fully exited the insertion sheath.

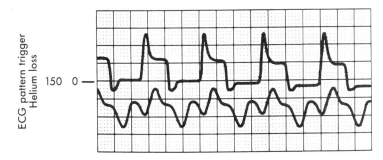

Fig. 28-6. Possible helium leak alarm with corresponding balloon pressure waveform.

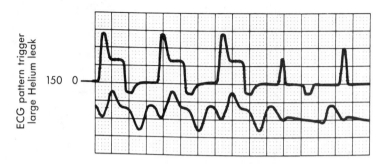

Fig. 28-7. Large helium leak alarm with corresponding balloon pressure waveform.

Any evidence of blood leakage within the IAB assembly warrants immediate IAB removal.

Select another trigger mode.

Perform leak test.

Alarm: large helium leak (Fig. 28-7)

Possible causes:

Leak in balloon connections, catheter, and vent hole

Possible internal balloon leak

Corrective actions:

Check all connection points including catheter tubing and balloon connector.

Cover purge (vent) hole with the rubber sleeve.

Perform leak test.

Alarm: purge failure (Fig. 28-8). Possible causes:

Leaks

Low helium level

Loss of trigger

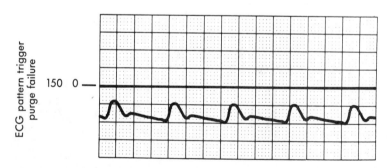

Fig. 28-8. Purge failure alarm with corresponding balloon pressure waveform.

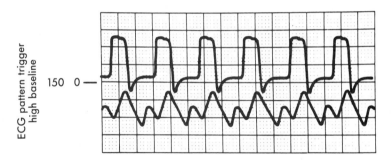

Fig. 28-9. High baseline alarm with corresponding balloon pressure waveform.

Corrective actions:

Cover purge (vent) hole with rubber sleeve.

Replace or reinsert full helium tank.

Adjust ECG gain to reestablish triggering.

Check electrode contacts.

Select another trigger mode.

Connect balloon connector to console.

   Alarm: high baseline (Fig. 28-9). Possible causes:

Kinked catheter

Partially wrapped balloon

   Corrective action:

Find kink and straighten out catheter; be sure that the IAB membrane has fully exited the insertion sheath.

Notify physician; connect a 50- or 60-cc syringe to balloon connector and manually inflate and deflate several times.

   Alarm: high pressure (Fig. 28-10). Possible causes:

Kinked catheter   Balloon too large

Partially wrapped balloon

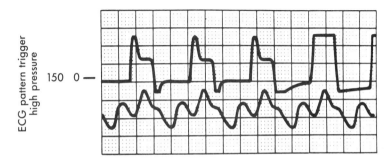

Fig. 28-10. High pressure alarm with corresponding balloon pressure waveform.

Corrective actions:

Find kink and straighten out catheter; be sure that the IAB membrane has fully exited the insertion sheath.

Notify physician; connect a 50- or 60-cc syringe to balloon connector and manually inflate and deflate IAB several times.

Decrease IAB volume until the balloon pressure waveform (BPW) returns to normal configuration. NOTE: Do not reduce the IAB volume to less than two thirds of the balloon's capacity. To prevent thrombus formation, pump the balloon at its maximal capacity for 5 minutes every hour.

GUIDELINES FOR USE OF THE IABC IN AIR AMBULANCE TRANSPORT

Transport pump: KAAT II (Kontron Air Ambulance Transport)

Weight: 118 lb (including wheelbase)

Securing pump: Use FAA cargo-mounting procedure based on clinical placement and follow FAA regulations and STCs. NOTE: Removal of the wheelbase allows the console to be mounted easily onto aircraft brown line track system.

Pump surge power requirements: 4 A

Pump maintenance requirements: 2 A

Battery time: 3 hours

Battery charging status displayed on screen:

CHRG BAT: HI

CHRG BAT: LO

CHARGING BAT

Alarms pressure or volume sensitive:

Both

In-line pressure transducer with continually displayed balloon pressure waveform

Recommendations for purging with change in altitude:

Beat-to-beat assessment of helium pressure and volume

Purging with altitude change is not necessary

Sao_2 monitoring capabilities:

Yes

Digital display on screen

RESOURCE

For further information on the Kontron Model 7000 or KAAT II intraaortic balloon pumps contact:

Kontron Instruments, Inc.
9 Plymouth Street
Everett, MA 02149
(617) 389-6400 or 1-800-343-3297
24-hour Customer Support Center: 1-800-447-6961

CHAPTER 29

Boston Scientific Corporation Cardiac Assist Series 3001

Kathleen Rolston and Tom Wrublewski

The Series 3001 is an advanced, clinically proven intraaortic balloon pumping system. It is simple to operate and offers the flexibility necessary for hospital and mobile use. The superior console design, shown in Fig. 29-1, provides reliability and numerous physiological benefits for the patient requiring mechanical cardiac support. Its compact, lightweight design makes transport convenient and safe.

SYSTEM SPECIFICATIONS AND COMPONENTS
Electrical requirements

AC power	Factory configured for 115 or 230 V, 50/60 Hz
Auxiliary power	24-V DC input for direct connection to aircraft power or to external battery pack
Battery type	Sealed lead-acid
Battery time	*Standard:* up to 1.25 hours running time
	Optional: up to 2.5 hours running time
Operating current	4 Amps for 115 V AC.
	2 Amps for 230 V AC.
	9.5 Amps for 24 to 28 V DC.

Physical structure

Weight (including helium tanks)	131 lbs without batteries (59.4 kg)
	158 lbs with 1.25-hour batteries (71.7 kg)
	175 lbs with 2.5-hour batteries (79.4 kg)
Width	32 inches (81.2 cm)
Depth	16 inches (40.6 cm)
Overall height	
	35.75 inches (90.8 cm)

Patient safety

Environmental	Designed to meet relevant AAMI and UL standards
Operating diagnostics	The console performs a self-check when power is turned ON;

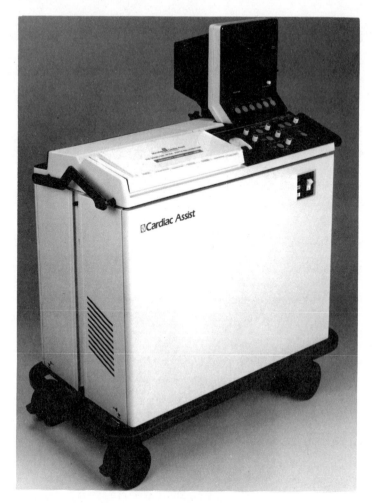

Fig. 29-1. Boston Scientific Corporation Cardiac Assist Division Series 3001 intraaortic balloon pump.

	automatic calibration of pressure and leak parameters takes place with each PURGE cycle every 2 hours. Video information center messages and on-line tutorials indicate and explain alarm and precautionary conditions
Patient leak current	Less than 10 microamperes at 115 V AC

Balloon inflation characteristics

Shuttle gas	Helium, medical grade
Helium system	Closed type, filled during controlled system purge; software-based check and display of purge status

Video information center (VIC) display

Type	Nonfade memory scope with freeze of selected traces
Display trace sweep	25 mm/sec; two channel with freeze capability
ECG trace	Up to 4 seconds of information displayed
Arterial pressure	0 to 100 mm Hg or 0 to 200 mm Hg display calibrated for transducer input
AUG pressure	Peak assisted pressure
SYS pressure	Peak systolic pressure
DIA pressure	Diastolic pressure
MEAN pressure	Mean pressure
Heart rate	Derived from R-wave trigger or AP trigger
ECG trigger	
Real time timing	Start of deflation is adjustable from 0.0 to 0.030 second after R wave; start of inflation is adjustable from 100 ms after the trigger event to 75% of the cardiac period
Conventional timing	Start of deflation is adjustable from 0.28 second before the trigger event to the trigger event; the start of inflation is adjustable from 100 ms after the trigger event to 75% of the cardiac period
Telewire input	FM (frequency modulated) transmitter with coaxial cable connection to console
High level input Pacemaker pulse rejection	100 mV to 3 V, ¼-inch standard phone jack system recognizes and rejects pacer artifact as a trigger signal (when artifact filter is activated)

Arterial pressure trigger

Transducer sensitivity	5 mV/V/mm Hg
Calibration	Automatic for offset of ± 150 mm Hg
High level input	100 mm Hg/V, typical
Input offset	0 mm Hg = 0 V
Sensitivity range	0.1 V/100 mm Hg to 10 V/100 mm Hg
Trigger	Computer examination of pressure waveform based on waveform slope (trigger event is the rise in systolic pressure); variable trigger level (14 mm Hg minimum pulse pressure required)
Timing	Inflation is adjustable from 0 to 0.9 second after the trigger event; deflation is adjustable from 0.2 second after inflation to 1.0 second after the trigger event

Internal trigger

Trigger	Signal internally generated at operator-selected rates of 40 to 212 beats/minute

COMPONENTS
Video information center (VIC)

The video information center is illustrated in Fig. 29-2.

CRT monitor: The video information center has a 7-inch CRT monitor that displays

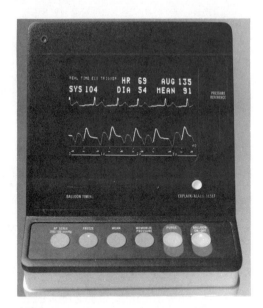

Fig. 29-2. Video information center (VIC).

patient ECG and arterial pressure waveforms and pertinent information about balloon and console operation.

Pressure reference slide control: This slide control causes vertical movement of a horizontal pressure reference line on the screen.

Explain/Alarm reset button: Pressing this button during an alarm condition silences the audio alarm; when the button is pressed, the alarm condition appearing on the VIC is erased and a corrective action message is displayed.

Inflate and deflate slide controls: These slide controls are used to set the inflate and deflate times—movement to the right results in later activation; to the left, earlier activation.

Video information center panel controls

See Fig. 29-2.

Wean button: With this control, assist frequency can be selected in incremental steps from 7 of 8 to 1 of 8.

Freeze display button: Pressing this button freezes the ARTERIAL PRESSURE, ECG, and BALLOON DYNAMICS INDICATOR displays; the display remains frozen until the button is pressed again.

Arterial pressure scale selection button: This is used to select either the 0 to 200 mm Hg or the 0 to 100 mm Hg arterial pressure scale.

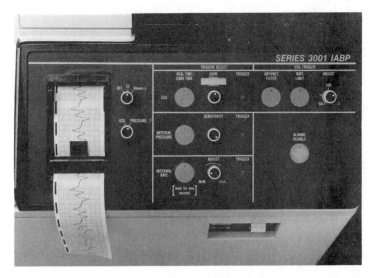

Fig. 29-3. Console main control panel.

Balloon On/Off button: Balloon pumping is started and stopped by pressing this button.

Purge button: When this button is pressed, the console will evacuate the balloon and refill the SAFETY DOME with fresh helium; the cycle requires approximately 11 seconds.

Memorize pressure button: Depressing this button will freeze (memorize) the arterial pressure waveform of the first cardiac cycle, beginning with the next full sweep; to clear the MEMORIZED WAVEFORM, simply press the button again.

Main control panel

The main control panel is illustrated in Fig. 29-3.

ECG controls

ECG trigger select button: Pressing this button will engage ECG-triggered operation; pressing this button will toggle between conventional time and real time.

ECG gain control: This control sets the gain; adjust so that the light bar is in the center of the green zone.

Artifact filter button: This feature is used to eliminate competing pacemaker spikes.

AP controls

Arterial pressure trigger select button: Pressing this button will select the ARTERIAL PRESSURE waveform as the triggering signal; a light on the button will indicate this trigger mode has been activated.

Arterial pressure sensitivity control knob: Clockwise rotation of this knob increases the sensitivity of the ARTERIAL PRESSURE trigger mode.

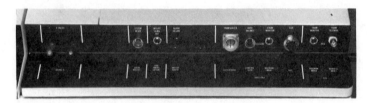

Fig. 29-4. Rear input/connector panel.

Internal rate controls

Internal rate trigger select button: Pressing this button and holding it for 1 second activates the INTERNAL RATE trigger mode.

Internal rate adjust control: This controls adjusts the internal rate over a range of 40 to 210 beats/minute.

Alarms disable button: When this button is pressed, an ALARMS DISABLED message will appear on the VIC screen.

Patient/console connections

The patient/console connections are illustrated in Fig. 29-4. Direct patient ECG signals can be obtained by using the five-lead ECG cable, TELEWIRE CABLE; standard skin electrodes and lead wires are attached to the patient and then connected to the TELEWIRE CABLE.

ECG from monitor input: This ¼-inch phone jack permits input of the ECG from the patient monitor via a connector cable.

Arterial pressure from monitor input: This ¼-inch phone jack input accepts an arterial pressure signal from the patient monitor via a connector cable.

Pressure transducer input connector: This is used for the direct input of a pressure signal from a pressure transducer.

SET-UP INSTRUCTIONS

Setting balloon volume: Push the VOLUME RELEASE button and set BALLOON DISPLACEMENT SYRINGE to the appropriate volume; connect the console to the patient balloon.

H or helium: Open tank and regulator; check helium tank pressure gauge.

E or ECG signal: Acquire from skin leads via TELEWIRE or slave from monitor.

A or arterial pressure: Direct transducer connection (use auto balance) or slave from monitor (use size control).

R or R wave: Use gain to establish R wave as the trigger signal.

T or timing: Set deflation at the R wave and inflation at the dicrotic notch on AP wave.

P: Purge the IABP after connecting to catheter.

U: Unassisted pressure signal should be calibrated.

M: Memorize unassisted pressure.

P: Pump on.

TIMING THE SERIES 3001 CONSOLE

Timing the Series 3001 can be achieved in 1:1 assist by using the memorized pressure feature. The augmented cardiac cycle can be compared with the unaugmented cycle by pressing the MEMORIZE PRESSURE button when the balloon is OFF (this will cause the first unaugmented pressure waveform to remain on the left side of the VIC screen) and then turning the balloon ON. The BALLOON ON tracing will then be superimposed over the memorized, unaugmented BALLOON OFF waveform so that hemodynamic changes can be assessed in the 1:1 mode.

ECG triggered real time timing mode: To engage, press the ECG button in the trigger select area of the console. In this mode, the R wave should appear at the left edge of the screen. Balloon deflation should be adjusted to occur with the R wave. Balloon inflation should be initially adjusted to start at the dicrotic notch. Initiate balloon assist, and slowly move the inflate control so that the upstroke of the balloon augmentation wave coincides with the dicrotic notch.

ECG triggered conventional timing mode: Press the ECG trigger button to engage. In this trigger mode, the R wave should appear at the left edge of the screen. Balloon deflation should be adjusted to occur before or with the R wave. Balloon inflation should be initially adjusted to start at the dicrotic notch.

Arterial pressure triggered timing: Arterial pressure triggering is used when the ECG signal is inadequate or unavailable as a trigger source. Adjust the sensitivity control until a systolic upstroke consistently appears as the trigger signal. Balloon inflation should be initially adjusted to start at the dicrotic notch. Balloon deflation should be adjusted to occur well before the next systolic upstroke. Once balloon assist is initiated, the inflation slide control should be adjusted so the upstroke of the balloon augmentation wave coincides with the dicrotic notch of the unassisted AP waveform. The deflation control should be adjusted for optimal systolic unloading.

Internal rate triggered timing: This mode of operation does not integrate balloon function with cardiac performance. The DEFLATE SLIDE CONTROL is inoperative in this mode; deflation occurs at the internally generated trigger. Adjust the INFLATE SLIDE CONTROL to produce the desired duration of inflation.

ALARMS, INTERPRETATION, AND RESPONSES

Alarms, interpretations, and responses are described in Table 29-1.

Table 29-1. Alarm conditions

Alarm	Explain message	Console response
NO R-WAVE TRIGGER	None; self-explanatory	If the condition occurs with balloon on, a continuous beep sounds, the balloon deflates, and pumping stops; resumes pumping when an R wave is detected
NO AP TRIGGER	None; self-explanatory	If the condition occurs with the balloon on, a continuous beep sounds, the balloon deflates, and pumping stops; resumes pumping when a systole is detected
VOLUME LOSS	Possible leak; check connections, twisted balloon, kinked catheter	Continuous beep; balloon deflates; pumping stops
VOLUME GAIN	Check balloon connection Possible diaphragm failure	Intermittent 1-second beep; pumping not interrupted
LOW AUGMENTATION	Augmentation below minimum alarm limit; verify AP; check CATH/AP for kinks, disconnects; adjust alarm	Intermittent 1-second beep; pumping not interrupted
IABP DISCONNECTED	None; self-explanatory	If the condition occurs with the balloon on, a continuous beep sounds and the pumping stops; connection must be reestablished and the balloon purged; if the condition occurs during purging, the connection must be reestablished and the balloon purged; console will not alarm
ALARMS DISABLED	None; self-explanatory	

Advisory and alarm messages

Alarm messages are displayed in the upper field of the VIC screen. Four alarm conditions are associated with a continuous beep when the balloon is on:

- Volume loss
- No R-wave trigger
- No AP trigger
- IAB disconnected

These four alarms immediately halt balloon pumping. All other alarms are advisory and are associated with an intermittent beep. The other alarms do not interrupt balloon pumping. Table 29-1 is a partial listing of the alarms and their responses.

TROUBLESHOOTING

Clinical

Electrosurgical interference

Use TELEWIRE ECG lead select switch to provide the best ECG signal.

Connect TELEWIRE to epicardial or endocardial pacing wires by attaching alligator clip cables from pacemaker wires to the LA and RA inputs of TELEWIRE (lead I).

Use electrode tip of cardiac assist sidewinder balloon by connecting red electrode connecting wire to the RA input of TELEWIRE (lead I). Position other skin electrodes as far away as possible and connect to other TELEWIRE leads.

Use AP trigger when ECG trigger cannot be established.

Pacemaker artifact

When atrial or AV sequential pacing causes double triggering.

Activate artifact filter to reject the pacer artifact.

Adjust ECG gain if necessary to provide a trigger at the beginning of the QRS.

The rate limit control may be used to reject competing triggers by rotating the rate adjust control counterclockwise until double triggering eliminated. Adjust timing appropriately.

Trigger from pacer spikes can be ensured by attaching alligator clip cables from pacemaker terminals to the LA and RA inputs of TELEWIRE (lead I).

Cardiac arrest

Internal trigger: Adjust rate for CPR rate; adjust inflation time with inflate control; the flashing square on the VIC indicates deflation and time to compress.

AP trigger: Trigger from pressure generated by CPR; time balloon to be inflated between compressions.

Dysrhythmias

Deflation is triggered by the R wave in arrhythmias. Consistent tracking of dysrhythmias occurs if the ECG trigger source is dependable. Assist ratio of 1:1 is recommended for maximal LV workload reduction and augmentation of coronary perfusion.

Technical

Volume loss alarm

Check the intraaortic balloon catheter. The appearance of blood in the catheter tubing indicates a leak in the balloon and requires immediate changing of the balloon.

Purge the console. If blood is not seen in the catheter and a balloon leak is not suspected, then press BALLOON ON and resume pumping.

WARNING: DO NOT OPERATE THE CONSOLE WITH THE ALARMS DISABLE ENGAGED FOR A PROLONGED PERIOD WITHOUT DETERMINING THE CAUSE FOR THE ALARM.

Volume gain alarm

Check all pneumatic connections. The most likely cause is a loose or disconnected catheter. Press PURGE, then resume pumping.

Check for possible leak in the replacement diaphragm.

THE REPLACEMENT DIAPHRAGM

The replacement diaphragm in the safety dome should be replaced as needed or every 250 hours of console running time.

BALLOON DYNAMICS INDICATORS

Balloon dynamics indicators are illustrated in Fig. 29-5, *A*. The time it takes to inflate and deflate the balloon can be assessed by observing the balloon dynamics indicators (BDI) on the VIC screen. The BDI is a graphic illustration of the time required for gas motion into and out of the balloon catheter. The indicator is displayed on the VIC screen below the arterial trace and consists of two figures: inflation and deflation.

Prolonged inflation

In Fig. 29-5, *B*, note that the inflation segment is connected to the deflation segment. This can mean that the inflation time is overly long, indicating the following: The balloon may be partially wrapped.
The console drive pressure may be too low.
The VOLUME DISPLACEMENT may be too high.
The SAFETY DOME may not be properly filled or calibrated (air in system).
The system may require purging.
The balloon may be positioned too low in the aorta.

Verify complete balloon unwrap by fluoroscopy or portable chest x-ray examination, and make sure that the catheter and all connection tubings are free of kinks.

Prolonged deflation

The appearance of a long tail on the deflation segment (Fig. 29-5, *C*) indicates the time of deflation is excessive. The following list of potential causes should be investigated:
The balloon catheter may be kinked.
The balloon may be partially within the introducer sheath.
The balloon connector tubing may be too long.

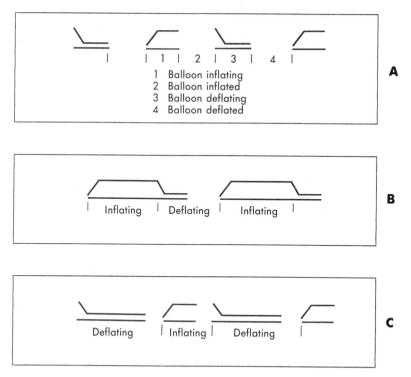

Fig. 29-5. A, Balloon dynamics indicators (BDI); **B,** BDI—slow inflation time; **C,** BDI—slow deflation time.

The SAFETY DOME may not be properly filled or calibrated.
The system may require purging or have excessive moisture.

TRANSPORT OPERATION

The Series 3001 console will operate on internal batteries when the power is ON and the pump is not connected to an AC power source. Switching will be automatic and will be accompanied by a single beep tone if the AC plug is removed from a wall outlet or AC power is lost during operation. When the BATTERY LOW message appears on the VIC screen, accompanied by an intermittent beep, approximately 10% of the maximal battery operating time remains.

Battery type	Operating time with full charge
Standard	1.25 hours
Optional	2.50 hours

AIR TRANSPORT CONSIDERATION

Changes in altitude result in barometric pressure changes. This change will affect balloon displacement volume (Boyle's law); therefore system purging is recommended for every 2000-foot change in altitude. Ensure that all air is eradicated from the volume displacement system before takeoff.

RESOURCES
For further information, consult the following organization and/or publication:

Cardiac Assist
135 Forbes Blvd.
Mansfield, MA 02048
or call 1-800-842-0996

Cardiac Assist, Boston Scientific Corporation: Series 3001 Intraaortic Balloon Pump Operating Manual, Boston Scientific Corporation, Mansfield, MA, August 1991.

CHAPTER 30

Bard H-8000

Patricia C. Garison and **Theresa M. Gaffney**

The Bard H-8000* intraaortic balloon pump (Fig. 30-1) control unit is a compact, lightweight, portable system, designed to achieve intraaortic balloon counterpulsation (IABC) in a number of settings, including the operating room, cardiac catheterization laboratory, and critical care units and in transport situations. In addition to operating the unit in its four-wheeled, multiposition cart, the H-8000 can be carried by hand or mounted on a footboard or bedrail to facilitate intrahospital transport.

SYSTEM SPECIFICATIONS AND COMPONENTS

The Bard H-8000 intraaortic balloon pump console combines advanced microprocessing technology with mechanical and pneumatic systems to shuttle a preselected volume of gas into and out of the intraaortic balloon. It maintains precise inflation and deflation and automatically adjusts to a wide range of physiological states. The console's comprehensive surveillance system notifies the operator of changes in the patient's condition and any malfunctions within the balloon catheter or the console itself.

System specifications†
Dimensions

Console size: 18.2 in × 23.5 in × 9.0 in (55.5 cm × 68.75 cm × 22.5 cm)
Console weight: 50 lb (22.7 kg) with standard battery; 54 lb (24.5 kg) with optional
   extended life battery
   Power
   AC
Power input: Factory set is 100 V AC, 115 V AC, 220 V AC, or 240 V AC (50 Hz or
   60 Hz)

---

*Bard is a registered trademark of C.R. Bard, Inc.
†Specifications are subject to change without notice.

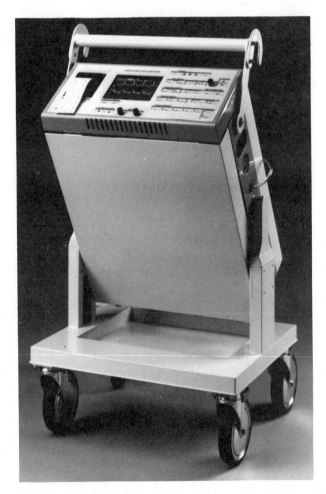

Fig. 30-1. Bard H-8000 intraaortic balloon pump control unit.

Peak current: 5 A

Fuses: 3 A for 115 V; 1.5 A for 220 V

Common mode isolation rejection: >90 dB all leads (at 60 Hz)

ECG input protection: Protected against defibrillator shocks to 360 J. Protected against electrocautery voltages; electrocautery filter on all selectable low-level leads

   Battery

Running time: With standard battery, 1 hour with 40-cc balloon at 120 beats/minute; with optional extended life battery, 2.5 hours with 40-cc balloon at 120 beats/minute, up to 3 hours with 40-cc balloon at 75 beats/minute

Recharge time: With standard battery, 7 to 8 hours; with extended life battery, 12 hours

Environmental

Operating temperature: 5° C to 35° C

Operating humidity: 15% RH to 80% RH

Storage temperature: −15° C to 40° C

Shock and vibration: Designed to meet MIL STD 810E method 514.4 (basic transportation) ECRI Class 5, subclass B

Pneumatics

Gas volumes

Pumping volume: 20 to 50 cc; operator set to ± 2 cc, using regulator dial on LEFT-SIDE PANEL; with on-screen read-out

Pumping range: 30 to 200 beats/minute

Gases

Shuttle gas: Helium; *Drive gas:* air

Tank size: 95 cc, 1800 psi, disposable

Alternate source: "D" cylinder; 3000 psi; connector on bottom panel

Balloon pressure waveform

Continuous monitoring of inflation pressure and volume.

Leak detection

Measured on a beat-to-beat basis at the balloon side of the VOLUME CONTROL isolation diaphragm.

System responses: ALARM and SHUTDOWN at < -10 mm Hg

On mode: Access by pressing the ON key on the PUMP CONTROL PANEL; activates the inflate/deflate cycle; system is pumping without AUTOPURGE and AUTOFILL and without the following alarms: gas leakage, poor deflation, ECG detected

Auto mode: Access by pressing the AUTO key on the PUMP CONTROL PANEL; activates the automatic system surveillance and all alarms; system automatically purges every 2 hours, and AUTOFILLS on a beat-to-beat basis

Patient signal acquisition

ECG

Low-level input: Obtained via patient cable: six-pin, AAMI, three-lead, low noise, filtered; input located on the RIGHT-SIDE PANEL

High-level input: ECG phono-phono input located on LEFT-SIDE PANEL (1 V); minimal detected QRS complex: 0.18 mV

Arterial pressure

Low level input: Transducer: Precalibrated, disposable-type, 5 μV/V/mm sensitivity recommended; cable: six-pin male connector—AAMI; input located on the RIGHT-SIDE PANEL

High level input: Phono-phono cable 100 mm Hg/V; input on the LEFT-SIDE PANEL

   Triggering

ECG mode:

Trigger	Recognition criteria
R wave	QRS only
Peaks	QRS or pacer spikes
A/V Pace	V-pacing spikes

   Minimum 200 V QRS signal

Pressure mode: Uses arterial pressure upstroke; trigger point is approximately 50% of the systolic maximum; the system suspends augmentation every 64th beat to examine the arterial pressure tracing morphology for changes in upstroke or pressure

Internal mode: Asynchronous 75 beats/minute

   Assist ratios

   1:1, 1:2, 1:3, 1:4, 1:8

System components

   Display screen. The display screen is in the center of the control panel (Fig. 30-2) between the function control keys and the recorder. The flat screen is a dot-matrix, vacuum-fluorescent type with dual-trace capabilities.

Channel 1: Displays the ECG with an assist signal represented as a line graph between the ECG and the pressure channels

Channel 2: Displays either the arterial pressure or the balloon pressure

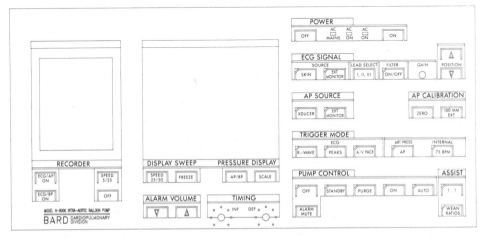

Fig. 30-2. Bard H-8000 intraaortic balloon pump control panel illustrated.

At the top of the screen above the ECG trace are three display lines:

- The first line provides a flashing, visual alarm status message.
- The second line displays the balloon volume, battery voltage, heart rate, assist ratio, and the ECG lead in use.
- The third line is a digital display of hemodynamic values during pumping and weaning.

Recorder. Located on the far left of the control panel is the two-channel strip-chart recorder, which allows the operator to obtain a permanent record of two synchronous traces, either ECG and arterial pressure (AP) or ECG and balloon pressure (BP). The balloon inflation/deflation timing markers are inserted between the ECG and pressure tracings. The recorder also prints the digital values of heart rate, peak systolic pressure, peak diastolic pressure, end diastolic pressure, and mean arterial pressure.

Operating panel and keyboard. The function control keys allow selection of all operating parameters for the IABP. On the right side of the panel are five groups of keys; each group controls a separate function and each key is individually labeled:

Power (on/off): Indicator lights describe the power source: AC MAIN/ AC ON/ DC ON

ECG signal: ECG source, lead selection, transport filter, gain, and position

AP source: Arterial pressure source; arterial pressure calibration

Trigger mode: ECG/arterial pressure/internal

Pump control: OFF/STANDBY/PURGE/ON/AUTO; ASSIST RATIO: 1:1/WEAN RATIOS: 1:2, 1:3, 1:4, 1:8 ALARM MUTE

Bed mount. The lightweight console with integrated handles can be carried or secured to a bed mount, footboard, or siderails.

Wheel cart. The four-wheeled cart is designed for positioning the console at either a 45-, 75-, or 90-degree angle to optimize viewing in a variety of clinical situations.

THEORY OF OPERATION

The Bard H-8000 IABP system is an electromechanical device designed to inflate and deflate intraaortic balloon catheters to a known, user-selectable volume. The H-8000 system consists of six major subsystems that work simultaneously to provide precise operation and maintenance of aortic counterpulsation. These six subsystems are the power control system, operator interface, patient input panels, triggering, pneumatic control, and system surveillance.

Power control system

The H-8000 can be operated in either AC or DC power. Light emitting diode (LED) lights in the POWER section of the keypad indicate the mode in which the unit is operating. AC operation is always recommended unless operation in transport or during a power failure becomes necessary.

Operator interface

The operator interface contains the keypad and timing controls; the display for monitoring ECG and pressure waveforms, and pumping status; and the strip-chart recorder for obtaining hard copy of displayed information and parameters.

Patient input panels

Patient data input—specifically, ECG and arterial pressure waveforms—can be acquired from either direct (low-level), indirect (high-level), or both sources (Fig. 30-3). These inputs provide the electronic cues for detection, recognition, and issuance of trigger signals, as well as the numeric value of heart rate and arterial pressure.

Triggering

The H-8000 contains five triggering options that use the patient's ECG or arterial pressure waveforms for recognizing appropriate trigger events. An internally generated, fixed-rate trigger is available for use during periods of cardiac standstill. To enhance the quality of trigger signals, there are display filters and gain and pressure size controls.

Pneumatic control

The pneumatic system generates the necessary volume, pressure, and vacuum to shuttle helium into and out of the catheter. Inflation volume is set according to balloon size and can be adjusted using the volume control. The helium-filled IAB catheter and pneumatic tubing are then attached to the IAB console isolation assembly, forming a closed, closely monitored system.

The isolation assembly is composed of the following internal elements:

Segregating diaphragm: Separates the patient/catheter side from the internal pneumatic system

In-line pressure transducer: Relays pressure status to the system, producing a characteristic balloon pressure waveform

Fill and vent valves: Regulate the helium volume within the balloon

Leak-detection safety circuits: Analyze volume and pressure on a beat-to-beat basis, ensure constant volume delivery, and cause system shutdown when a pressure threshold is exceeded

System surveillance

The H-8000 uses two electronic surveillance systems. One system monitors and controls helium delivery, and the other monitors signals for triggering and timing

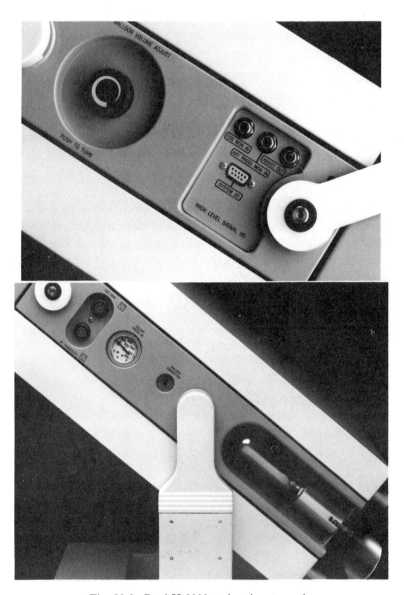

Fig. 30-3. Bard H-8000 patient input panels.

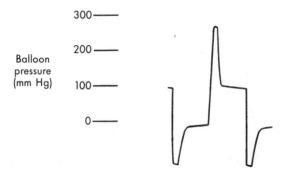

Balloon
pressure
(mm Hg)

300 ——
200 ——
100 ——
0 ——

Fig. 30-4. Depiction of Helium surveillance by a balloon pressure waveform.

circuits. Helium is under constant surveillance to ensure precise volume delivery under circumstances of varying pressure and heart rate. Helium surveillance is depicted by a balloon pressure waveform (Fig. 30-4), which has characteristic morphology consisting of a baseline, inflation limb, plateau, and deflation limb.

STEPS TO OPERATION

The following is a summary of the steps involved in setting up and initiating counterpulsation with the Bard H-8000.

I. Inspect the system.
Power
1. Check that the detachable power cord is securely seated in the main power receptacle on the bottom panel.
2. Plug the system line cord into a grounded, three-prong AC receptacle marked HOSPITAL GRADE.
3. Check that the AC MAINS switch on the bottom panel of the console is in the "on" position.
4. Press the ON key on the power control panel.
5. Check that the AC MAINS and AC ON indicator lights on the front panel are illuminated.
    Supplies
1. Inspect the helium tank gauge for a minimal gas pressure of 200 psi.
2. Check that there is an adequate paper supply for the strip-chart recorder.
3. Have ECG skin cable, pressure transducer, and phone-phone jack cables available for patient inputs.

II. Connect an ECG source

The ECG is the most easily obtained and reliable trigger source. Every effort should be made to obtain a clean, interference-free ECG signal from the patient skin electrodes. In situations where a direct skin electrode connection is not feasible or desirable, a high-gain signal from an external monitor (1 V) can be used. *Many operators find it advantageous to have both monitor and direct skin leads on the patient, for maximal flexibility and backup during pumping.*

Direct (low-level) ECG

1. Carefully prepare the patient's skin and apply electrodes to the selected sites according to standard hospital procedure. Site selection depends on the quality of the trigger signal and on the environment in which the control system is used. For example, during surgery, electrodes should be placed where they will not interfere with the operation but will remain dry and free of mechanical interference (e.g., backs of the shoulders or posterior chest).
2. Attach the six-pin patient cable to the ECG INPUT SKIN connector in the right hand panel. The Bard H-8000 IABP and its cables have built-in filters and suppressors to help reduce electrosurgical interference.
3. Press the SKIN key on the ECG SIGNAL SOURCE on the function control panel.
4. Press through the LEAD SELECT key on the control panel to choose the lead configuration (Lead I, Lead II, Lead III) that provides the largest, most reliable QRS complex for the trigger source.
5. Adjust the GAIN dial if necessary to increase the ECG amplitude. If you do not get a high-quality ECG, check the electrode skin contact to be sure that the electrodes are firmly seated in the cable or change the electrodes.

External (high-level) ECG

1. Prepare the skin and apply the monitor electrodes according to standard hospital procedure.
2. Connect the phone-phone cable between the external monitor (1 V) and the ECG MON IN on the left-side panel of the console.
3. Select an appropriate lead for triggering on the patient monitor, not the balloon console.
4. Press the EXT MONITOR key on the ECG SIGNAL SOURCE on the function control panel.

III. Connect an arterial pressure source

Direct arterial monitoring

1. Connect the transducer: Connect a compatible six-pin transducer cable or a transducer adapter to the AP TRANSDUCER input on the RIGHT-SIDE PANEL of the console.

2. Calibrate the transducer to zero:
   a. Press AP/BP key under the display screen to select arterial pressure (AP) signal.
   b. Press SCALE for the pressure range of 0 to 150 mm Hg.
   c. Open the transducer stopcock to air.
   d. Press ZERO key under AP CALIBRATION and hold until the mean pressure digital readout shows zeroes and the pressure trace is at the zero line on the monitor.
3. Calibrate to 100 mm Hg pressure:
   a. Precalibrated transducer:
      (1) Press 100 MM EXT calibration button under AP CALIBRATION.
      (2) Hold until the digital mean pressure reads 100 mm Hg and the pressure trace is at the 100 mm Hg line on the monitor.
   b. Uncalibrated (strain-gauge) transducer:
      (1) Apply 100 mm Hg pressure with a mercury manometer to the transducer.
      (2) Press 100 MM EXT calibration button until the mean pressure digital mean readout reads 100 mm Hg and the pressure trace is at the 100 mm line on the monitor.
4. Select a pressure display range. Press the SCALE key on the control panel to select the pressure range of 0 to 60, 0 to 150, or 0 to 300 mm Hg. Selection of the display range depends on the patient's blood pressure, the quality of the waveform, and whether you are monitoring arterial or balloon pressure.
5. Complete the arterial line assembly using standard hospital protocol for arterial pressure line assembly and maintenance.
6. Close the pressure transducer to air.
7. Check the arterial pressure waveform to ensure that there is a clearly discernible dicrotic notch. Check that the digital readout is registering systolic, diastolic, and mean pressures.

External monitor arterial pressure input
1. Connect a phono-phono cable between the high level arterial pressure output from the monitor and ART PRESS MON IN on the left-hand panel of the console. The input should be 100 mm Hg/V.
2. Proceed with steps 4 through 7 above.

Displaying the balloon pressure. The balloon pressure waveform is used to assess the status of the intraaortic balloon and the function of the pneumatic system. The balloon pressure is derived from a built-in pressure transducer attached to the patient side of the closed system.
1. Press the AP/BP key of the PRESSURE DISPLAY under the display sweep screen to select balloon pressure (BP).
2. Adjust the display range to accommodate the size of the balloon pressure waveform.

IV. Select a trigger

1. Review all the triggering options and select the most appropriate one for your patient. Consider a second reasonable option as well. In the event that your primary trigger is no longer usable, you can quickly switch to another reliable source.
2. Press the appropriate key on the TRIGGER MODE panel.
3. Check for triggering: The LED in the selected key will flash with detection of each trigger.
4. Should you lose the trigger signal, the system will sound an alarm, display the alarm message NO TRIGGER, deflate the balloon, and shut the system down. You may need to find a new trigger source.
5. Set the *approximate* points of inflation and deflation according to the ECG. Adjust the inflation control dial to situate the inflate marker just beyond the peak of the T wave. Adjust the deflation control dial to situate the deflate marker just before the subsequent R wave. The ECG is used to set the *approximate* inflate/deflate points *only*. You must use the arterial pressure tracing to adjust inflation and deflation precisely.
6. Set the WEAN RATIO to 1:2.
7. Adjust the BALLOON VOLUME ADJUST dial to correspond to the displacement volume of the selected balloon. The BALLOON VOLUME ADJUST dial is located on the LEFT-SIDE PANEL of the console. While you turn the dial, watch the display screen for the balloon volume. Turn the dial until the desired volume is achieved.

V. Connect the balloon

1. Connect the end of the PVC tubing to the BALLOON CONNECTION port located in the RIGHT-SIDE PANEL.
2. Press STANDBY on the PUMP CONTROL panel to prepare the system for operation, and add helium to the system.
3. Press PURGE on the PUMP CONTROL panel to evacuate the remaining air and load the system with helium. Press PURGE again to fully flush the system and fill it completely with helium.
4. Select BALLOON PRESSURE on the DISPLAY SCREEN.
5. Press the PUMP CONTROL ON key. The balloon will begin inflating and deflating. In the ON mode, many alarms will be operative but the full surveillance system will not.
6. Verify the balloon pressure waveform for characteristic morphology.
7. Select ARTERIAL PRESSURE on the screen.
8. Adjust the timing using a 1:2 assist ratio.
9. Assess the hemodynamic effects of timing.
10. Press the ASSIST key control to 1:1.

11. Assess the counterpulsation and its effect on hemodynamics.
12. Press AUTO on the PUMP CONTROL PANEL to activate the automatic surveillance system and alarms.

SETTING INFLATION AND DEFLATION WITH THE BARD H-8000

This section describes features and controls of the H-8000 that are used to adjust inflate and deflate timing of the system. The reader should refer to Part Three of this book for a comprehensive discussion of the hemodynamic assessment of proper and improper IABP timing.

Timing refers to an operator-controlled action that varies the inflation and deflation cycles of the balloon relative to the synchronized trigger signal. The objective of balloon inflation is to increase intraaortic pressure during diastole. Therefore the operator must time the inflation to occur immediately after the aortic valve closes. The objective of balloon deflation is to decrease myocardial oxygen demand by causing a sudden reduction in intraaortic pressure immediately before the onset of systole, thus reducing resistance to left ventricular ejection. To achieve this, the operator must set balloon deflation to occur during isovolumetric contraction, just before the aortic valve opening.

With the Bard H-8000 the preliminary inflate/deflate settings are performed with the pump "OFF". The *approximate* points of inflation and deflation can be set according to the ECG and the arterial pressure waveform before initiating counterpulsation. Line graphs representing the balloon inflation and deflation commands are displayed just below the ECG channel. The line graphs are present whenever the system is triggering. Corresponding to the adjustment of inflation and deflation controls, the H-8000 highlights the arterial pressure trace from the beginning of diastole (the arterial pressure point where inflation would begin) to the beginning of systole (the point where deflation would end) (Fig. 30-5).

To set preliminary inflate/deflate positions, do the following:
1. Adjust the inflation control dial to situate the inflate marker just beyond the peak of the T wave.
2. Adjust the deflation control dial to situate the deflate marker just before the subsequent R wave
3. Begin counterpulsation by using the STANDBY, PURGE, ON sequence.

The arterial pressure tracing *must* be used to adjust the timing of inflation and deflation and assess the hemodynamic effects of counterpulsation. Perform the following steps to refine the preliminary inflation/deflation settings as necessary:
1. Press the AP/BP key to display the arterial pressure waveform on the display screen.
2. Select an assist ratio of 1:2 using the WEAN RATIO key. This allows the operator to view both the assisted and unassisted arterial pressure waveforms.

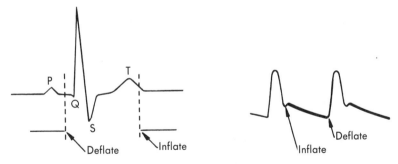

Fig. 30-5. Bard H-8000 highlights the arterial pressure trace from the beginning of systole.

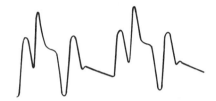

Fig. 30-6. Inflation and deflation timing using the arterial pressure waveform and a 1:2 assist ratio.

3. Slowly rotate the inflation dial until inflation occurs at the closure of the aortic valve. (This is usually the dicrotic notch, but the point may vary depending on the anatomical location of the arterial pressure line.)
4. Slowly rotate the deflation dial until the desired aortic end-diastolic pressure is achieved.

Fig. 30-6 illustrates an example of inflation and deflation timing using the arterial pressure waveform and a 1:2 assist ratio.

Once a reliable trigger source has been selected and the timing has been set, the control system of the Bard H-8000 will automatically sense and adjust for a wide range of heart rates and rhythms without operator input.

SYSTEM SURVEILLANCE: ALARM SYSTEMS AND CONTROLS

There are three automatic surveillance/alarm systems in the H-8000. Gas surveillance and alarms, control system surveillance and alarms, and safety circuit shutdown are described in Table 30-1.

Table 30-1. Surveillance systems

Alarm message	Condition	Detection criteria
Gas system surveillance and alarms		
GAS LEAKAGE	Leak in balloon line	Balloon pressure after deflation < -10 mm Hg in AUTO mode
POOR DEFLATION	Slow or no deflation pulse as seen in balloon pressure	Balloon pressure >50 mm Hg in AUTO MODE 80 msec after deflation command
FILL PRESSURE	High helium pressure in balloon line	Helium pressure during fill, or after deflation while pumping >24 mm Hg
KINKED LINE	Kink in balloon line	Balloon pressure just before deflation: >250 mm Hg, provided that assist interval >200 msec in AUTO mode; alarm occurs on fifth consecutive occurrence
BAL DISCONNECT	No pressure in balloon line, or balloon line not connected	Balloon pressure <120 mm Hg, 70 msec after inflation in AUTO mode
Control system surveillance and alarms		
ECG DETECTED	ECG detected while pumping in INTERNAL	Detects four consecutive ECG complexes
NO TRIGGER	No trigger signal detected for 5.12 sec	No trigger signal detected for 5.12 sec
LOW AIR DRIVE	Insufficient air drive pressure to inflate the balloon	Pressure at compressor tank <4 psi

Table 30-1.   Surveillance systems—cont'd

Alarm message	Condition	Detection criteria
LOW VACUUM	Insufficient vacuum	Pressure at vacuum tank >-2.0 psi
HIGH AIR DRIVE	Drive pressure exceeds 9 psi	
NOISY ECG	Oscillatory baseline noise in ECG	32 noisy segments: If <32 segments of noise, the system resets when the problem ceases
SET TIMING	Assist interval set too short to inflate the balloon	Inflation and deflation points are set at the same place, or the difference between the deflation point and the inflation point is <80 msec
HELIUM LOW	Insufficient helium supply pressure	Pressure at LOW PRESSURE REGULATOR <45 psi
ARRHYTHMIA	Time interval variation	Detects a large beat-to-beat variation in time interval for 8 cycles out of the last 16 beats
BAT LOW	Battery voltage low; nearing the end of discharge	Voltage at battery <22.5 V

Safety circuit: The purpose of the **SAFETY CIRCUIT** is to prevent prolonged balloon inflation (i.e., a balloon pressure greater than 50 mm Hg for longer than 2 seconds) and to warn the operator in case of interrupted operation. The system will deflate the balloon and shut down. This safety circuit is operated independent of the system computer.

TROUBLESHOOTING GUIDELINES

Maintaining optimal patient-input signals and ensuring the integrity of all pneumatic connections will help to prevent most system problems. Interruptions in continuous pumping can occur that are either console or catheter related. Tables 30-2 and 30-3 are guides to troubleshooting system alarms and common operational problems.

Table 30-2. Troubleshooting alarm messages

Alarm message	Possible condition	Operator action
BAL DISCONNECT	Balloon line not connected No pressure in balloon line	Check for disconnected PVC tubing at console or between balloon catheter and PVC tubing. SERVICE-REQUIRED SOURCES: • Balloon pressure transducer • Inflate or deflate valve • Power supply • Computer board
FILL PRESSURE	High helium pressure in balloon line	Check that the volume control is correctly set for the balloon size used. SERVICE-REQUIRED SOURCES: • Possible overfill by fill valve • Fill valve fails to close • Vent valve fails to open
GAS LEAKAGE	Loose connection	Check the connections at console and at catheter to ensure they are firmly seated. If it is a stretch at the connector, remove the connector, cut off a small segment of the connector, and replace.
	Leak in balloon line: catheter or PVC tubing	Small leak in tubing: wrap with non-porous tape. Large leak: change catheter or PVC tubing.

Table 30-2.   Troubleshooting alarm messages—cont'd

Alarm message	Possible condition	Operator action
	Blood in PVC tubing	Discontinue pumping; notify physician; remove and replace balloon catheter.
HIGH AIR DRIVE	Drive pressure exceeds 9 psi	SERVICE-REQUIRED SOURCES: • Pressure switch malfunction • Balloon volume control is loose or malfunctioning
HELIUM LOW	Insufficient helium supply pressure	Check gauge and replace tank if necessary. Check that the helium tank is properly seated. Ensure that supply valve is open.
KINKED LINE	Kink in balloon catheter or PVC tubing	Find the kink or twist in the catheter or tubing and straighten out.
LOW VACUUM	Insufficient vacuum	SERVICE-REQUIRED SOURCE: • Vacuum malfunction
BAT LOW	20 minutes or less of battery operation remain	Attach power cord to AC supply as soon as possible to recharge battery and maintain pumping.
NO TRIGGER	Loose or disconnected ECG leads	Check leads and connections.
	ECG gain too small	Use GAIN knob to increase size of ECG. Change lead selection; change trigger source.
	Monitor input disconnected	Check input from monitor and secure.
	If using AP, arterial line damped, disconnected, or turned off	Check arterial line tracing, flush line; change to ECG trigger; check transducer or monitor input.
	Patient's cardiac activity ceased	CHECK PATIENT FOR CARDIAC ACTIVITY. Switch to INTERNAL TRIGGER if no cardiac activity is present.

Continued.

Table 30-2.   Troubleshooting alarm messages—cont'd

Alarm message	Possible condition	Operator action
NOISY ECG	Patient muscle activity	Change position of ECG leads. Check all connections and leads and secure or change. Select another trigger mode. Select another lead.
	Electrocautery in use	Switch to direct ECG if on EX-TERNAL.
	Possible faulty ground in the AC outlet	Change AC source.
ECG DETECTED	Cardiac activity detected while pumping in INT mode	Switch trigger mode according to patient's rhythm. Readjust timing.
POOR DEFLATION	Slow or no deflation	Check balloon pressure wave-form.
	Kinked line	Check catheter and PVC tubing for kink.
	Possible occlusion in the catheter	Change catheter if necessary.
	Possible vacuum malfunction	SERVICE REQUIRED
SET TIMING	Assist interval set too short to inflate balloon	Press WEAN RATIO to 1:2 to evaluate timing. Readjust timing.
No Message	Failure to fill in STANDBY	Check helium gauge. Replace bottle if helium is empty.
	Balloon pressure remains below zero in standby mode	SERVICE-REQUIRED SOURCES: • Fill valve failure • Low pressure regulator miscalibrated

Table 30-3. Troubleshooting common operational problems

Problem	Possible cause	Probable alarm or message	Correction
No power or AC MAINS does not illuminate	Power cord not connected to AC power Fault in the AC power source AC switch in bottom panel is not on Console fuse is blown	BAT LOW (if AC has not been on and battery has run down)	Change AC power source; check connections. Check AC power switch. Change fuse.
No audible alarm	Alarm volume key has been turned to its lowest volume tone		Increase volume tone.
No ECG	Improper connections	NO TRIGGER	Check which ECG signal you are using—SKIN or EXT MONITOR—and that you have made the proper connections.
	Poor electrode contact Improperly placed electrodes		Change the electrodes. Ensure that all connections are secure.
Wandering ECG baseline	Transport	ARRHYTHMIA	Engage the transport filter.
	Respiratory variant		Change the electrodes.
No AP waveform	Balloon pressure has been selected for display Defect in the arterial pressure system	NO TRIGGER (if triggering in AP mode) No hemodynamic values are present on line three of the display	Select AP for display. Check patency of the arterial line: • Flush as needed. • Check stopcocks. • Replace transducer.
Transducer cannot be calibrated	Defective transducer		Check calibration procedure. Replace transducer.

AIR TRANSPORT

IABP consoles may be used in an air-transport capacity in both helicopters and fixed-wing aircraft. Because of the wide variety of aircraft in use today, it is beyond the scope of this chapter to describe operating information germane to each type. We do, however, suggest the following guidelines when operating an IABP system in air-transport situations:

1. Have all the items necessary for operation (i.e., cables, helium, recorder paper).
2. Have an alternate power source in the aircraft to avoid consuming DC power.
3. Have a predetermined method of securing the IABP console in the aircraft to prevent accidental movement in transport and to protect the system itself.
4. Always operate the IABP system in an alarms-active mode to ensure that the gas surveillance system is in constant operation. This mode will notify the clinician of changes in the helium supply that could be secondary to changes in barometric pressure.

RESOURCE

For further information about the Bard H-8000 IABP system, please contact the Bard Cardiopulmonary Division, One Park West, Tewksbury, MA 01876, 1-800-782-9003.

PART SIX

IABC IN SPECIAL SITUATIONS

CHAPTER 31

Ambulatory IABC

Susan J. Quaal

A shortage of donor hearts frequently results in a prolonged period of intraaortic balloon counterpulsation (IABC) before the patient receives a heart transplantation. Standard intraaortic balloon (IAB) insertion through the femoral artery severely restricts patient mobility. Therefore a patient who is already compromised is placed at risk for further complications such as pneumonia and embolism due to this imposed immobility. McBride and associates[1] at St. Louis University have used a left or right axillary artery insertion technique (Chapter 12) without the use of a graft, thus allowing the patient full mobility (Fig. 31-1).

PATIENT MANAGEMENT

Patient management is identical for those patients whose IAB is transfemorally inserted. The IABs inner cannula is used for pressure monitoring; radial and femoral arterial lines are not used because of mobility limitations. Because of the partial obstruction of the axillary artery proximal to the site of insertion, radial artery monitoring on the ipsilateral side of IAB placement will most likely be inaccurate. Timing principles are the same as for transfemoral IAB placement.

Anticoagulation therapy consists of dextran sulfate or heparin. Antibiotic coverage is listed in the box. If an infection is suspected at the IAB insertion site, the IAB should be removed and reinserted on the contralateral side. Because these patients were not intubated they were maintained on a high caloric, regular diet; appetite and caloric intake improved after initiating IABC.[2]

Balloon removal is usually accomplished in the operating room. The incision is reopened and proximal and distal control are again obtained. After complete balloon deflation, the IAB is withdrawn through the arteriotomy and vascular clamps are applied proximal and distal to the site. Each clamp is briefly removed in turn to flush any intraarterial thrombus out through the arteriotomy. The artery is then closed with a 5-0 polypropylene suture. No complications have been encountered when using this approach.[1]

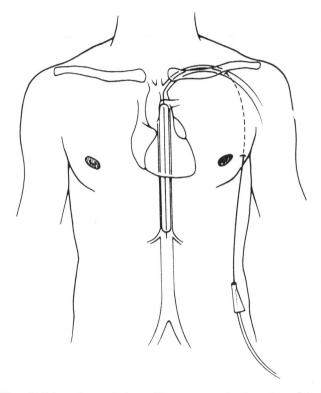

Fig. 31-1. Axillary IAB insertion technique. The most proximal portion of the IAB is located just beyond the origin of the left subclavian artery. This results in the distal end being located at the second or third lumbar vertebral body. (From McBride LR, Miller LW, Naunheim KS et al: *Ann Thorac Surg* 48:874, 1989.)

RECOMMENDED ANTIBIOTIC COVERAGE PROTOCOL
FOR AMBULATORY IABC PATIENTS

1. Cephalosporin only (no preoperative infection in the hospital <5 days).
2. Add aminoglycoside if in the hospital >5 days.
3. If infection is present before device insertion, continue preoperative antibiotics.
4. Stop prophylactic antibiotics after 3 doses if no infection is present.
5. Treat only cultured, clinically significant organisms.

From Reedy JE, Ruzevich SA, Noedel NR et al: Nursing care of the ambulatory patient with a mechanical assist device, *J Heart Transplant* 9:97, 1990.

LIMITATIONS

This technique has now been suspended at St. Louis University because of air leaks in the catheter probably as a result of patient mobility. Discussions are in process regarding redesigning the IAB to prevent air leaks.[3,4]

REFERENCES

1. McBride LR, Miller LW, Naunheim KS et al: Axillary artery insertion of an intraaortic balloon pump, *Ann Thorac Surg* 48:874, 1989.
2. Reedy JE, Ruzevich SA, Noedel NR et al: Nursing care of the ambulatory patient with a mechanical assist device, *J Heart Transplant* 9:97, 1990.
3. Reedy J: Personal correspondence, June 19, 1990.
4. Swartz MT: Personal correspondence, October 10, 1991.

CHAPTER 32

Pulmonary artery balloon counterpulsation

Bernice Coleman

At the completion of cardiopulmonary bypass (CPB), adequate biventricular function is required for successful weaning and postoperative recovery. Often cardiac surgical patients have some degree of left heart ventricular dysfunction in the operating room that may require treatment with inotropic medications, potassium repletion, volume replacement, pacing, correction of acidosis, and/or use of intraaortic balloon counterpulsation (IABC). However, a less described occurrence of right ventricular dysfunction that is observed in the operating room is significant enough to impede weaning from CPB, and persists after termination of CPB has been reported.[1-4] Significant ventricular dysfunction during the early postoperative phase has sometimes warranted the use of a right ventricular assist device to help in weaning from CPB and assist the dysfunctional right ventricle until it recovers. It is not uncommon for patients in the intensive care unit (ICU) to be supported with such a device until the right ventricle recovers. However, using a pulmonary artery balloon counterpulsation (PABC) model as a right ventricular assist device can pose quite a nursing challenge. This chapter reviews the operative causes for postpump right ventricle dysfunction (PPRVD), pathophysiology, indications, balloon placement, mechanism of action, timing, weaning, and nursing considerations specific to patients undergoing PABC.

CAUSES OF POSTPUMP RIGHT VENTRICULAR DYSFUNCTION

To appreciate how an intraoperative right ventricle injury affects left ventricle volume loading, a brief overview of normal right ventricular function follows. Generally, RV coronary perfusion is accomplished through the right coronary artery (RCA) and, to a lesser extent, the left coronary artery. The importance of this dual blood supply is most evident in the septum. The septal upper two thirds is perfused by the left anterior descending (LAD) coronary branch and the lower one third by the RCA. Anatomically, the septum is thought to be functionally a part of the left ventricle (LV). This is extremely important, because septal function is directly related to an intact pericardium and a normally functioning LV. In addition to these factors which support normal RV contractility, the complex manner in which RV tension and output are generated is also important. Three contractile phases normally must occur for adequate RV output to be maintained. First, there is a ringer motion of the figure eight muscles. Second, the RV free wall moves toward the interventricular septum (IVS). Lastly, LV tension is transferred through the IVS to the right ventricle and assists with propelling RV output into the pulmonary circuit. Therefore RV output is dependent on normal LV function. Alterations in any of these factors can occur with cardiac surgery, causing a decrease in RV cardiac output. However, elevation in pulmonary vascular resistance (PVR) is the major impedance to RV output, particularly when all other variables are normal. Many alterations in normal RV function may already be present before the patient arrives in the operating room. These risks range from coronary artery disease, myocardial damage, decreased contractility, to hypertrophy. Compounding such risks are insults resulting from the cardiac operation, which may include elevation in pulmonary vascular resistance,[1-6] opening of the pericardium,[7,8] extended time on CPB,[9] interventricular septal dysfunction,[10-12] biventricular failure,[13,14] perioperative myocardial infarction,[14,15] and problems associated with the delivery of cardioplegia via the native coronaries.

PATHOPHYSIOLOGY

Typically, the first diagnostic indication of RV dysfunction is observed in the operating room with concomitant LV dysfunction. It is characterized as a dilated right atrium with an associated elevation in volume and pressure, decreased right ventricular contractility, low left atrial volume and pressure, and poor left ventricle contractility and output. This clinical picture is commonly called biventricular failure (Fig. 32-1). RV dysfunction can also occur in isolation with the same clinical presentation, but LV filling pressures are low and contractility by direct visualization is good (Fig. 32-2).

INDICATIONS FOR PABC

The literature describing clinical use of PABC is limited to case reports and therefore lacks clinical trials to offer research-based indications. Therefore indications for use are based on experimental research using the concepts for IABC.[16-19] The key issue associated with PABC is an inability to quantify the degree of RV injury both intrinsically and extrinsically.[5,13] This issue is important, because a major indication for use is that RV injury should not be so severe that the RV is completely unable to pump its stroke volume toward the pulmonary circulation. In an

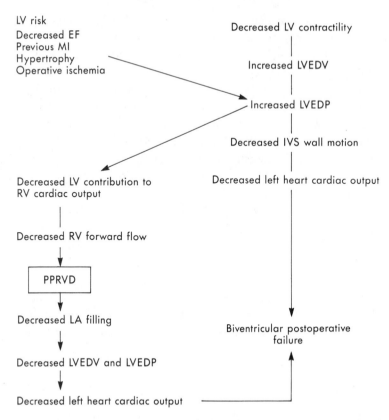

Fig. 32-1. Pathophysiology of postpump right ventricular dysfunction (PPRVD). (From Coleman B: *Crit Care Nurs Clin North Am* 1(2):379, 1989.)

attempt to further clarify the degree of RV dysfunction and which patients would benefit from PABC, Spence et al.[6] defined the extrinsic degree of injury to the RV as changes in cardiac output relative to baseline values. This injury was described as extreme failure, 0% to 20%; severe failure, 20% to 40%; and 40% to 60% of baseline as moderate injury. These investigators also found that the use of PABC with moderate RV dysfunction restored adequate systemic pressures. No change was demonstrated when PABC was used with a RV injury of less than 60% of baseline.[6] The importance of this study is the demonstration that when injury to the RV is greater than moderate, a RV assist device should be used instead of PABC.

Presently, use of PABC is limited to postpump cardiac surgical patients, because the current model is initiated in the operating room. Patients who are typically candidates are those who are not responsive to typical treatments intended to improve ventricular filling and cardiac output. There are two conditions in which right-sided

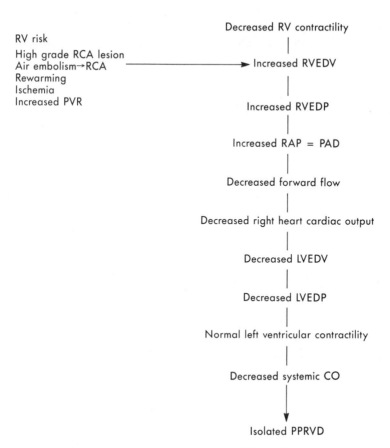

Fig. 32-2. Pathophysiology of postpump biventricular failure. (From Coleman B: *Crit Care Nurs Clin North Am* 1(2):379, 1989.)

cardiac output is diminished and PABC is used, one of which is transient elevation in PVR with isolated RV dysfunction associated with diminished forward flow and good LV contractility. The other involves patients with biventricular failure and elevated PVR who are not responsive to acidosis correction, pacing, pharmacological agents, and/or the use of IABC; these patients are also candidates for PABC.

Experimental studies with PABC

Wittnich, Spence, and Salerno[20] nicely delineated past experimental studies using PABC. Kralios et al.[16] reported the first experimental studies with PABC, using a model of pulmonary hypertension (homologous blood thrombi and cornstarch suspension injected into the pulmonary artery of dogs). PABC greatly increased cardiac output and decreased right atrial pressure. Spotnitz et al.[17] used a reciprocating piston pump (similar to the present day pulsatile assist device) in a dog model in which the pulmonary artery was occluded by a clamp. Right ventricular failure improved during PABC, with an increase in cardiac output and a decrease in right ventricular systolic and diastolic pressures.

A study by de la Rivere et al.[21] demonstrated improved cardiac output with a pulsatile assist device in a dog model that excluded the right ventricle from the circulation by closure of the tricuspid valve and interposition of a valved conduit between the right atrium and pulmonary artery. In a goat model of right heart failure, Gaines Pierce, and Prophet[22] assessed PABC during bypass of the left side of the heart. The effect of PABC in this study, however, was not as pronounced as in the studies in which peripheral vascular resistance was increased. Jett et al.[23] demonstrated beneficial effects from PABC in a lamb model of right ventricular failure caused by pulmonary artery banding and damage to the right ventricle. Studies by Opravil, Gorman, and Krejcie[19] confirmed the beneficial effect of PABC in a dog model of pulmonary hypertension (embolization and serotonin infusion). These investigators also attempted to develop a percutaneous PABC device.

In 1984 Spence, Weisel, Easdown et al.[24] reported on use of PABC and its mechanism of action when used in cases of right ventricular failure during bypass of the left side of the heart. By inserting a flow probe in the pulmonary artery, these researchers demonstrated that balloon inflation resulted in flow through the pulmonary circulation, whereas ventricular systole resulted in filling of the graft. They noted that during ventricular fibrillation, inflation and deflation of the balloon resulted in a to-and-fro movement of blood in the pulmonary artery branch, without any net forward flow augmentation. Thus it appears that at least 50% residual right ventricular function is necessary for PABC to be effective. During PABC, right ventricular cardiac output doubled, from 520 ml/min during failure to 1.1 L/min with PABC.

PULMONARY ARTERY BALLOON PLACEMENT

Despite past and current experimental animal use of an intrapulmonary balloon for initiation of PABC,[25] the clinical model employs placement of an extrapulmonary balloon for output counterpulsation of the right side of the heart. It requires that the sternum and pericardium be opened. The surgeon anastomoses a 20- to 22-mm Dacron graft onto the main pulmonary artery, just distal to the pulmonic valve.[1,4,6,26] A conventional IAB catheter is placed within the conduit. The distal conduit end is ligated with heavy suture to include the catheter distal to the end of the balloon (Fig. 32-3). Just before ligation, one must ensure that the graft is void of all air and stretched to prevent a recoil motion when the conduit is filled with blood. Conduit slack will prevent any net gain in forward flow through the pulmonary circulation and defeat the effects of PABC.[6] The catheter is then attached to an IAB

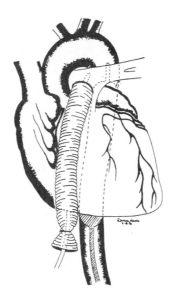

Fig. 32-3. A 20-cm Dacron graft anastomosed to the main pulmonary artery; a 40-cc intraaortic balloon (IAB) catheter was inserted into the graft, which was closed distally by heavy ligation. A 40-cc IAB catheter is also pictured in the descending aorta. (From Miller DC et al: *J Thorac Cardiovasc Surg* 8:760, 1980 and Coleman B: *Crit Care Nurs Clin North Am* 1(2):380, 1989.)

console. It exits the sternotomy incision through the base. The sternum is left open, but both subcutaneous tissue and skin are typically closed. A large sterile dressing is applied, which is changed by the surgeon.

Percutaneous technique

The surgical implantation technique described previously requires additional surgery for balloon and graft removal, a procedure that carries a significant risk of morbidity and mortality. Researchers at the University of Toronto[20] have developed a technique for inserting a PABC balloon into the pulmonary artery via the outflow of the right ventricle. A banana-shaped Datascope 20-ml balloon is inserted percutaneously via the femoral vein and guided into the pulmonary artery via the right side of the heart. After 24 hours of PABC, however, morphological damage has been noted in the heart and lungs, including focal myocardial and valvular hemorrhage with thrombus formation, as well as focal myocardial necrosis.

Anticoagulation

The issue of anticoagulation use while the patient undergoes PABC is a curious one. The literature does not report its use but does pose the question of its efficacy.

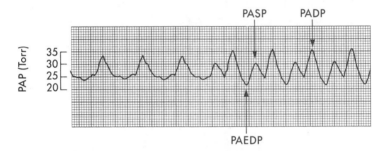

Fig. 32-4. Pulmonary artery pressure waveform. *PASP*, pulmonary artery systolic pressure; *PADP*, pulmonary artery diastolic pressure; *PAEDP*, pulmonary artery end diastolic pressure. (From Miller DC et al: *J Thorac Cardiovasc Surg* 8:761, 1980.)

In our limited experience, anticoagulation was not used and no clot in the diverticulum was found at balloon removal on postoperative day five.[27]

TIMING CONSIDERATIONS

No clinical research exists offering direction for exact timing of PABC, especially when used in conjunction with IABC. However, what is known is extrapolated from experimental animal trials and IABC concepts. Consistently, the literature demonstrates that once the PABC balloon catheter is placed within the conduit, it is connected to a counterpulsation console, which is triggered from an upright R wave. Timing is achieved by using the pulmonary artery waveform. Inflation is set to occur at pulmonic valve closure, while deflation is set to occur just before pulmonic systole[19] (Fig. 32-4). If PABC and IABC are used together, it is recommended that PABC inflation be timed to occur just a bit later than IABC, because the RV normally empties a bit later than the LV.[2,21,22] There are many unanswered questions about PABC timing in isolation and in conjunction with IABC. For instance, What is the normal delay time for a signal to travel from the tip of the pulmonary artery catheter to the transducer? When both IABC and PABC are in use, is there an additional delay time? When two catheters are being used for counterpulsation of the left and right sides of the heart, which usually work in concert and are manipulated by two consoles, what effects should be compensated for with respect to timing?[22] Further research in this area will offer answers to these important questions.

MECHANISM OF ACTION OF PABC

Positive effects of PABC using the current clinical model are achieved only if the dysfunctional RV can pump its stroke volume into the conduit above the outflow

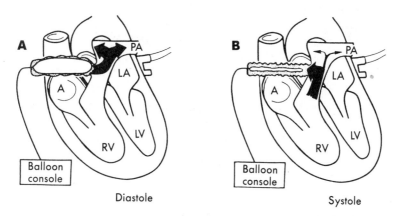

Fig. 32-5. The mechanism of action of pulmonary artery balloon counterpulsation is demonstrated. **A,** In diastole, balloon inflation ejects blood from the graft through the pulmonary circulation. **B,** During systole, the right ventricle fills the graft after the balloon deflates. There is almost no flow through the pulmonary circulation in systole. (From Spence P et al: *Surg Clin North Am* 65:694, 1985.)

tract. During RV systole, the pulmonic balloon within the conduit is deflated and right-sided cardiac output is pumped into the conduit, which fills with blood. During RV diastole, the pulmonic balloon inflates and augments forward flow by propelling stroke volume into the pulmonary circulation, which then fills the left side of the heart (Fig. 32-5).

As long as the patient remains in normal sinus rhythm and maintains at least moderate right ventricular contractility, the pulmonic balloon will function as previously stated and improved hemodynamics are observed. Benefits of augmented forward flow using PABC are (1) increase in RV stroke work index, (2) decrease in PVR, (3) decrease in peak systolic pulmonary pressure, (4) increase in pressure gradient across the pulmonary vasculature, (5) increase in LV preload, and (6) no direct change in coronary perfusion.

Conditions in which PABC through a conduit approach would be ineffective are atrial fibrillation, ventricular fibrillation, and pulmonary hypertension. In these conditions the conduit is filled by retrograde filling from the pulmonary circulation. This occurs in atrial fibrillation and ventricular fibrillation because RV forward flow is extremely diminished and does not fill the conduit. In the case of pulmonary hypertension, high pressures within the pulmonary circulatory beds cause retrograde filling.

WEANING CONSIDERATIONS

The patient's clinical picture will provide the best guide to timing for PABC weaning. The literature and clinical experience have supported using the typical sequence of 1:1, 1:2, and so on used for IABC weaning. In the case where both IABC and PABC are in use, it is of benefit to wean the patient from IABC first. This allows for close monitoring of both LV function and recovery while assessing the impact of IABC weaning on RV function and recovery. In addition, monitoring of oxygenation, cardiopulmonary hemodynamics, mentation, urine output, and the patient's requirements for inotropic and chronotropic medications will all serve to provide a complete picture of the patient's response to weaning.

NURSING MANAGEMENT SPECIFIC TO PABC

Nursing management of patients with PABC is similar to management of a recovering postoperative cardiac surgical patient. This section focuses on three nursing diagnoses specific to the care of PABC patients.

Alteration in cardiac output

Major considerations for maintaining an adequate cardiac output are monitoring rhythm, timing of the balloon(s), volume replacement, biventricular contractility, and potential for bleeding. Extremely crucial to proper functioning of the balloon(s) is the presence of normal sinus rhythm (NSR). These patients are at risk for developing dysrhythmias secondary to low serum potassium levels, hypoxemia, and conduction system trauma caused by surgery. Anticipate these potential problems, and plan for appropriate interventions. Recognize that any changes in cardiac rhythm will affect balloon timing. Monitor and obtain a timing-pattern hard copy at the beginning of the shift, with rhythm changes and PRN. Volume replacement for these patients will be individualized and specific to the cardiopulmonary hemodynamics. Recovery patterns of each ventricle will vary. RV recovery, although unpredictable, is dependent on the degree of injury, cause, and reversibility.[4] However, in the absence of persistent pulmonary hypertension, recovery can occur within 3 to 5 days.[14,21] The LV may take longer and is reported to recover within 8 to 11 days, depending on the injury sustained.[14] Close monitoring of the resistances (PVR and SVR) and the patient's clinical presentation will assist in determining ventricular recovery. When the patient is being weaned from the balloon(s), continue to monitor ventricular function, stroke work indices, and filling pressures of the right side of the heart as an indication of weaning tolerance. Lastly, patients will have a decrease in platelet count from balloon counterpulsation. Close monitoring of all clotting indices is essential. In addition, monitor for the signs and symptoms of cardiac tamponade or excessive bleeding from chest tubes. Because of the potential for bleeding, patients may not be anticoagulated during counterpulsation.

Impaired gas exchange

Because of balloon placement and the open sternum, the patient's mobility, secretion clearance, and gas exchange will be somewhat impaired. Reposition the patient if his or her condition allows every 2 hours. Provide good skin care, because alteration in tissue perfusion from diminished cardiac output predisposes the skin to break down. Always preoxygenate, because pulmonary hypoxemia causes an increase in PVR, which can lead to a decrease in forward flow secondary to elevated resistance.

Mental status changes

The great challenge of managing these patients is a balance between caring for the physical and psychosocial needs. Expect that these patients will have a great deal of sensory input from both machinery and personnel in their room. Monitor their mental status closely both as an indication for intensive care psychosis and the potential for embolic events. Encourage the family as much as possible to visit, touch, and talk with the patient. Provide clear information for the family in understandable terms.

SUMMARY

PPRVD is a clinical problem frequently encountered in the operating room. Its treatment with the use of PABC during the perioperative period can be initiated with a conventional IABP catheter and console. The care of these patients poses quite a challenge for nurses as we balance high technology with high touch care.

Wittnich, Spence, and Salerno[20] summarized the current state of PABC as follows:

Further developments in technology are needed before the technique can be introduced for wide clinical use. Although current knowledge indicates that PABC is useful in patients who have reduced right ventricular function, its long-term effects on the lungs and heart need to be evaluated, especially when it is performed via the percutaneous route. Earlier reports of difficulties have been related to the design of the balloon and implementation of the technique. Enormous strides have been made in addressing a number of these issues and with further refinements, PABC may eventually become available in most cardiac operating rooms.

REFERENCES

1. Miller D, Cabal-Moreno R, Stinson E et al: Right ventricular failure: observation of interrelationships affecting RV failure after aortocoronary bypass, valve surgery and congenital heart defects repair, *Cardiovasc Clin* 17:45, 1987.
2. Moran J, Opravil M, Gorman A et al: Pulmonary artery balloon counterpulsation for right ventricular failure. II. Clinical experiences, *Ann Thorac Surg* 38:254, 1984.
3. Fledge J, Wright C, Reisinger T et al: Successful balloon counterpulsation for right ventricular failure, *Ann Thorac Surg* 37:167, 1984.
4. Symbas P, McKean R, Santera A et al: Pulmonary balloon counterpulsation for treatment of intraoperative right ventricular failure, *Ann Thorac Surg* 39:437, 1985.

5. Morris J, Wechssler A: Right ventricular function: the assessment of contractile performance, *Cardiovasc Clin* 17:3, 1987.
6. Spence P, Baylis C, Peniston C et al: Right ventricular failure associated with left ventricular failure, *Cardiovasc Clin* 17:239, 1987.
7. Ross T: Acute displacement of diastolic pressure-volume curve of the left ventricle, *Circulation* 59:39, 1979.
8. Mangano D: Biventricular function after myocardial revascularization in humans: deterioration and recovery patterns during the first 24 hours, *Anesthesiology* 62:571, 1985.
9. Edmunds L, Stephenson L: Cardiopulmonary bypass for open heart surgery. In Geha A, Glenn W, Hammond G et al, eds: *Thoracic and cardiovascular surgery*, New York, 1983, Appleton-Century-Crofts.
10. Gray R, Maddahi J, Raymond M et al: Cardiac dysfunction and interventricular relationships immediately after coronary bypass. In Roberts A, ed: *Coronary artery surgery: application of new technologies*, St Louis, 1983, Mosby–Year Book.
11. Kerber R, Litchfield R: Postoperative abnormalities of interventricular septal motion: two dimensional and M-mode echocardiographic correlation, *Am Heart J* 104:263, 1982.
12. Righetti A, Crawford M, O'Rourke R: Interventricular septal motion and left ventricular function after coronary bypass surgery, *Am J Cardiol* 39:372, 1977.
13. Mills N, Ochsner J: Right ventricular failure: observation of interrelationships affecting RV failure after aortocoronary bypass, valve surgery and congenital heart defect repair, *Cardiovasc Clin* 17:45, 1987.
14. Pennington G, Merjavy J, Swartz M: The importance of biventricular failure in patients with postoperative cardiogenic shock, *Ann Thorac Surg* 39:16, 1985.
15. Balderman S, Bhayana T, Steinbach J: Perioperative myocardial infarction: a diagnostic dilemma, *Ann Thorac Surg* 30:370, 1980.
16. Kralios A, Swart H, Moulopoulos S et al: Intrapulmonary artery balloon pumping, *J Thorac Cardiovasc Surg* 60:215, 1970.
17. Spotnitz H, Berman M, Reis R et al: The effects of counterpulsation of the pulmonary artery and right ventricular hemodynamics, *J Thorac Cardiovasc Surg* 61:167, 1971.
18. Jett K, Picone A, Clark R: Circulatory support for right ventricular dysfunction, *J Thorac Cardiovasc Surg* 94:95, 1987.
19. Opravil M, Gorman A, Krejcie J: Pulmonary balloon counterpulsation for right ventricular failure. I. Experimental results, *Ann Thorac Surg* 38:242, 1984.
20. Wittnich C, Spence PA, Salerno TA: Pulmonary artery balloon counterpulsation for the management of right heart failure, *Counterpulse* 2:408, 1992.
21. de la Rivere AB, Haasler G, Malm JR et al: Mechanical assistance of the pulmonary circulation after right ventricular exclusion, *J Thorac Cardiovasc Surg* 85:809, 1983.
22. Gaines WE, Pierce WS, Prophet GA: Pulmonary circulatory support: a quantitative comparison of four methods, *J Thorac Cardiovasc Surg* 88:958, 1984.
23. Jett GK, Siwek LG, Picone AL et al: Pulmonary artery balloon counterpulsation for right ventricular failure, *J Thorac Cardiovasc Surg* 86:364, 1983.
24. Spence PA, Weisel RD, Easdown J et al: Pulmonary artery balloon counterpulsation and its mechanism of action in right ventricular failure during left heart bypass, *Surg Forum* 35:325, 1984.
25. Gonzales-Lavin L, Gu J, McGrath L et al: Pulmonary artery balloon counterpulsation for right ventriculotomy in the swine, *J Thorac Cardiovasc Surg* 99:153, 1990.
26. Spence P, Weisel R, Salerno T: Right ventricular failure, *Surg Clin North Am* 65:689, 1985.
27. Coleman B: Nursing implications for pulmonary artery balloon counterpulsation: a treatment for right ventricular dysfunction after cardiac surgery, *Crit Care Clin North Am* 1:373, 1989.

CHAPTER 33

Pediatric adaptation in balloon counterpulsation

L. George Veasy

While equipment for intraaortic balloon counterpulsation (IABC) has been adapted for pediatric use, this mode of circulatory support has found only limited acceptance for use in children.[1-5] The principal reason for its limited use is the small number of pediatric patients in any given institution who might benefit from its use. In pediatrics, as in the adult population, IABC has been employed perioperatively in roughly 70% of the cases. In the Hospital for Sick Children, Toronto, Canada, where intraaortic balloon pumping is available, it has been used in only 1.2% of open heart surgeries.[5] At Primary Children's Medical Center, IABC has been employed perioperatively in 1.6% of open heart procedures. Thus it requires a large volume of open heart procedures to use IABC with a frequency that would permit acquiring expertise in its use and justify the expense to establish and maintain such a service. Most busy pediatric services, even in larger centers, do not approach a volume that would predict IABC use in more than 6 to 8 cases yearly.

INDICATIONS

The indication for the use of IABC is essentially the same for infants and children as it is for adults. The sole indication is low cardiac output with two qualifications: (1) failure of low cardiac output to respond to maximum medical effort and (2) the basic cause for the low cardiac output is temporary and survival is likely.

The decision when "maximum" medical support has failed to ensure recovery of the patient should probably be made jointly by the surgeon, cardiologist, and intensivist. Each case has to be decided on its own merits. Objective criteria that can be used as guidelines in deciding to use IABC include: (1) persistently poor peripheral perfusion, (2) diminishing cardiac output below a cardiac index (CI) of 2.0, (3) a low or diminishing mixed venous oxygen under 30 mm Hg, (4) persistent metabolic acidosis, (5) urine output dropping under 1 ml/kg/min, (6) poor and diminishing cardiac function by echocardiography, and (7) increasing IO_2 requirements.

Because IABC is an invasive procedure, there is a natural tendency to delay its use as long as possible. Prolonged delay often occurs in pediatric patients because the only mode of introduction of the balloon catheter in pediatric patients requires a vascular surgeon. Mobilization of the surgical team and the operative procedure itself can result in an additional delay of 1 to 2 hours. All too often, a patient's cardiac output has continued to decrease below retrievable levels (CI = <1.2)[6] before IABC can be started.

BALLOON SIZE

Once a decision has been made and the surgical team is in place, selection of the appropriate size balloon must be made. The volume and length of the balloons currently commercially available are listed in Table 33-1. The length of the balloon that can be accommodated by the patient can be estimated by laying the balloon catheter in its clear, sterile packaging over the patient. The upper edge of the balloon should be positioned at the junction of the manubrium with the body of the sternum, which will approximate the origin of the left subclavian artery.[4] The balloon should not extend below half the distance between the xiphoid and the umbilicus, which will keep the balloon above the origin of the renal and superior mesenteric arteries. Balloon volume selection is limited by sizes available; an ideal size for each patient is not possible. The largest size that can be accommodated by the patient should be the first selection. It has been recommended that balloon volume should be at least half the patient's stroke volume. Cardiac output in such critically ill patients is often difficult to determine accurately. Consequently, an assumption can be made that the patient's CI would be 2.0 or less.[4] The following formula can be employed:

$$\frac{CI \times BSA}{HR} \times 0.5 = \text{balloon size}$$

If the prospective patient had a body surface area (BSA) of 0.4 M^2 and a heart rate (HR) of 140, stroke volume would then be 5.7 ml. Because a 3 ml balloon is not available, the 5 ml balloon should be selected.

Table 33-1.   Pediatric intraaortic balloon catheters*

Volume (ml)	Catheter (Fr)	Balloon length (cm)	Balloon diameter (mm)
2.5	4.5	10.7	6.0
5.0	5.5	12.8	8.0
7.0	5.5	14.2	9.0
12.0	6.5	15.8	10.0
20.0	7.5	17.8	12.0
(4.0 ml available by special order)			

*Datascope Corp., Paramus, NJ.

TIMING

Timing of balloon inflation and deflation is essentially the same as it is in adults. Balloon inflation should coincide with the dicrotic notch seen on the arterial pulse wave (Fig. 33-1). With low cardiac output, this marker is often difficult to see and is frequently noted low on the descending limb of the arterial pulse. Thus balloon inflation high on the descending limb of the arterial pulse contour may be more appropriate. We have recently used echocardiography with Doppler interrogation to determine when forward flow in the aorta from ventricular systole has ended and have inflated the balloon immediately thereafter. This gives an additional area of diastolic perfusion and increases the myocardial oxygen supply/demand ratio. In the ideal case, suprasystolic diastolic augmentation and lowered end-diastolic pressures should be achieved (see Fig. 33-1). Continuous monitoring and appropriate adjusting of balloon inflation and deflation are prime requirements for effective pediatric IABC.

NURSING CONSIDERATIONS

Institution of IABC significantly increases nursing demands. A single nurse can not manage a critically ill patient and the pumping module simultaneously. Pediatric patients who require IABC are usually so critically ill they are on mechanical ventilation. Thus any patient on IABC requires an additional nurse. The femoral area is

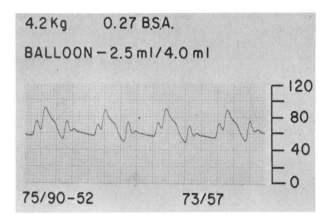

Fig. 33-1. Arterial pressure pulse in a small patient weighing 4.2 kg. The suprasystolic diastolic augmentation of pressure, the lowered end-diastolic pressure, and the lowered systolic pressure following the assisted pulse represent an "ideal" effect of IABC and dispel the concept that the arterial tree in infants and children is too compliant to permit effective IABC. Note also the low position of the dicrotic notch on the unassisted pulse and the inflation of the balloon occurring higher on the descending limb of the arterial pulse.

at high risk of contamination and sterile, watertight dressings are mandatory. Stringent measures to avoid contamination must be rigidly observed. The involved lower extremity demands continuous observation for ischemia. This is particularly true if MAST trousers are employed concurrently with IABC. It has been our experience that perfusion of the involved lower extremity improves when IABC is effective in increasing tissue perfusion elsewhere. Because the balloon catheters extend beyond the site of cutdown for such a short distance and the attachment to the pumping module is relatively close to the patient, vigilant care must be exercised to prevent patient movement from dislodging or crimping the thin-walled balloon catheter. The patient must be immobilized either by sedation or by physical restraint, and extra precaution to protect the catheter should be undertaken during special nursing procedures such as chest therapy.

SUMMARY

While the use of IABC cannot be as easily or as readily employed in children as it is in adults, it unequivocally can be and should be used in selected cases where its use may save a patient who otherwise could be lost.

REFERENCES

1. Pollock JC, Charlton MC, Williams WG et al: Intraaortic balloon pumping in children, *Ann Thorac Surg* 29:522, 1980.
2. Veasy LG, Blaylock RC, Orth JL et al: Intra-aortic balloon pumping in infants and children, *Circulation* 68:1095, 1983.
3. Annela J, McCloskey A, Viewig C: Nursing dynamics of pediatric intraaortic balloon pumping, *Crit Care Nurse* 10:24, 1988.
4. Veasy LG, Webster HF, McGough EC: Intra-aortic balloon pumping: adaptation for pediatric use, *Crit Care Clin* 2:237, 1986.
5. Del Nido PJ, Swan PR, Benson LN et al: Successful use of intraaortic balloon pumping in a 2-kilogram infant, *Ann Thorac Surg* 46:574, 1988.
6. Bolooki H: *Clinical application of intra-aortic balloon pumping*, ed 2, New York, 1984, Futura Publishing.

CHAPTER 34

Air transport

Gary B. Mertlich and Susan J. Quaal

Air transport of the intraaortic balloon counterpulsation (IABC) patient offers a rapid and efficient means of interhospital transfer and has now been successfully undertaken by several medical flight teams.[1-3] Conditions for which the IABC patient has been transported to a tertiary facility are listed in the box on p. 536.[4-6]

Decreased transport time, balloon-pump consoles that are designed to accommodate size and weight restrictions of aircraft, and expansion of aeromedicine as a specialty have greatly increased air transport of IABC patients. Air transport teams need to develop policies, procedures, and training programs that incorporate flight physiology principles. To develop criteria that facilitate safe patient transport, the nurse must understand how altitude and associated reduced barometric pressures affect the counterpulsating IAB catheter.

PHYSIOLOGY OF FLIGHT
Altitude

Barometric pressure, which is the pressure exerted by gases within ambient air, decreases with increasing altitude, giving rise to physiological effects associated with flight. Between 0 and 12,000 feet, barometric pressure decreases from 760 mm Hg to 483 mm Hg; the human body is usually able to adapt this change. Between 12,000 and 50,000 feet, barometric pressure drops from 396 to 87 mm Hg. Physiological adaptation may be impossible, depending on altitude achieved and rate of ascent. However, problems with evolved and trapped gases may occur at any altitude proportionate to change in elevation and rate of ascent.[7-8]

Helicopter flights usually do not exceed an altitude greater than 10,000 feet because they are not pressurized. Fixed-wing flights with pressurized cabins are within the range of 12,000 to 50,000 feet because of increased fuel efficiency at higher altitudes.

Parts of this chapter from Mertlich G, Quaal SJ: Air transport of the patient requiring intra-aortic balloon pumping, *Crit Care Nurs Clin North Am* 1(3):443, 1989.

CONDITIONS FOR WHICH THE IABC PATIENT HAS REQUIRED INTERFACILITY TRANSPORT

1. Accelerating angina (patient transported to a cardiac facility for bypass surgery).
2. Ischemic or idiopathic cardiomyopathy when cardiac transplantation is an option.
3. Emergency structural defects, such as mitral valve regurgitation or ventricular septal defect, that necessitate surgical repair.
4. Hemodynamic instability during a cardiac catheterization.
5. Need for advanced pharmacological therapy, necessitating transfer to a tertiary care facility.
6. IAB pump–dependent patient has exhausted the resources of the referring facility.

Cabin pressurization is a variable that must be defined for each aircraft. An aircraft flying at 24,000 feet, for example, may reach a cabin-pressurization state that is equivalent to an altitude of 7000 feet and its associated barometric pressure. Air-transport monitoring of the IABC patient requires that the operator understands effects of barometric-pressure change on balloon gas volume associated with both "unpressurized" cruising altitude and "pressurized" cabin altitude.[9]

Pressurized cabins were designed to prevent physiological problems associated with high altitudes. The need for supplementary oxygen in healthy individuals is eliminated by maintaining a "mechanically" produced cabin altitude (pressurized cabin) below 8000 feet.

Cabin pressurization is achieved by bleeding off air from engine compressors and directing it into the cabin through the air conditioning system. Rate and amount of pressurization are regulated by the pilot with valves that control cabin leak until the desired cabin altitude or pressure differential is obtained. Pressure differential is a function of the difference between cabin pressure and ambient air. Thus occupants are still subjected to a mediated barometric pressure change between ground altitude and cruising altitude. This is demonstrated by equalization of eustachian tubes during ascent and descent on commercial flights.

Each aircraft is rated according to a maximum pressure differential related to its structural design, which determines rate of pressurization and maximum cabin altitude for each individual aircraft.[10] Fig. 34-1 lists cabin altitudes obtainable for various flight altitudes specific to aircraft with a maximum differential between 4 to 9 psi. An aircraft cabin, with a pressure differential of 6 psi, undergoes a 7000-foot change in altitude when ascending from sea level to a flight altitude of 24,000 feet.

Gas expansion associated with decreasing barometric pressure (flight ascent): application of Boyle's law. Hydrostatic forces within the body only slightly modify transmis-

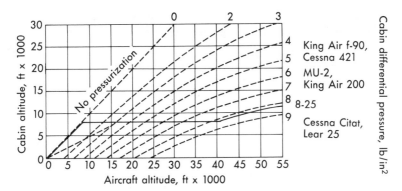

Fig. 34-1. Graph illustrating relationship between aircraft altitude, cabin altitude, and cabin differential pressure, as approximated for various air ambulances. (Modified from Brown HHS: Cabin pressure. In Gillies JA, ed: *A textbook of aviation physiology*, New York, 1965, Pergamon Press.)

sion of changes in barometric pressure. Water and other body fluids are considered to be incompressible; therefore they transmit pressure rather than resist or yield to it.[11] This action is exemplified by a hydraulic break line.

Physical laws of fluids state that if pressure is exerted on an enclosed fluid, it will be transmitted to all parts of that fluid.[12] Soft body tissues act as a fluid, transferring increases or decreases in barometric pressure. Since gas is compressible, unless completely encapsulated by an unyielding structure, any amount trapped within the body is directly affected by changes in pressure outside the body.[13] Helium gas within the IAB is therefore affected by changes in barometric pressure, which are transmitted through body tissues to the balloon.[14]

Gas expansion within body cavities poses a potential complication associated with exposure to lower barometric pressures, which is an inverse relationship to increasing altitude. Boyle's law expresses the relationship between gas volume (*V*) and pressure (*P*): If temperature remains constant (as within the body), gas volume varies inversely to the pressure acting on it.[15] As pressure decreases, gas expands and vice versa. Expressed as an equation, Boyle's law is:

$$\frac{*P_1V_1}{\text{Temperature}} = \frac{P_2V_2}{\text{Temperature}}$$

Consider a patient with air in his chest, abdominal cavity, or cranial vault. Boyle's law expresses the consequences of subjecting the patient to higher altitudes with associated lower barometric pressures. Potential expansion of these chamber-

---

*Pressure must be expressed in absolute units.

Table 34-1. Theoretical estimates of changes in balloon volume with increased altitudes calculated from the table of US standard atmosphere

Altitude (ft)	Volume of unrestrained gas (cc)	Barometric pressure (mm Hg)
0	40	760
2000	43	706
4000	46	656
6000	50	609
8000	54	565
10000	58	523
12000	63	484
14000	68	446

$$\frac{P_1V_1 + 80 \text{ mm Hg MAP}}{\text{Temperature}} = \frac{P_2V_2 + 80 \text{ mm MAP}}{\text{Temperature}}$$

trapped gases should be eliminated with chest tubes, nasogastric tubes, or prevented by minimizing changes in altitude during flight.

The effect of altitude on helium gas within the IAB is an important component of patient monitoring during air transport. Helium within the IAB is affected by barometric pressure, which is transmitted through body tissues to the balloon. As the aircraft ascends, reduction in barometric pressure will result in a gradient between inside and outside the IAB. Balloon-gas volume, in an unrestricted state, can expand from 40 cc at sea level to as much as 51.7 cc at 7000 feet, representing a 23% change in volume. Table 34-1 lists theoretical changes in 40 cc volume, according to Boyle's law, as the unrestrained gas is subjected to decrease in barometric pressure on ascent from 0 to 14,000 feet. Gas within the IAB is restricted by the elasticity of the balloon's polyurethane polymer, thus partially absorbing the effect of decreased pressure external to the IAB invoked by changes in altitude. Therefore an increase in altitude provokes an altered amount of balloon gas expansion.

Effect of increased IABC pressure on catheter volume: relationship to changing altitude. Mertlich and Quaal[16] evaluated the resistive qualities of IAB membranes in response to increasing intracatheter pressure. A static compliance test was performed to assess the effect of internal pressure on IAB compliance (simulating helium gas within the IAB affected by barometric pressure). Testing consisted of incrementally increasing pressure within eight percutaneous intraaortic balloons from four leading manufacturers. Results for all trials showed a curvilinear relationship between intracatheter pressure and balloon volume. Clinically significant balloon expansion data were obtained by indexing results to associated barometric pressures that occur with changes in altitude. Manufacturer variation was only observed at moderate-to-high pressures. Study findings could then be used to make recommendations for IAB purging during ascent and descent.

Gas compression associated with increasing barometric pressure (flight descent).
During descent, barometric pressure increases. Less density, or moles per cubic centimeter, is required to occupy the same volume at decreased barometric pressures. At 18,000 feet, for example, barometric pressure is approximately 379 mm Hg. Helium molecules occupy a space of 40 cc at that altitude and pressure, but occupy only 19.9 cc when the aircraft descends to sea level or a barometric pressure of 760 mm Hg. Balloon contraction on descent is therefore inversely proportional to gas expansion, true to Boyle's law.

Decreased gas volume caused by increased barometric pressure will not be mediated by balloon structure, which occurs with ascent and decreasing barometric pressure. Decreases in balloon volume can therefore be directly computed from Boyle's law (absolute pressure should be used). For example, if barometric pressure is 609 mm at 6000 feet, adding 80 mm MAP yields a total absolute barometric pressure of 689 mm Hg. Total barometric pressure at 6000 feet, multiplied by 40 cc of balloon gas volume, should equal total barometric pressure at sea level (760 + MAP of 90 mm Hg = 850 mm Hg) multiplied by 32.423 of balloon gas volume, which corresponds to the amount of balloon contraction. Balloon gas contraction is approximately 1.5 cc per 1000 feet descent (averaged from standard atmosphere tables for 40 cc volume).

Recommendations for purging during flight. "Purging" of a pressure-sensitive IAB pump references the transducer to altitude appropriate gas density. This transducer, positioned between the helium source and balloon catheter, senses changes in barometric pressure and adjusts the helium gas charge delivered into the balloon. "Purging" with altitude changes, therefore references the transducer to changing barometric pressure and prevents possible balloon expansion. The results of Quaal and Mertlich's research[16] suggest that purging should be done every 1000 feet of altitude ascent or descent. Because of cabin pressurization, purging should be accomplished through use of an in-cabin altimeter. This recommendation does not exclude the possible need for more frequent purging as necessitated by patient or environmental circumstances or console alarms. Once cruising altitude is attained, routine purging is no longer necessary.

It is important that alarms are left "ON" during flight so that potential balloon gas volume expansion activates an alarm. A console alarm triggered by balloon gas expansion may prompt purging by an operator who is actually unaware of the intrinsic changes within the balloon. During fixed-wing flight, if the IABP console alarm is inactivated or unable to sense changes in volume or pressure associated with sudden rapid decompression, the operator should wear prophylactic oxygen. In the event of unexpected decompression, this will allow the operator to place the console on standby immediately rather than having to obtain oxygen first to avoid the effects of hypoxia. It is also the clinician's responsibility to know individual balloon pump manufacturer's alarm system capabilities. Each manufacturer's alarm system responds differently based on specific algorithms and computer designs.

Acceleration

Acceleration, although not a major problem in many disease states, can cause complications in cardiac patients with minimal reserve. Acceleration research has been confined to observations in healthy individuals. Unlike rotor-wing aircraft, fixed-wing aircraft must accelerate to a certain speed to become airborne, then maintain an angle of climb for greatest efficiency. This will subject the patient in a supine position to two forms of acceleration: (1) positive, in which G forces are directed through the long axis of the body from head to feet, and (2) negative, in which the opposite occurs and forces are from feet to head. Both negative and positive acceleration have been associated with alterations in cardiac output and disturbances in rhythm.[17-18]

During take-off, decreased preload may occur when the patient is positioned with his head toward the front of the aircraft (positive acceleration). This position can have a profound effect on circulation through redistribution of blood below the diaphragm, resulting in decreased cardiac output and stroke volume by as much as 38% at +2.4 G.[19]

Likewise, when the patient's position is reversed, a subsequent increase in preload is seen (negative acceleration). Increased preload because of blood being forced toward the heart from the lower extremities produces cardiac failure only after prolonged exposure.[20]

Rhythm disturbances were noted only in extreme episodes of positive acceleration up to +7 G.[18] Immediate marked bradycardia has been associated with negative acceleration. Animal model studies suggest that bradycardia is caused by stimulation of carotid baroreceptors as negative acceleration redistributes blood to the upper body.[17] Heart rates below 40 beats per minute have been seen along with sinus pauses of 3 to 5 seconds at −2 to 2.5 G.[21]

Acceleration directed through the anteroposterior axis of body (transverse) rather than the long axis (positive and negative) appears to be well tolerated. Transverse positioning induces minimal hemodynamic changes when compared with positive or negative positioning.[22] This maneuver would require a large, expensive aircraft that would be unable to gain access to many cities with smaller landing fields. The impact of changing G forces as described would most likely occur only during emergency aircraft maneuvers with commercial flights.

Compensation for the hemodynamics of flight can be accomplished in several ways: (1) flight angles can be adjusted to some degree if the pilot is informed ahead of time; (2) judicious use of vasoactive drugs prior to take-off; (3) providing for adequate intravascular volume, maximizing IAB capabilities, and appropriate pharmacological support; and (4) close observation and early intervention during critical periods of take-off and landing may avert a crisis. Placement and light inflation (10 to 20 mm below diastolic blood pressure) of the lower-extremity portion of pneumatic antishock garments, similar to the action of G suits, have been proposed as a preven-

craft should be customized to accommodate the IAB pump. Dispatching an aircraft readied for transport of the IABC patient for a non-IABC transport obviously makes the aircraft unavailable for transport of the IABC patient. Nurse and dispatcher therefore need to be involved in aircraft selection in response to calls for patient transport.

If airport-to-hospital ground shuttle is needed, ambulance size and inverter capabilities should be assessed. Ambulance companies may have vehicles well suited for emergency medical systems (EMS) requirements but not for critical-care transport.

The referring hospital must be contacted to determine software brand in use, thus facilitating proper interface with transport biomedical equipment. Preparations must also be made for the patient's arrival at the receiving hospital, including (1) procurement of a critical care bed; (2) notification of the admitting physician; (3) having an IAB pump available for the patient's use in the critical care unit and appropriate connectors if the patient arrives with an IAB that is a different brand than the facility's balloon-pump console.

Extra helium tanks should be on hand at all times. Depending on length of transport, changes in altitude and interruptions in pumping can cause helium to be quickly consumed. Projected use of helium during transport should be guided by the manufacturer's specifications. Plan for all the helium that could possibly be used plus one extra tank. This is to guard against unforeseen drains on the helium source and accidental discharge of a tank.

Accessory biomedical equipment needs vary with each individual flight. Every patient must have an arterial line; some patients will also have a pulmonary artery catheter line. Monitoring of ECG and arterial pressure waveforms can be accomplished throughout the balloon pump console monitor. It is recommended that ECG and hemodynamic pressure signals also be monitored with a separate transport monitor. These signals can then be slaved into the balloon pump monitor via a telephone jack connector. Redundant monitoring of ECG and arterial pressure provides multiple signals as balloon triggering options in the event that one monitored signal is disengaged or internal console circuitry malfunctions in flight. Aircraft vibration can interfere with the ECG signal. Recommended signals for console triggering are therefore prioritized as follows: (1) arterial pressure direct to console; (2) arterial pressure slaved to console; (3) ECG direct to console; and (4) ECG slaved to console.

Intravenous pumps are the next most frequently needed item because pharmacological support is frequently necessary. The number of intravenous pumps required will, of course, be governed by quantity of drips infusing. Type and size of intravenous pumps vary greatly, along with accuracy rates. It is therefore advantageous to employ pumps and tubing with which the flight nurses are comfortable, provided they meet aircraft size and power requirements. Using a familiar pump minimizes potential for error when administering intravenous medications.

The patient may require other supportive interventions, such as pacemaker, ventilator, or defibrillation. Proficiency in using a temporary pacemaker generator is encouraged; extra batteries should be carried. An external pacemaker has also proved beneficial during actual patient transport. If an external pacemaker is employed, the IAB pump operator must understand that both milliamps and pacemaker current output duration may interfere with ECG balloon console trigger. Therefore it is recommended that an arterial trigger source be used in conjunction with external pacemaking.

Defibrillation can be cumbersome in a crowded aircraft cabin. Use of remote defibrillator pads allows for greater maneuverability to carry out the defibrillation procedure.

Accessory monitoring equipment, such as Dopplers and arterial saturation monitors, may also be utilized. Small items, such as electrodes, tape and syringes, are best assembled and stored in a readily accessible transport pack (Table 34-2). An in-cabin, hand-held altimeter is mandatory.

Table 34-2. Contents of air transport IABC flight bag

Count	Description
1	Altimeter
2	60 cc Luer-Lok syringe
2	3-cc syringe
2	10-cc syringe
1	2-in cloth tape
1	2-in plastic tape
1	Roll elastoplast
1	Small tool set
1	Multidose vial of heparin
1	IAB catheter for testing
2	Packages of ECG monitoring electrodes
3	Pressure bags
3	500-cc bags of normal saline
3	Pressure line kits
4	Stopcocks
1	Assorted balloon connector
1	3-ft length balloon extension tubing
1	6-ft length balloon extension tubing
1	3-way connector
2	Packages of wrist restraints
1	Balloon pump operator's manual
1	Flight instructions
1	IAB flowsheet
3	Slave cables
2	Disposable helium tanks
2	Pressure monitoring cables
1	ECG monitoring cable

A daily check of equipment is recommended to verify the battery charged status of the transport balloon pump and to determine that the IABP is complete and functional with all its component parts. Such inspection is particularly crucial if various services within the institution share an IABP. The key to an uneventful transport is prior planning and functional, dependable biomedical equipment.

Arrangement of patient, transport team, and biomedical equipment within the aircraft also requires prior planning. Four factors are of specific importance: (1) access to patient; (2) assess to console; (3) placement of the console in relation to the patient; and (4) movement within the cabin.

Importance of patient access is generally taken for granted. Access can, however, easily be impeded by invasive lines, cables, and layers of blankets. Patient access can be facilitated by (1) coiling and labeling lines and cables; (2) arranging a central opening bedding envelope; and (3) proper positioning of the console within the aircraft for safety an accessibility.

The medical attendant must be able to remain seat-belted when making any adjustments on the IAB pump. Also, the console should not be positioned more than 5 feet away from the patient because falsely triggered balloon alarms have been noticed with use of greater than 6 feet of extension tubing.

Ability to move freely within the cabin is also an FAA requirement. Tubing and cables that must cross the center aisle should do so without restricting movement. Figs. 34-2 and 34-3 illustrate medically retrofitted aircraft interiors. Note positioning of the medical crew's seats in relation to the patient and balloon console. The patient is easily reached by two members of the crew; IAB pump is close to the patient, separated from the aisle and patient but still accessible to a third crew member.

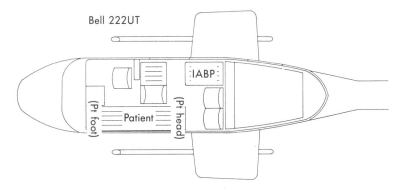

Fig. 34-2. Interior medical configuration of a Bell 222 UT helicopter with reference to IABP placement. (Original photo courtesy Marius Burke, Jr, Director of Operations, Air Methods, Englewood, Colo; Original photo redrawn by Ken Hulme, Department of Computer Science, University of Utah; from *Crit Care Nurs Clin North Am* 1:453, 1989.)

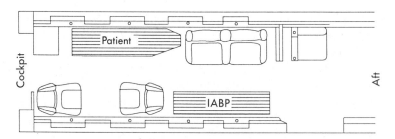

Fig. 34-3. Interior medical configuration of a Mitsubishi MU-2B-60 fixed-wing turbo prop aircraft with reference to IABP placement. (Courtesy Marius Burke, Jr, Director of Operations, Air Methods, Englewood Colo; original photo redrawn by Ken Hulme, Department of Computer Science, University of Utah; from *Crit Care Nurs Clin North Am* 1:453, 1989.)

Before any transport, a mock loading and unloading of the actual console with a simulated patient, and performance of procedures, such as defibrillation, fitting of the IAB, and altimeter measurements should be undertaken. This will yield valuable information as to how equipment, personnel, and aircraft will interface in emergency situations. A test flight is essential before any actual patient transport to fully activate all biomedical equipment in conjunction with the IAB pump to determine exact power requirements and effects of noise and vibration on this specialized instrumentation. While flying en route to the patient, the medical team can test all equipment and inverters, practice monitoring altitude changes with the altimeter, and make any final preparations for receipt of the patient.

PATIENT AND PERSONNEL CONSIDERATIONS WHEN AIR TRANSPORTING THE IABC PATIENT

1. Transport personnel should be completely familiar with the function of the IABP console; capable of handling bleeding at the balloon site, should it occur, and delivering intravenous medications, CPR, and ACLS; and proficient in operation of the ventilator, hemodynamic monitoring, and aerohemodynamics.
2. All patients must be stabilized before transfer. Appropriate management of hemodynamic instability and/or respiratory distress should be undertaken before beginning transport.
3. Medical personnel delivering care must transfer patients into and out of transport vehicles with minimal interruption of IABP.
4. Health care professionals present during transport should be thoroughly familiar with the patient's medical status and anticipated complications.

NURSE REQUIREMENTS FOR AIR TRANSPORT OF THE IABC PATIENT

Air transport of the IABC patient requires a high level of skill and competence. The nurse caring for the IABC patient must be experienced in balloon pumping in a variety of settings (catheterization laboratory or operating room) and during unstable hemodynamic conditions, such as dysrhythmias, pacemakers, severe cardiogenic

Patient name					Date						
Received from:					Balloon size and insertion site:						
Time onto console		Trigger Source		Mode	vs Augmented		BP	HR		Rhythm	
					Unaugmented		BP	HR			
Transfers	Time Disconnected		Reconnect	Alarms		Hand Pump				Comments	

Time	Heart Rate	Rhythm	Pas/Pad Pcwp	Trigger Mode	Assist Ratio	Distal Pulse	Pressures 1:2 Ratio Assist					Comments
							1	2	3	4	5	

KEY Balloon On ¹ Balloon Off (waveform with points 2, 4, 5, 3, 2)

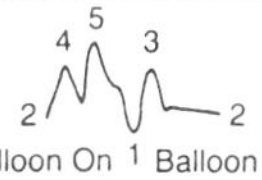

1 = Balloon-Assisted Aortic End-Diastolic Pressure
2 = Patient Aortic End-Diastolic Pressure
3 = Assisted Systole
4 = Patient Systole
5 = Peak Diastolic Augmented Pressure

Purged Ascent (Q 2000 ft)		Altitude			Total Change in Altitude						
Purged Descent (Q 1000 ft)		Altitude							Total Change in Altitude		
Final destination						Receiving Nurse					
Time of	vs Augmented		BP		HR	Rhythm					
	Unaugmented		BP		HR						

Notes _____

RN Signature _____

Fig. 34-4. Air transport IABP flowsheet. (From *Crit Care Nurs Clin North Am* 1:456, 1989.)

shock, and cardiac arrest. The nurse must be trained in all aspects of console operation and troubleshooting.

Evanston Hospital, Evanston, Illinois, put forth several important recommendations for ground transport of the IABC patient, which we have incorporated into our air transport protocol (see box on p. 548).

Documentation of IABP performance during air transport is essential and can be an addendum to a standard critical care unit flowsheet (Fig. 34-4).

REFERENCES

1. Campbell P: Air transport of the IABP-dependent patient, *Aeromed J* 1:5, 1986.
2. Kramer RP, Snow NJ: Technical considerations for transporting patients by air ambulance with intra-aortic balloon pumps, *J Extra-Corpor Technol* 18:145, 1986.
3. Wedige-Stetcher T: In-flight cardiac support. Aero-medical transport of IABP and LVAD patients, *Aeromed J* 3:16, 1988.
4. Gottlieb SO: Mobile intra-aortic balloon pumping: expanding horizons for the community, *Cardiac Assists* 2:1, 1985.
5. LoCicero J III, Hartz RS, Sanders JH, et al: Inter-hospital transport of patients with ongoing intra-aortic balloon pumping, *Am J Cardiol* 56:59, 1985.
6. Singh JB, Connelly P, Kocot S, et al: Interhospital transport of patients with ongoing intra-aortic balloon pumping, *Am J Cardiol* 56:59, 1985.
7. Bancroft RW: Medical aspects of pressurized equipment. In Armstrong HG, ed: *Aerospace medicine*, Baltimore, 1961, Williams & Wilkins.
8. Federal Aviation Regulations, Custom's Guide for Private Flyers: *Airman's information manual*, Seattle, 1988, ASA Publications Inc.
9. Luft VC: Physiological aspects of pressure cabins and rapid decompression. In Boothby WM, ed: *Handbook of respiratory physiology*, Randolph Air Force Base Texas School of Aviation, USAF, San Antonio, Tex, 1959.
10. Heimbach RD, Sheffield PJ: Protection in the pressure environment: cabin pressurization and oxygen equipment. In Dehart RL, ed: *Fundamentals of aerospace medicine*, Philadelphia, 1985, Lea & Febiger.
11. Sears FW, Xemansky MW: *University physics*, ed 4, Boston, 1970, Addison-Wesley.
12. Office of Federal Register National Archives and Code of Federal Records Administration Regulations: *Part 23 and 25*, Washington DC, 1988, Government Printing Office.
13. Weast RC, Astle MJ, Beyer WH: *Handbook of chemistry and physics*, ed 6, Boca Raton, Fla, 1986, CRC.
14. Miles S, Mackey DE: *Underwater medicine*, ed 4, Philadelphia, 1976, JB Lippincott.
15. Shilling CW, Werts MF, Schandelmeier NR: *The underwater handbook: a guide to physiology and performance for the engineer*, New York, 1976, Plenum Press.
16. Mertlich G and Quaal SJ: Effect of increased intra-aortic balloon pressure on catheter volume: relationship to changing altitude, *Crit Care Med* 20:297, 1992.
17. Lamb LE: Cardiopulmonary aspects of aerospace medicine. In Randel HW, ed: *Aerospace medicine*, ed 2, Baltimore, 1971, Williams & Wilkins.
18. Sidney D, Leverett J, Whinney JE: Biodynamics: sustained acceleration. In DeHart RL, ed: *Fundamentals of aerospace medicine*, Philadelphia, 1985, Lea & Febiger.
19. Howard P: The physiology of positive acceleration. In Gillies AJ, ed: *A textbook of aviation physiology*, Long Island City, 1965, Pergamon Press.
20. Christy RL: Effects of radial and angular acceleration. In Armstrong HC, ed: *Aerospace medicine*, Baltimore, 1961, Williams & Wilkins.
21. Ryan GEA, Derr WK, Franks WR: Some physiological findings on normal men subjected to negative G, *J Aviat Med* 21:173, 1950.

22. Wood EH, Sutterer WS, Marchall NW: *Technical report 60-636*, Wright Air Development Division, 1960.
23. Guignard JC: Vibration. In Gillies AJ, ed: *A textbook of aviation physiology*, Long Island City, 1965, Pergamon Press.
24. Lederer LG: Civil aviation medicine. In Armstrong HC, ed: *Aerospace medicine*, Baltimore, 1961, Williams & Wilkins.
25. Henning E, Nixon CE: Vibration, noise and communication. In DeHart RL, ed: *A textbook of aviation physiology*, Long Island City, 1965, Pergamon Press.
26. Brown HHS: The cabin pressure. In Gillies VA, ed: *A textbook of aviation physiology*, Long Island City, 1965, Pergamon Press.
27. Hegy DE: Supervisor/Airworthiness Section, Federal Aviation Administration: *Personal correspondence*, January 23, 1989.
28. Federal Aviation Regulations. Custom's Guide for Private Flyers. *Airman's information manual*, Seattle, 1988, ASA Publications, Inc.
29. Office of Federal Register National Archives and Code of Federal Records Administration Regulation. *Part 23 and 25*, Washington, DC, 1988, Government Printing Office.
30. US Department of Transportation, Federal Aviation Administration: *Action Notice A 8300.20*, May 7, 1987.
31. Johanson BC, Dungca CU, Hoffmeister D et al: Standard no. 24. In *Standards for critical care*, ed 2, St. Louis, 1985, Mosby–Year Book.

CHAPTER 35

Balloon pumping and beyond

Spyridon D. Moulopoulos

Boston surgeon Dwight D. Harken's initial presentation of the counterpulsation principle[4] to the Third World Congress of Cardiology in Brussels (September 1958) started a new era in the treatment of heart diseases. It indicated that mechanical assistance to the failing heart does not mean only the availability of a second energy source. The time sequence of the events and the cardiac cycle of the pulsatile heart activity were to be "exploited" for assistance purposes. What remained was to devise a technique to demonstrate the practicability of the principle.

In 1957 another giant in the field, Willem J. Kolff, started an ambitious project, intended to replace the heart with an intrathoracic mechanical pump. Kolff gave ample opportunity to many younger prospective investigators from all over the world to be indoctrinated and work in this field. Although many of them (including this writer) recognized the magnitude of the project, they were hesitant to commit themselves to what seemed at the time a very long-range and dubiously attainable target. They discussed what could be an easier and earlier goal—partial replacement of the heart action.

The idea of the intraaortic balloon emerged from these two ideas: the need for partial replacement of the heart and the possibility of using phases of the cardiac cycle to that effect.

THE INTRAAORTIC BALLOON AND THE INDICATIONS

The first publication in 1962 described a balloon on a catheter introduced into the aorta, inflated during the diastolic phase of the heart's action, and deflated shortly before the next systole.

Since then a large number of publications established the technique as a useful therapeutic tool. Strangely enough, the main clinical indications for use were—and still are—post–open heart surgery and post–myocardial infarction shock but not heart failure in general, as initially intended. Why were the indications changed? Is it because the method is beneficial only in these conditions?

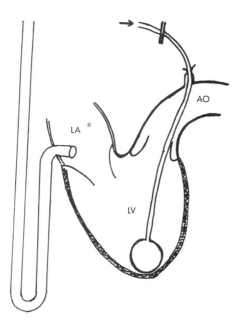

Fig. 35-4. A small balloon in the left ventricle inflated during late systole to increase the reduced compliance of the ventricle. (From Moulopoulos S. In Unger F, ed: *Assisted circulation,* ed 3, Berlin, 1989, Springer Verlag.)

Similar results were obtained by introducing a small balloon into the ventricle or pumping via a catheter introduced into the left ventricle. In fact, with brief pulses of 90 msec, coronary flow increased by 18.8% ± 3.7% but aortic flow increased by 18% ± 4.9% (Fig. 35-4). This larger effect on aortic flow suggests the possibility of positive outcome by interfering with left ventricular hemodynamics during systole.

End-systolic counterpulsation. During reduced left ventricular compliance, which is not uncommon, end-systolic counterpulsation into the left ventricle has been found to be beneficial. End-systolic pumping reduces left ventricular residual volume after cardiac systole and increases left ventricular capacity for the next inflow period. Ventricular chamber compliance is then increased, even if myocardial compliance remains the same.

A small balloon inserted in the left ventricle was inflated for 100 msec during late systole in a reduced ventricular compliance animal model.[11] The result was an increase in aortic flow and pressure, as well as in myocardial contractility. A further development of this technique resulted in an end-systolic left ventricle to inferior vena cava bypass.

In a low-compliance, low-contractility experimental preparation, such a shunt operating for a brief time (80 to 100 msec) during late systole—with the help of an

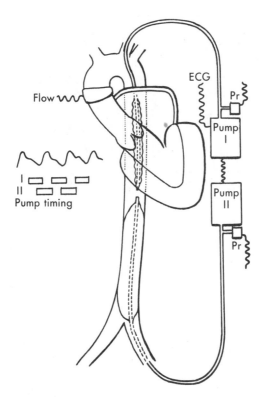

Fig. 35-5. Two balloons in the aorta, operating at a phase difference. The second *(lower)* balloon serves as an outlet valve to the space of the aorta, in which the first *(upper)* balloon operates. (From Moulopoulos S. In Unger F, ed: *Assisted circulation,* Berlin, 1989, Springer Verlag.)

R wave–triggered valve—produced a reduction in left ventricular end-diastolic pressure by 7.21 ± 1.07 mm Hg and an increase in contractility (dp/dt) by 1.78 ± 0.32 mm Hg.sec^{-1}.

A "ventricularized" aorta. Obstructing the descending aorta by an intraaortic balloon has been used by Kuhn et al.[5] during extracorporeal circulatory support of the lower part of the body.

Bregman, Parodi, and Malm[3] used "unidirectional," dual-chambered IABC with the intent to promote preferentially coronary blood flow.

Another technique employed two balloons in the descending aorta[8] (Fig. 35-5). The distal balloon was inflated during cardiac systole, providing an "outlet valve" and producing a "closed" space between the aortic valve and the distal balloon in which the proximal balloon could operate. Thus a part of the descending aorta was in a way ventricularized, because a "closed" space was formed with a pumping device in it and an inlet (aortic) and an outlet (balloon) valve.

With this technique, aortic flow increased by 31.6% ± 8.73%. The idea was to use the technique in situations in which the IAB was inefficient because of very low (below 60 mm Hg systolic) aortic pressure. In fact, the intraaortic balloon was inefficient under such low pressure, because it operated in a space (aorta) with an inlet (aortic) but without an outlet valve. Therefore if systolic aortic pressure was low, blood pumped out of the aorta by the IAB "regurgitated" into the aorta from peripheral vessels, thus rendering pumping inefficient. The second peripheral balloon helps correct this situation.

The bridging devices

Cardiac transplantation gave great impetus to the use of mechanical assist or replacement devices. The best candidates for cardiac transplantation are patients who will otherwise die from an acute myocardial infarction, most often caused by cardiogenic shock or occurring after open-heart surgery. These are usually otherwise healthy individuals, as far as other systems besides the heart are concerned. Patients in chronic heart failure, however, demonstrate significant deterioration in lung, kidney, or liver function. Transplantation is not recommended for this latter population, because of the long time frame required to match the candidate with a suitable donor heart.

The so-called bridging devices are intended to support or even replace the heart during the period required until a donor heart becomes available. It is anyone's guess as to how long a wait this may be—from a few days to over 6 months. Therefore appropriate mechanical support devices should offer the possibility of "chronic" assistance, extended to a period of 6 months. The hope that properly functioning assist devices will sometimes be used for permanent support lies in the back of the investigator's mind, in view of donor scarcity and the numbers of people dying while awaiting for a transplant. A large number of devices are available for bridging to transplantation. Three categories have mostly been used: the hemopump, the pneumatic displacement pump, and centrifugal and roller pumps.

The hemopump. The hemopump, an achievement of modern technology, consists of a catheter inserted into the left ventricle via a femoral artery. The catheter is supplied with a rotor that "sucks" blood from the left ventricle into the descending aorta. It is estimated that 2.5 to 3.0 L/min can thus be pumped out of the left ventricle. There is no pulsatile flow from this system (Fig. 35-6).

The hemopump has been used by Wampler et al.[13] in 41 cases of cardiogenic shock with an impressive 41% 30-day survival rate. There are sometimes difficulties in inserting the large catheter through the femoral artery. Particular attention should be paid to optimal catheter positioning. If it is pushed deeply into the ventricle, cardiac output may be reduced. If it is slightly withdrawn, it may be placed in the aorta and out of the ventricle. It is also difficult to assess the exact flow produced by the system.

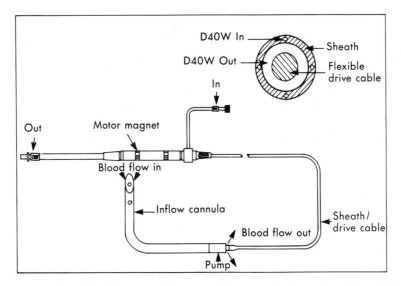

Fig. 35-6. Diagram of the "hemopump" system. The motor is situated at the position designated as PUMP. The motor is out of the body. (From Rutan P, Rountree W, Myers K et al: *Crit Care Nurs Clin North Amer* 1:527, 1989.)

The pneumatic displacement pump. Pneumatic displacement pumps have been used clinically for many years. A sac made of plastic is divided into two chambers: the blood chamber and the air chamber. The blood chamber usually has two valves, and blood is pumped by air compression. Energy is provided by a pneumatic driving system positioned outside the body.

Other investigators have used membranes, pusher plates, or pistons to separate blood and air chambers. In some devices the driving system is electromechanical.

Different pump shapes have been tried to minimize intrathoracic fitting procedures. A "soft shell" housing is a recent development in this direction (Kolff, personal communication).

Paracorporeal pneumatic systems have also been tried, with pumps positioned outside the body. Tubes are introduced through the chest to the left ventricle and aorta for left bypass and to the right atrium and pulmonary artery for right bypass.

Left ventricular assist has been used more often than has right ventricular assist. Bypassing both ventricles or excising the heart and inserting the "total artificial heart" has also been tried in a considerable number of patients.

Some of these cases were successfuly transplanted. Mortality rates of patients bridged to transplant with a paracorporeal pneumatic system are far higher than the usual heart transplant mortality rates.

Centrifugal and roller pumps. Centrifugal and roller pumps are tried in cases in

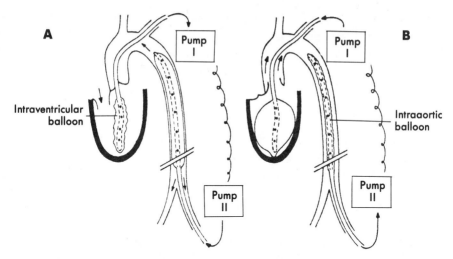

Fig. 35-7. A, Intraventricular balloon is deflated, and intraaortic balloon is inflated. **B,** Intraventricular balloon is inflated, and intraaortic balloon is deflated.

which brief operation periods are anticipated. They are easy to operate and sterilize and contain no valves.

Roller pumps have a high hemolysis, and therefore their operation time is limited to hours. Centrifugal pumps produce thrombi at the shaftseal and need heat dissipation. Flow is nonpulsatile, although this has not definitively proven to be a disadvantage.

There are scattered data on clinical results with pneumatic or mechanical pumps.[6] Among 155 cases of postinfarction cardiogenic shock from a clinical registry, 10% of the patients were weaned and survived without a transplant and 45% survived when a pneumatic or centrifugal device was used as a bridge to transplantation. In another series of 52 patients in whom a device was used as a bridge, 23 were transplanted and 17 were discharged.

The intraventricular balloon. All efforts until now were aimed at assisting, replacing, or bypassing the heart. The intraventricular balloon is the first attempt to insert a pumping system within the heart for "total" replacement[11] (Fig. 35-7).

In an arrested or fibrillated heart, a proper size balloon inserted into the left ventricle produces an output of between 70% and 100% of the resting output of the experimental animal with a venous pressure of 15 to 16 cm H_2O. This device can be driven with an IAB pump-driving system. It has an optimal pumping rate of 70 to 90 beats/min.

Clinical use is limited by the fact that dying hearts are usually large and dilated. Therefore a large balloon—9 cm diameter—is needed, and there are technical problems with balloon insertion. Insertion through the apex after a limited thoracotomy has been tried in one patient.

It is of interest that the combination of an intraventricular balloon and a counterpulsating intraaortic balloon produces the highest cardiac output.

SUMMARY

The extensive clinical use of IABC has demonstrated the effectiveness of the system, mostly in cases of cardiogenic shock.

Other techniques operating during cardiac diastole, such as an intraaortic balloon with an out of the body compliance chamber or an intraventricular balloon pumping at the end of diastole, have been subjected to limited experimental or clinical trials.

Helping the heart during systole was tried by copulsation into the pericardial sac or a pericardial cup. Mid-systolic or end-systolic counterpulsation in the ascending aorta or the left ventricle were shown experimentally to improve coronary circulation and increase ventricular compliance. The possibility of using two balloons in the aorta operating at phase difference was suggested for severe cases where a single balloon is ineffective.

Devices used for bridging to transplantation are being more and more extensively used. Roller pumps, centrifugal pumps, and pneumatic or electromechanical pumps were tried with moderate success. A large intraventricular balloon was used experimentally in the left ventricle of a fibrillating heart and was shown to be experimentally effective in maintaining the circulation.

Mechanical assistance to the circulation is a promising, rapidly developing field, because such treatment constitutes a rational approach to help an ailing hydraulic system.

REFERENCES

1. Anstadt E, Blakemore W, Baue A: A new instrument for prolonged mechanical cardiac massage, *Circulation* 32(suppl II):43, 1965.
2. Benzini A, Parda P: The pneumomassage of the heart, *Surgery* 39:375, 1956.
3. Bregman D, Parodi E, Malm J: Left ventricular and unidirectional intraaortic balloon pumping, *J Thorac Cardiovasc Surgery* 68:677, 1974.
4. Harken D: *Assisted circulation, III Europe Congr Cardiol* Brussels, 1958 (syllabus).
5. Kuhn L, Gruber F, Frankel A: Hemodynamic effects of balloon obstruction of the abdominal aorta and superior vena caval-distal aortic shunting in dogs with myocardial infarction and shock, *Am J Cardiol* 7:218, 1961.
6. Kunst E, v.Alste J: Heart assist and replacement technology. Report of the Commission of the European Communities, 1990.
7. Moulopoulos S: Systolic counterpulsation. In Unger F, ed: *Assisted circulation*, Berlin, 1989, Springer Verlag.

8. Moulopoulos S, Stamatelopoulos S, Petrou P: Intraaortic balloon assistance in intractable cardiogenic shock, *Eur Heart J* 7:396, 1986.
9. Moulopoulos S, Topaz S, Kolff W: Diastolic balloon pumping (with carbon dioxide) in the aorta—a mechanical assistance to the failing circulation, *Am Heart J* 63:669, 1962.
10. Moulopoulos S et al: Left intraventricular "pseudoaugmentation." A new principle of mechanical assistance, *Trans Am Soc Artif Intern Organs* 17:588, 1981.
11. Moulopoulos S et al: Intraventricular plus intraaortic balloon pumping during intractable cardiac arrest, *Circulation* 80(suppl III):167, 1989.
12. Sideris D et al: Intraaortic balloon assistance without a pump, *Eur Heart J* 4:536, 1983.
13. Wampler R et al: Treatment of cardiogenic shock with a hemopump left ventricular assist device, *Ann Thorac Surg* 52:506, 1991.
14. Willerson J, Frazier O: Reducing mortality in patients with extensive myocardial infarction, *N Engl J Med* 325:1166, 1991.

Index

A

Abdominal aortic aneurysm
  as contraindication, 144
  surgery for, 138, 139
Acceleration during air transport, 540-541
Acetazolamide, 67, 72
Actin, 31
Actin cross-bridges, 34
Action potential, myocardial cell, 7
Acute heart failure, 47
Adenosine triphosphate, 32
Adrenergic receptors, 59-60
Adult learners, 380
Afterload
  cardiac output and, 13
  cardiac transplantation and, 132
  reduction of, 105-107
Age
  heart failure and, 42
  as risk factor for complications, 147-148
Air embolism, 157
Air transport, 535-551
  aircraft characteristics for, 542-544
  Bard H-8000 device and, 514
  Boston Scientific Corporation devices
    and, 494
  Datascope systems and, 460-461
  Kontron Instruments, Inc., devices and,
    482
  patient management in, 544-550
  physiology of flight and, 535-542
  St. Jude Medical control system and, 444
Alarm, during air transport, 539
Alarms
  in Bard H-8000 device, 507-509
  in Datascope systems, 457-458
  in Kontron Instruments, Inc., devices,
    477-478
  St. Jude Medical, Inc., control system,
    442-443

Albutamol, 78
Allen test, 327-328
Altitude, of air transport, 535-539
Ambulance; *see* Transport
Ambulatory intraaortic balloon counterpul-
    sation, 517-519
Amiloride
  dosage and side effects of, 72-73
  pharmacology of, 72-73
Amrinone, 80
Anacrotic limb, 247
Anasarca, heart failure and, 62
Anemia, risk for, 325
Aneurysm, aortic
  as contraindication, 144
  surgery for, 138, 139
Angina, unstable, 121
Angioplasty, percutaneous transluminal
    coronary, 128-130
Angiotensin, heart failure and, 57-59
Angiotensin-converting enzyme inhibitor,
    84-86
Ankle-arm index, 324
Ankle-brachial index, 149-150, 158
Anrep effect, 109
Antegrade insertion of balloon, 189-192,
    333, 335
Antibiotic, for ambulatory patient, 518
Anticoagulation, 525-526
Anxiety, 338
Aorta
  length of, 208-209
  ventricularized, 558-559
Aortic aneurysm
  as contraindication, 144
  surgery for, 138, 139
Aortic arch, removal of balloon from, 191
Aortic dissection, 153-154, 326
Aortic end-diastolic pressure
  afterload and, 13

Aortic end-diastolic pressure—cont'd
  balloon-assisted, 253, 257-258
Aortic insufficiency, 144
Aortic pressure, 298
Aortic sinuses of Valsalva, 19
Aortic valve, 249
Arch
  aortic, 191
  dicrotic, 247
Arrhythmia
  cardiac output and, 321
  heart failure and, 44, 62
  real timing and, 283-284, 291, 293
Arterial circulation, coronary, 19-21
Arterial helium embolism, 156
Arterial pressure
  counterpulsation's effect on, 98-99
  mean, 317, 319
  nitroprusside and, 81
Arterial pressure waveform, 229, 233-237
  normal, 247-248
  real timing and, 287
  timing and, 246-259; *see also* Timing
Artery
  coronary; *see* Coronary *entries*
  dimensions of, 210
  femoral; *see* Femoral artery
  mesenteric, 334
  pulmonary; *see* Pulmonary artery *entries*
  renal, 113
Artifact, pacemaker, 491
Ascending aorta, 189-192
Ascites, heart failure and, 62
Assessment
  educational needs, 379-381
  preflight, 544
Atrial fibrillation, 459
Atrial kick, 4
Atrial natriuretic factor, 59
Atrial overload, 83
Atrioventricular node, 7
Atrium, anatomy of, 6
Augmentation, diastolic, 98-99, 283
  concept of, 411-412
  inflation and, 113-115
Augmented arterial pressure, 296-297
Augmented diastolic pressure, 248
Autonomic nervous system, 14

Autoregulation
  of coronary blood flow, 23
  heterometric and homeometric, 107-110
Axillary artery, 193, 195, 196
Axis, phlebostatic, 219

B

Backward heart failure, 48-49
Balloon
  in Boston Scientific devices, 492-493
  deflation of, 253-254; *see* Deflation of
    balloon
  fabrication of, 418, 420
  inflation of, during diastole, 248-253
  insertion of; *see* Insertion of balloon
  intraventricular, 561
  materials for, 171-172
  removal of, 174
  sheathless insertion of, 199-206
  volume of, air flight and, 537
  without pump, 554
Balloon plateau pressure
  high, 300-303
  low, 300
Balloon pressure waveform, 294-308
  abnormal, 299-308
  augmented arterial pressure and,
    296-297
  normal, 294-296
  variations of normal in, 297-299
Balloon-assisted aortic end-diastolic
    pressure, 253, 257-258, 317
Band, Z, 28
Bard H-8000 device, 495-515
  air transport and, 514
  alarms in, 507-509
  components of, 498-499
  inflation and deflating settings in,
    506-507
  set-up of, 502-506
  specifications for, 495-498
  theory of operation of, 499-502
  troubleshooting guidelines for, 510-513
Barometric pressure, 535-539
Baroreceptor, 110, 111
Baseline pressure, balloon, 303-308
Bedside providers, 374-375
Beta-adrenergic agonist, 78-79

Beta-adrenergic blocking agent, 86
Beta-adrenergic receptors, heart failure
    and, 59-60
Bleeding, thrombolysis and, 127
Blood flow
    cardiac arrest and, 131
    cardiac physiology and, 9
    effects of intraaortic balloon
        counterpulsation on, 103-105
    ocular, 165-170
    phasic coronary, 23
    renal artery, 113
    retrograde, 257-258
    through series circuit, 5
Blood pressure
    baroreceptors and, 110
    documentation of, 317-320, 322
Blood transfusion, thrombolysis and, 127
Boston Scientific Corporation devices,
    483-494
    alarms in, 489-490
    balloon dynamics in, 492-493
    components of, 485-488
    set-up instructions for, 488-489
    specifications for, 483-485
    timing in, 489
    transport and, 493-494
    troubleshooting in, 491-492
Bowel complications, 332
Boyle's law, 536-537
Bradycardia
    balloon pressure waveform and, 297
    heart failure and, 44
Brain, air embolism to, 157
Bridging devices, 559-561
Bubble, air, 157
Bubble blowing phenomenon, 115
Bumetanide
    dosage and side effects of, 68-69
    pharmacology of, 74
Butopamine, 78
Bypass
    cardiopulmonary, 135-136
        intraaortic balloon counterpulsation
            after, 135-136
        pulmonary artery balloon
            counterpulsation and, 520-529
    coronary artery, 165-170

C

Cabin pressurization of aircraft, 536
Calcium
    adrenergic receptors and, 59
    depolarization and, 32-35
Calcium-sensitizing agent, 80
Capillary gas, 234
Capillary refill time, 159
Carbon dioxide, diastolic augmentation
    and, 115
Cardiac arrest
    Boston Scientific device and, 491
    Datascope systems and, 459
    resuscitation after, 131
Cardiac cycle, normal, 8-9
Cardiac output
    decreased, 316-317
    factors influencing, 9-14
    potential alteration, 321
    pulmonary artery balloon
        counterpulsation and, 528
Cardiac surgery, 134-135
Cardiac transplantation, 132-134
    bridging devices and, 559-561
Cardiogenic shock, 122
Cardiopulmonary bypass
    intraaortic balloon counterpulsation
        after, 135-136
    pulmonary artery balloon
        counterpulsation and, 520-529
Cardiopulmonary circulation
    normal, 3
    physiology of, 19-24
Cardiopulmonary resuscitation, 131
Case studies, 343-356
Catheter
    insertion of, 171-189; *see also* Insertion
        of balloon catheter
    kinked, 306
    malposition of, 159
    in mesenteric artery, 334
    problems with, 156-157
    pulmonary artery
        placement of, 229-231
        pulmonary artery capillary pressure
            and, 233-237
        right atrial pressure and, 233
        right ventricular pressure and, 233

Catheter—cont'd
 volume of, air flight and, 537
Cell membrane, function of, 26
Centrifugal pump, 560-561
Cerebral blood flow, 131
Certification guidelines, 374, 375
Chart, flow, 393-394
Chemoreceptor, 110
Chest pain, 322
 case studies of, 343-345
Child
 balloon pressure waveform in, 298-299
 intraaortic balloon counterpulsation in, 531-534
Chloride, diuretics and, 72-74
Chlorothiazide, 68-69
Chlorthalidone
 dosage and side effects of, 68-69
 pharmacology of, 73
Chronic heart failure, 48
Circulation, coronary, 19-24
Circulatory vs. heart failure, 42
Clinical skills lab test, 385
Clinical training, 376-377, 378
Clinical training record, 386
Clot, 151-152
Coefficient, damping, 222, 223
Collateral coronary circulation, 23-24, 104-105
Comfort of patient, 330, 332
Community hospital setting, 357-368
 case histories concerning, 360
 clinical applications in, 358-359
 financial considerations in, 364-366
 ground transport and, 359-360
 nursing care in, 361-364
 quality management in, 369-371
 technological developments and, 358
Compartment syndrome
 as complication, 152-153
 nursing care for, 325
Compliance, Starling curve and, 52
Concentric hypertrophy, 55
Conduction system, anatomy of, 6-7
Consciousness, level of, 337
 pulmonary artery balloon counterpulsation and, 529
Console, pump, 98, 99

Contractility, factors affecting, 13-14
Contraction
 isometric, 37
 isotonic, 37
 isovolumic, 13
Conventional timing, 246-280; see also Timing, conventional
Convoluted tubule, 65
Coronary angioplasty, percutaneous transluminal,128-130
Coronary artery, left main, 135-136
Coronary artery bypass, 165-170
Coronary circulation
 collateral, 23-24
 physiology of, 19-24
Coronary perfusion, 103-105
Coronary vein, 20, 21, 23
Cost of procedure, 364-367
Cough, left ventricular failure and, 61
Counterpulsation
 end-systolic, 557-558
 intraaortic balloon; see Intraaortic balloon counterpulsation
 midsystolic, 556-557
Course outline, 382-384
Creatinine phosphokinase, 153
Cross-bridges
 formation of, 35
 relaxation of, 34
Curve, Starling, 12
 compliance and, 52-54
Cycle
 counterpulsation, 99
 Krebs', 37
Cyclothiazide, 68-69

D

Damping coefficient, 222, 223, 225-227
Datascope systems, 447-461
 air transport and, 460-461
 alarms in, 457-458
 pacers in, 455-456
 set-up instructions for, 452-454
 specifications for, 450, 451
 theory of operation of, 447, 450-451
 timing in, 456-457
 triggers for, 454-455
 troubleshooting and, 458-460

Defibrillation, during air transport, 546
Deflation of balloon
  conventional timing of, 96-97
    incorrect, 257-259
    landmarks of, 253-254
  real timing of, 284
    incorrect, 288
Delirium, 158
Denopamine, 78
Depolarization
  calcium and, 32-35
  physiology of, 7
Depression, of balloon baseline pressure,
    304-308
Dextran, low molecular weight, 186
Diabetes mellitus
  case studies of, 345-346
  heart failure and, 45-46
  as risk factor for complications, 148-149
Diagnosis, nursing; *see* Nursing diagnosis
Diastasis, period of, 9
Diastole
  assistance during, 554-555
  balloon inflation and, 103-105
  deflation and, 96-97
  electrocardiography and, 247
  inflation during, 281-282
  normal, 247-248
  ventricular, 8-9
Diastolic augmentation, 98-99, 248, 283
  concept of, 411-412
  inflation and, 113-115
Diastolic heart failure, 46-47
Diastolic pressure time index, 101, 102
Dicrotic arch, 247
Dicrotic limb, 247
Dicrotic notch
  adjusting for, 249
  in incorrect inflation, 256-257
Digitalis, 77-78
Direct bedside providers, 374-375
Director
  medical, 371-372
  nursing, 372-373
Disk, intercalated, 28
Displacement pump, pneumatic, 560
Dissection, aortic, 153-154
Distal compartment, 95

Distal convoluted tubule, 65
Diuretics, 65-74
  glomerular filtration and, 67
  mechanisms of, 65-67
  moderate, 73
  potent, 74
  reabsorption and secretion and, 67
  weak, 67, 72-73
Dobutamine, 319
  pharmacology of, 75-76
Documentation
  of balloon insertion, 391-393
  of blood pressure, 317-320, 322
  of nursing care, 313
Dopamine, 319-320
  pharmacology of, 76
Doppler technology in vascular
    assessment, 158-159
Dorsalis pedalis pulse, 324
Drug therapy, 65-89
  diuretic, 65-74; *see also* Diuretics
  inotropic, 74-79
  phosphodiesterase inhibitor and, 79-80
  withdrawal of, 121
Dual-chambered balloon, 421
Dynamic work, 39-40, 106-107
Dyspnea, in heart failure, 60-61
Dysrhythmia
  Boston Scientific device and, 491
  heart failure and, 44

E

Eccentric hypertrophy, 55
Echocardiography, transesophageal, 400
Ectopy, 459
Edema
  pulmonary; *see* Pulmonary edema
  systemic, heart failure and, 62
Education, 377, 379-381
Ejection fraction, 241-242
  systolic heart failure and, 46
Electrical cardiac events, 281
Electrical power during air transport,
    543-544
Electrocardiography
  air transport and, 545
  in heart failure, 44-45
  timing and, 254, 255

Electrocardiography—cont'd
   trigger, 246-247, 322, 332-333
   weaning and, 401, 402
Electrochemical activity, normal, 7
Embolism
   air, 157
   helium, 156
   pulmonary, series circuit pressure
     changes in, 51
Embolus, risk for, 326
End-diastolic pressure
   afterload and, 13
   balloon-assisted aortic, 253, 257-258
   real timing and, 285-286
End-diastolic volume, 11
Endocardial viability ratio, 103
End-systolic counterpulsation, 557-558
Energy
   kinetic, 9
   myocardial, 37-40
Enoximone, 80
Entrapment of balloon, 155-156
Epinephrine, 77
Epinine, 79
Equipment, 376-377, 378
   air transport and, 546-547
Ethacrynic acid, 70-71, 74
Exercises, practice
   for conventional timing, 260-280
   for real timing, 289-293
Exertional dyspnea, in heart failure, 60
Exhaustion, heart failure and, 61
External work, cardiac, 37, 39
Extremity; see Limb
Eye, ocular pneumoplethysmography in,
   165-170

F

Facilitator, nurse manager as, 395
Family of patient, 335-336, 339
Fasciotomy, for compartment syndrome,
   153
Fast-flush test, 223-228
Fatigue, heart failure and, 61
Federal Aviation Administration
   certification, 542-543
Femoral artery
   entry through, 93

Femoral artery—cont'd
   percutaneous insertion in, 180-181
   sheathless insertion of balloon in, 201-202
   surgical cutdown in, 172-178
Fiber, myocardial, 11, 13
Fibrillation, ventricular, 459
Filament, myosin, 31
Filtration, glomerular, 67
Financial considerations, 364-367
First responders, team, 373-375
Flight, physiology of, 535-542
Flow chart
   intraaortic balloon counterpulsation, 393-
     394
   nursing care, 314-315
Forward heart failure, 48, 49-50
Fraction, ejection, 241-242
Framingham study, 44
Frank-Starling law, 9, 11-13
Frequency ratio weaning, 401, 403
Furosemide
   dosage and side effects of, 70-71
   pharmacology of, 74

G

G protein, 60
Gangrene, limb ischemia and, 151
Gas
   air transport and, 536-537
   for balloon, 115
   capillary, 234
Gas exchange, impaired, 329
Gender, as risk factor, 147
Glomerular filtration, 67
Glycoside, digitalis, 77-78
Ground transport, 359-360, 364
   air transport and, 545
Guidewire
   in percutaneous technique, 180-185, 187
   Seldinger technique for, 192
   for sheathless insertion of balloon,
     201-202, 203

H

H zone, 30
Heart
   physiology of
     blood flow and, 9

Heart—cont'd
  physiology of—cont'd
    cardiac output and, 9-14
    conduction system of, 6-7
    coronary circulation and, 19-24
    depolarization and repolarization in, 7
    left atrium and, 6
    left ventricle and, 6
    oxygen use and, 14, 16-19
    right atrium and, 4, 6
    vascular resistance and, 14
    ventricular systole and diastole in, 8-9
  transplantation of, 132-134
    bridging devices and, 559-561
Heart failure, 41-89
  acute, 47
  age and, 42
  backward vs. forward, 48-50
  causes of, 43-44
  chronic, 48
  compensatory mechanisms of, 52-60
    atrial natriuretic factor and, 59
    beta-adrenergic receptors and, 59-60
    G proteins and, 60
    mitochondrial function and, 60
    renal, 57-59
    Starling regulation and, 52-54
    sympathetic nervous system and, 54
    ventricular remodeling and, 54-57
  definition of, 43
  diastolic, 46-47
  indications of, 44-45
  low and high output, 50, 52
  pharmacological management of, 65-89
    angiotensin-converting enzyme
      inhibitors for, 84-86
    beta-adrenergic blocking agents for,
      86
    calcium-sensitizing agents for, 80
    diuretics for, 65-74; see also Diuretics
    inotropic agents for, 74-79
    phosphodiesterase inhibitors for,
      79-80
    vasodilators for, 80-84
  rate of, 42
  risk factors for, 45-46
  signs and symptoms of, 60-62
  systolic, 46

Heart rate
  balloon pressure waveform and, 297
  cardiac output and, 10
  effect of intraaortic balloon
    counterpulsation on, 110
Height, aortic segment related to, 209
Helicopter flight, 535; see also Air
    transport
Helium, 93
  air transport and, 545
  balloon pressure waveform and, 294
  diastolic augmentation and, 115
Helium embolism, 156
Helium leak alarm, 346-347
Hematologic changes, 156
Hemodynamics
  of intraaortic balloon counterpulsation,
    101-117
    afterload reduction and, 105-107
    baroreceptor response and, 110
    chemoreceptor response and, 110, 112
    diastolic augmentation and, 113-115
    heterometric-homeometric regulation
      and, 107-110
    inflation in diastole and, 103-105
    lactate and, 112-113
    myocardial oxygen and, 101-103
    oxygen supply and demand in,
      101-103
    Poiseuille law's and, 112
    preload and heart rate and, 110
    renal function and, 113
  monitoring of, 217-245
    accuracy factors in, 221
    derived indices in, 238-241
    dynamic factors in, 221-223
    ejection fraction and, 241-242
    fast-flush test and, 223-228
    oxygen and, 242
    pressure waveforms and, 229-237
    static factors in, 217-220
    of venous oxygen saturation, 242-243
  nursing care and, 316
  weaning from IABC and, 399
Hemopump, 559
Heparin, 186
Heterometric-homeometric regulation,
    107-110

High density lipoprotein, 45-46
Humidity, during air transport, 541-542
Hydralazine, 81
Hydrochlorothiazide
  dosage and side effects of, 68-69
  pharmacology of, 73
Hydroflumethiazide, 68-69
Hydrolysis, adenosine triphosphate, 32
Hypertension, 45
Hypertrophy, 54
Hypotension, 107

I

Ibopamine, 79
Indapamide
  dosage and side effects of, 68-69
  pharmacology of, 73
Index
  ankle-arm, 324
  ankle-brachial pressure, 149-150
  stroke volume, 238-240
  ventricular stroke work, 240-241
Indolamine derivatives, 68-69
Infant as patient, 531-534
Infarction
  myocardial, 120-121
  spinal cord, 152
Infection
  as complication, 154, 159
  risk for, 325
Inflation of balloon
  conventional timing of, 115, 281-282
    during diastole, 248-253, 281-282
    incorrect timing of, 256-257
  real timing of, incorrect, 288
Injury
  high risk for, 325
  local, 154
Innervation, of heart, 15
Inotropic agent, 74-79
Insertion of balloon catheter
  antegrade, 189-192, 333, 335
  hematologic changes and, 156
  percutaneous, 178-189, 199-200
  as risk factor for complications, 149
  sheathless, 199-206
  subclavian, 193, 194
  surgical cutdown for, 172-178

Insertion of balloon catheter—cont'd
  techniques for, 171-197
    surgical cutdown for, 172-178
  transaxillary, 193, 195-196
Intercalated disk, 28
Intraaortic balloon assistance without
    pump, 554
Intraaortic balloon counterpulsation
  abdominal aortic aneurysmectomy and,
    138, 139
  ambulatory, 517-519
  basic principles of, 93-100
  cardiac surgery and, 134-135
  catheter design for, 207-210
  for child, 531-534
  in community hospital, 357-368
  complications of, 146-164
    nursing and, 158-159
    predisposing factors for, 147-150
    vascular, 150-158
  contraindications to, 144-145
  heart transplantation and, 132-134
  hemodynamics of, 101-117; see also
    Hemodynamics
  history of, 411-431
    biological auxiliary ventricle and,
      413-414
    clinical modality and, 418-421
    diastolic augmentation and, 411-412
    further advances and, 421-427
    permanent assist and, 417-418, 424
    temporary cardiac assist and, 414-417
  indications for, 118-120
  insertion techniques for, 171-197
    antegrade, 189-192
    percutaneous, 178-189
    sheathless, 199-206
    subclavian, 193, 194
    surgical cutdown for, 172-178
    transaxillary, 193, 195-196
  instrumentation for
    Bard H-8000 device and, 495-514; see
      also Bard H-8000 device
    Boston Scientific Corporation devices
      for, 483-494
    Boston Scientific devices for; see also
      Boston Scientific Corporation
      devices

Pressure waveform—cont'd
  arterial—cont'd
    timing and, 246-259; *see also* Timing
  balloon, 294-308
Presystolic pressure, 285
Propranolol, 86
Protein
  G, 60
  troponin, 31
Proximal compartment, 95
Proximal convoluted tubule, 65
Pseudoaugmentation, left intraventricular,
      555
Pulmonary artery balloon
      counterpulsation, 520-529
  indications for, 521-524
  mechanism of action of, 526-527
  nursing care for, 528-529
  pathophysiology and, 521
  placement of, 524-526
  right ventricular dysfunction and,
      520-521
  timing and, 526
  weaning from, 528
Pulmonary artery capillary pressure,
      233-237
Pulmonary artery catheter, 229-237
  placement of, 229-231
  right atrial pressure and, 233
  right ventricular pressure and, 233
  troubleshooting for, 229-230
Pulmonary artery pressure, 233
Pulmonary artery wedge pressure
  Frank-Starling law and, 11, 13
  measurement of, 223
Pulmonary edema
  backward heart failure and, 49
  dyspnea and, 61
  pathophysiology of, 51
Pulmonary embolism, 51
Pulse
  dorsalis pedalis, 324
  loss of, 150
  tibial, 324
Pump
  centrifugal, 560-561
  pneumatic displacement, 560
  purging of, during flight, 539

Pump—cont'd
  roller, 560-561
  in St. Jude Medical, Inc., system, 433,
      434
Pump console, 98, 99
Purging of pump, during flight, 539

Q

Quality assurance in hemodynamic
      monitoring, 217-229; *see also*
      Hemodynamics, monitoring of
Quality management program, 368-397
  education and training for, 377-381
  equipment and support services for,
      376-377
  issues in, 381, 387-395
  nurse manager in, 395
  policies and procedures for, 375-376
  scope of, 369-371
  team for, 371-375
Quinethazone
  dosage and side effects of, 68-69
  pharmacology of, 73

R

Radial artery pressure, 81
Ratio, endocardial viability, 103
Reabsorption, renal, 67
Real timing, 259, 281-293
  benefits of, 284-286
  cardiac electrical and mechanical events
      and, 281
  conventional timing vs., 281-282
  principles of, 283
  process of, 286-288
  tutorial exercises about, 290-293
Referral hospital, 371
Refill time, capillary, 159
Regurgitation, mitral, 123-126, 358, 360
Relaxation, repolarization and, 35
Remodeling, ventricular, 54-55, 56
Renal artery, 113
Renal embolism, 152
Renal function
  diuretics and, 65-67
  effect of intraaortic balloon
      counterpulsation on, 113
  heart failure and, 57-59

Renal function—cont'd
  nursing diagnosis about, 329
Renal-angiotensin-aldosterone, 57-59
Reocclusion, after thrombolytic therapy,
      130-131
Repolarization
  physiology of, 7
  relaxation and, 35
Resistance, vascular
  diastolic augmentation and, 114
  factors affecting, 14
Resuscitation, 131
Reticulum, sarcoplasmic
  function of, 31-32
  illustration of, 27
Retrograde flow, incorrect deflation and,
      257-258
Right atrial pressure, 233
Right atrium, anatomy of, 4, 6
Right ventricular dysfunction, 520-521
Right ventricular pressure, 233
Right ventricular stroke work index, 240-241
Right ventricular waveform, 229
Roller pump, 560-561
R-to-R interval, timing and, 254-255
Rupture of intraaortic balloon, 155-156
Rural hospital setting, 369

S

Safe timing, 255-256
Safety, of Datascope system, 447
St. Jude Medical, Inc., Cardiac Assist
      control system, 430-446
  in air transport, 444
  alarms in, 442-443
  components of, 430-437
  set-up instructions for, 441
  specifications for, 445-446
  theory of operation of, 438-439
  timing in, 439, 441
  troubleshooting guidelines for, 430, 444
Salbutamol, 78
Sarcolemma
  function of, 26
  illustration of, 27
Sarcomere
  function of, 28
  illustration of, 29, 30

Sarcomere—cont'd
  lengthened, 56
Sarcoplasmic reticulum
  function of, 31-32
  illustration of, 27
Sarcotubular system, function of, 31-32
Saturation, venous oxygen, 242-243
Secretion, renal, 67
Seizure, 157
Seldinger technique for guidewire
      placement, 192
Septal defect, ventricular, 123-126
Sheathless insertion of balloon, 199-206
  advantages of, 200-201
  clinical results of, 202-205
  contraindications to, 202
  technique of, 201-202
  unsuccessful, 202
Shock, cardiogenic, 122
Sinus, Valsalva, 19
Size considerations in intraaortic balloon
      counterpulsation, 205-214
  for child, 532
Skills lab test, 385
Skin, nursing care for, 335
Sodium
  diuretics and, 72-74
  renal function and, 67
Sodium nitroglycerin, 81
Sodium nitroprusside, 80-81
Spinal cord infarction, 152
Spironolactone
  dosage and side effects of, 70-71, 72
  pharmacology of, 72
Square wave response, 223, 225
Staffing, 387
Starling curve, 52-54
Starling response, 52
Static work, 39-40, 106-107
Stopcock, 220, 221
Stretching of myocardial fibers, 11, 13
Stroke volume, 238-241
  cardiac output and, 10
  sarcomeres and, 56
  vasoconstrictors and, 320
Stroke work index, 240-241
ST-T wave abnormality, unstable angina
      and, 121

Subclavian insertion of balloon, 193, 194
Sulfonamide
    dosage and side effects of, 68-69
    pharmacology of, 73
Sulmazole, 80
Surgery
    cardiac, 134-135
    noncardiac, 138, 140
Surgical cutdown for insertion of balloon, 172-178
Sympathetic nervous system
    heart and, 15
    in heart failure, 54
Syncytium, 28
Systemic vascular resistance, 114
Systole
    assistance during, 556-559
    electrocardiography and, 247
    normal, 247-248
    ventricular, 8-9
        blood flow during, 9
Systolic heart failure, 46
Systolic pressure, ophthalmic, 165-170
Systolic unloading, 284

T

T tubule
    function of, 31
    illustration of, 27
Tachycardia
    balloon pressure waveform and, 297
    heart failure and, 44
Teaching-learning process, 379
Team first responders, 373-375
Tension
    contraction and, 37
    intramyocardial wall, 19
Tension time index, 101, 102-103
Terbutaline, 78
Terminal cisternae, 32
Testing, clinical, 380, 385
Thiazide diuretics
    dosage and side effects of, 68-69
    pharmacology of, 73
Thoracic aortic aneurysm, 144
Thrombocytopenia, 325
Thromboembolism, 151-152
Thrombolysis, 126-128
    reocclusion after, 130-131

Tibial pulse, 324
Timing
    cardiac output and, 321
    for child, 533
    conventional, 246-280
        arterial pressure waveform and, 247-254
        definition of, 246-247
        of deflation, 96-97
        functional range of, 255-256
        incorrect, 256-259
        of inflation, 115
        practice exercises for, 260-280
        problems with, 281-282
    in Kontron Instruments, Inc., devices, 476-477
    pulmonary artery balloon counterpulsation and, 526
    real, 259, 281-293
        incorrect, 288
Tone, vagal, 110
Training
    clinical, 376-377, 378
    for nurses, 361-362
        cost of, 366
Transaxillary insertion of balloon, 193, 195-196
Transcranial Doppler diastole, 169
Transduced waveform; see Balloon pressure waveform
Transducer
    calibration of, with mercury, 221, 222
    zeroing and, 217-220
Transesophageal echocardiography, 400
Transluminal coronary angioplasty, percutaneous, 128-130
Transplantation
    bridging devices and, 559-561
    cardiac, 132-134
Transport
    air, 535-551
        aircraft characteristics for, 542-544
        Bard H-8000 device and, 514
        Boston Scientific Corporation devices and, 493-494
        Datascope systems and, 460-461
        Kontron devices and, 482
        patient management in, 544-550
        physiology of flight and, 535-542

Transport—cont'd
air—cont'd
St. Jude Medical control system and,
444
ground, 359-360, 364, 545
Triamterene
dosage and side effects of, 72-73
pharmacology of, 72
Trigger, 246-247, 332-333
in Bard H-8000 device, 500
in Kontron devices, 472-474
in St. Jude Medical system, 436-437
Trigger electrocardiography, 322
Trisegmental intraaortic balloon, 211
Tropomyosin, function of, 31
Troponin proteins, function of, 31
Tubule
convoluted, 65
T
function of, 31
illustration of, 27
Turbulence during air transport, 542
Tutorial exercises
for conventional timing, 260-280
for real timing, 289-293

U

Ulcer, limb ischemia and, 151
Underdamping, 225
Unidirectional intraaortic balloon, 211
Unloading, systolic, 284
Unstable angina, 121
Urinary symptoms, 62
Urine output, 113
U-shaped left ventricular assist device,
417-418

V

Vagal tone, baroreceptors and, 110
Valsalva, sinuses of, 19
Valve
aortic, balloon inflation and, 249
mitral, regurgitation of, 123-126, 358, 360
Vascular assessment, 158-159
Vascular complications, 323
Vascular disease, peripheral
compartment syndrome as, 152-153
as contraindication, 144-145

Vascular disease—cont'd
as risk factor for complications, 148
Vascular insufficiency, 151
Vascular resistance
diastolic augmentation and, 114
factors affecting, 14
Vasoactive agent, 319-320, 322
Vasodilation, balloon inflation in diastole
and, 103
Vasodilator, 80-84
pharmacology of, 80-84
Vasopressor agent, 319-320, 322
Velocity of blood flow
effect of intraaortic balloon counterpulsa-
tion on, 105
phasic, 23
Venous circulation, coronary, 20, 21, 23
Venous oxygen saturation, 242-243
Ventricular arrhythmia
heart failure and, 62
pulmonary artery catheter causing, 229
Ventricular assist device, U-shaped, 417
Ventricular diastole, 8-9
Ventricular dysfunction, right, pulmonary
artery balloon counterpulsation for,
520-521
Ventricular ejection pressure, left, real tim-
ing and, 284
Ventricular fibrillation, Datascope systems
and, 459
Ventricular function, normal, 4
Ventricular irritability, 123
Ventricular pseudoaugmentation, 555
Ventricular remodeling, in heart failure,
54-55, 56
Ventricular septal defect, 123-126
Ventricular stroke work index, 240-241
Ventricular systole, 8-9
blood flow during, 9
preload effects on, 12
Ventricularized aorta, 558-559
Vesicle, sarcolemma and, 26
Viability ratio, endocardial, 103
Vibration, during air transport, 541
Volume
balloon, 210-214
air flight and, 537
catheter, air flight and, 537

Volume—cont'd
stroke, 238-241
sarcomeres and, 56
volume, diastolic augmentation and, 114
Volume weaning, 403

W

Wall, ventricular remodeling and, 55
Wall tension, intramyocardial, 19
Water condensation, Datascope systems
and, 459-460
Waveform
arterial pressure, 229-237
conventional timing and, 246-259; *see
also* Timing, conventional
real timing and, 287
balloon pressure, 294-308
Weakness, heart failure and, 61
Weaning
from intraaortic balloon
counterpulsation, 398-410
readiness for, 399-400

Weaning—cont'd
from intraaortic balloon—cont'd
relapses from, 404
successful, 403
techniques of, 400-403
from pulmonary artery balloon
counterpulsation, 528
Wedge pressure, pulmonary artery
Frank-Starling law and, 11, 13
measurement of, 223
Wedging of catheter, spontaneous,
229
Windkessel effect, 9, 10, 109-110, 248
Work, cardiac, 37-40

X

Xamoterol, 78, 79

Z

Z band, 28
Zeroing, 217-220